Aging in Place
*Supporting the Frail Elderly
in Residential Environments*

AGING IN PLACE

Supporting the Frail Elderly in Residential Environments

**American Association of
Homes for the Aging
In association with
The Foundation on Gerontology**

Edited by

David Tilson

PROFESSIONAL BOOKS ON AGING
SCOTT, FORESMAN AND COMPANY
GLENVIEW, ILLINOIS   LONDON

Library of Congress Cataloging-in-Publication Data

Aging in place : supporting the frail elderly in residential
  environments / edited by David Tilson.
      p.   cm. — (Professional books on aging)
    "American Association of Homes for the Aging in association with
the Foundation on Gerontology."
  Includes bibliographical references.
  ISBN 0-673-24945-X
  1. Frail elderly — Home care — United States — Congresses. 2. Frail
elderly — Housing — United States — Congresses.   I. Tilson, David.
II. American Association of Homes for the Aging.   III. Foundation on
Gerontology.   IV. Series.
HV1465.A347   1989
362.6'1'0973 — dc20   89-10868
                                                      CIP

1 2 3 4 5 6 KPF 94 93 92 91 90 89

ISBN 0-673-24945-X

Scott, Foresman professional books are available for bulk sales at quantity
discounts. For information, please contact Marketing Manager, Professional
Books Group, Scott, Foresman and Company, 1900 East Lake Avenue, Glenview,
IL 60025.

Foreword

Recent directions in gerontological and public policy research have generally supported the concept that long-term-care services for the elderly should be provided to individuals in their own residences for as long as possible. Several public opinion polls and numerous surveys of older persons show very strong support for this idea.

Our definition of residence includes an individual's home or apartment as well as specialized environments for the elderly that provide varying amounts of supportive services: congregate housing, residential care facilities, and the residential portions of continuing care retirement communities. The essential point is that the environment be residential — rather than institutional — in nature. Although it would appear that many elected officials favor long-term-care policies that would enable most frail elders to continue living in residential environments as long as possible, at present the financing and service systems are strongly biased toward providing long-term care in nursing homes — that is, institutional settings.

This book is the outgrowth of a symposium on support of the frail elderly in residential environments held under the joint auspices of the Southmark Foundation on Gerontology and the American Association of Homes for the Aging at Airlie House, Warrenton, Virginia, in 1988. The symposium brought together notable individuals from the academic and research communities, public policy experts, and professionals from the fields of long-term care and housing for the elderly.

The project had its genesis in two related, yet distinct, undertakings by the sponsoring organizations. The Southmark Foundation on Gerontology,[1] established by the Southmark Corporation in 1986, is a nonprofit charitable foundation whose goal is to help develop ways to improve the quality of life of the elderly in their living environments. During the summer of 1986, the foundation's Scientific Advisory Board recommended that one of its initial projects be an invitational conference and book on support of the frail elderly in residential environments. The board envisioned a policy-oriented effort that would include commissioning papers by experts and inviting a balanced group of knowledgeable individuals who would analyze and discuss the topics addressed by the papers. The purpose was to increase understanding of the issues by the general public, the policymakers, and the professional communities.

At the same time, the American Association of Homes for the Aging (AAHA), which represents over 3,400 nonprofit sponsors of housing, health care facilities, and community services for the elderly, had undertaken a project designed to enhance understanding by the public policy community of the need for a rational and comprehensive approach to long-term care. This project involved a number of national aging organizations whose principal interest was to improve the quality of life for the elderly. Thus, when the foundation approached AAHA to discuss its project, there was an agreement to merge mutual interests and proceed with a jointly sponsored symposium.

Clearly, an undertaking of this magnitude required conceptual insight, leadership, and months of hard work and planning. David Tilson, executive director of the Southmark Foundation,[2] proposed the idea, planned the symposium, commissioned the papers, edited this book, and is principal author of the introduction. He was ably assisted by Monsignor Charles J. Fahey, director of the Third Age Center at Fordham University and a former president of AAHA, who chaired both the advisory committee and the symposium. The members of the *ad hoc* advisory committee, who met in

---

[1]The Southmark Foundation on Gerontology was renamed "The Foundation on Gerontology" in 1989.
[2]Mr. Tilson left the foundation in March 1989.

February 1987 to help plan the symposium, made important contributions. To the authors of the excellent commissioned papers that constitute Chapters 1 through 11 of this book, we owe a special vote of thanks.

Substantial public support is emerging for new policies that will enable local communities to organize in ways that meet the needs and desires of the frail elderly to age in place with dignity. Although nursing homes will continue to be necessary, the public policy bias favoring them as the main setting for long-term care should be changed. We recognize that such a major shift in policy direction is a complex matter that will take time. But adopting the right policy goal and starting to move in the right direction is essential.

We hope this book will help policymakers at all levels of government design better programs and services for dealing with the needs of an expanding elderly population. We also hope the book will be helpful to providers, developers, and the general public, enhancing their understanding of these complex issues.

Finally, we wish to express our appreciation to the W.K. Kellogg Foundation, which provided a grant that helped make this project possible.

Richard T. Conard, M.D.
President
The Foundation on Gerontology

Sheldon L. Goldberg
President
American Association of Homes
for the Aging

Contents

Contributors

The Reverend Monsignor Charles J. Fahey is Marie Ward Doty Professor of Aging Studies in the School of Social Service and Director of the Third Age Center at Fordham University.

Leslie A. Grant, Ph.D., is a research associate at the Institute for Health and Aging, University of California, San Francisco.

Claire E. Gutkin, Ph.D., is assistant director for management information systems in the Department of Social Gerontological Research at the Hebrew Rehabilitation Center for the Aged in Boston.

Brian F. Hofland, Ph.D., is vice president of the Retirement Research Foundation in Park Ridge, Illinois.

M. Powell Lawton, Ph.D., is director of behavioral research at the Philadelphia Geriatric Center. He is a former president of the American Gerontological Society.

John N. Morris, Ph.D., is associate director of the Department of Social Gerontological Research at the Hebrew Rehabilitation Center for the Aged in Boston.

Mark R. Meiners, Ph.D., is associate director for economics of aging and health, Center on Aging, University of Maryland. He is also director of the Robert Wood Johnson Foundation program to promote long-term-care insurance for the elderly.

Robert J. Newcomer, Ph.D., is professor and associate director of the Institute for Health and Aging at the University of California, San Francisco.

Sandra J. Newman, Ph.D., is associate director for research at the Institute for Policy Studies and Research Professor in the Department of Geography and Environmental Engineering at Johns Hopkins University.

Leon A. Pastalan, Ph.D., is professor of architecture and co-director of the National Center on Housing and Living Arrangements for Older Americans at the University of Michigan.

Jon Pynoos, Ph.D., is United Parcel Service Foundation Chair Associate Professor of Gerontology in the Department of Public Policy and Urban Planning at the Andrus Gerontology Center, and director of the Program in Policy and Services Research, at the University of Southern California.

Hirsch S. Ruchlin, Ph.D., is professor of health economics with joint appointments in the Departments of Public Health and Medicine at the Cornell University Medical College in New York.

Clarence C. Sherwood, Ph.D., is professor emeritus of sociology at Boston University.

Sylvia Sherwood, Ph.D., is director of the Department of Social Gerontological Research at the Hebrew Rehabilitation Center for the Aged in Boston.

Gordon F. Streib, Ph.D., is joint professor in the Department of Community Health and Family Medicine, College of Medicine, University of Florida. He is a professor emeritus at Cornell University and at the College of Liberal Arts and Sciences, University of Florida.

James T. Sykes is a senior lecturer at the Medical School and Senior Special Assistant to the Vice Chancellor for Health Sciences at the University of Wisconsin–Madison.

David Tilson is a policy analyst who directed and wrote a number of major studies at the National Academy of Sciences between 1974 and 1986, the most recent of which was "Improving the Quality of Care in Nursing Homes," a study of nursing home regulation that was published in 1986.

Introduction

DAVID TILSON   AND   CHARLES J. FAHEY

Mid pleasures and palaces though we may roam
Be it ever so humble there's no place like home;
A charm from the sky seems to hallow us there,
Which, seek through the world, is ne'er met with elsewhere.
Home, home, sweet, sweet home!
There's no place like home! There's no place like home!

The values implicit in these familiar words are as compelling today as when they were written by John Howard Payne in 1823.[1] Where one lives is a central factor affecting the quality of one's life. Housing not only touches the basic human need for shelter, but also expresses and affects psychological well-being. A house is the symbol of one's status in the community and an articulation of what one feels is significant in life. It is not only a functional place in meeting narrowly defined human needs, but also a place in which family and other significant relationships are experienced. One's home is intertwined with aspirations about family and friends. It is a place of memories and of hope. It is a place of identity. It is a manifestation of one's power to choose, to exercise autonomy.

This is as true for the very old as it is for the young, as true for the frail and disabled as it is for the well and independent. Surveys by the American Association of Retired Persons (AARP) have confirmed what everyone has known all along: Most older people prefer to remain in their own home (or in a retirement residence of their choice) as long as possible. Almost everyone wants to "age in place," but relatively few people understand the complex social and economic realities implied by the phrase.

What does "aging in place" mean? Jon Pynoos in Chapter 7 notes that it implies several concepts: the aging of the individual and the changes in functional, income, marital, and health status that are associated with aging; the aging of the residential environment, including both the residence itself and the neighborhood and community in which it is set; the changes over time in the "fit" of the individual to the residential setting; and an emerging social policy that implies a set of goals for long-term care, housing, and social service programs.

Despite the fact that most people prefer to age in place in a residential setting rather than be forced to move to a nursing home when they become too frail to manage by themselves, this value preference has not really influenced public policies concerning the frail elderly. True, there has been much public discussion of the desirability of maintaining frail people in their chosen residential environments, and programs that achieve this goal can be found in many parts of the country. But our public policies, at both the national and state levels, remain fragmented and largely biased in favor of institutional — that is, nursing home — care for those unable to function independently. As a result, apart from the informal support provided by family or friends, in most communities it is usually difficult — sometimes impossible — and expensive to obtain the adequate and reliable professional services needed to enable frail elders to remain in residential environments of their choice.

There is growing public awareness and concern about the inadequacies of the long-term-care financing and service systems. Elected officials at all levels of government are beginning to recognize that this is an important concern of most people, not just the elderly. The absence of satisfactory insurance or other financing mechanisms to enable a person (or family) of middle income to pay for long-term care in noninstitutional settings, and thus avoid the dreaded move to a nursing home and "spend-down" to Medicaid eligibility, is now widely understood.

Although some of the legislative proposals introduced in Congress in 1989 for financing of long-term-care services are designed to foster in-home care, none evidences real understanding of the critical relationships among housing, social service, and health policies. For the most part, they expand the Medicare program to include long-term health care services, including home health care. The implicit service paradigm they all seem to share is that the problem essentially can be solved within the current health system—a health insurance problem that can be solved by providing an effective financing arrangement to cover nursing home care and home health care so that the middle-class elderly will not be forced to liquidate their assets once they are admitted to a nursing home. Such proposals pose the serious danger of "medicalizing" long-term care through inflexible federally developed and administered regulations governing individual eligibility criteria, eligible providers who must have specified credentials to perform specific tasks, services eligible for reimbursement, and so on.

Long-term care should not be viewed as a health insurance problem alone, though health services are certainly important. Long-term care is a social issue of considerable complexity that can be dealt with more humanely and possibly more cheaply if it is *not* consigned to the formal health system. What is needed is a set of policies that incorporate the necessary linkages among housing, social service, income maintenance, health, welfare, tax, and zoning policies to foster aging in place. The policy mosaic must include financing systems—for both services and housing—and mechanisms that support these linkages and provide the proper behavioral incentives to the private sector, in both its for-profit and not-for-profit components. It must include appropriate consumer protection policies, including regulation of facilities and services, that are aimed at ensuring a reasonable quality of life for the frail elderly. The private sector should continue to be responsible for developing, managing, and providing the necessary housing and services and also have a role in financing them.

The roles played by federal, state and local governments and their relationships to the public and private sectors are a crucial element in the policy framework. These relationships should be structured to allow considerable state and local initiative, flexibility, and innovation in the organization and delivery of housing and services that fosters aging in place under widely varying local circumstances. The reality is that we are just beginning to understand the complex phenomena of aging and how best to support frail elderly in a variety of residential environments. The knowledge base is still slender. There is uncertainty about the dimensions of some aspects of the problem and even more uncertainty about the best ways to deal with them. Thus, drawing up a set of policies based on the assumption that any of the currently fashionable service paradigms should be set in the concrete of government regulations and prescribed for everyone everywhere would be certain to have unfortunate consequences.

This book is intended to provide some insights into several major aspects of aging in place. Part One, Dimensions of the Problem discusses the characteristics of the frail elderly population, including their needs for service, their residential circumstances, and how these are likely to change over time. Part Two, Current Residential Realities, reviews the main categories of residential environments in which the elderly now live and age in place. Part Three, The Policy Setting, examines the policy terrain, including financing, and analyzes the barriers that need to be overcome or bypassed. Part Four, Planning for the Future, explores some underlying factors that need to be addressed to effect improvements in long-term-care services and in housing for the elderly: implicit values and attitudes, architectural design, and our limited knowledge base.

The rest of this overview summarizes and comments on the main points discussed in Parts One through Four of the book.

Dimensions of the Problem

The current data on aging in place are inadequate, because neither the federal nor state governments have made any systematic efforts to conceptualize the kinds of information needed or to collect the data regularly. This situation undoubtedly stems from the fact that aging in place issues are not a priority of any major government bureaucracy. And since collection of data is expensive, no major government agency has made the necessary resource commitment. What we know about the numbers and characteristics of the frail elderly, the characteristics of their residential environments, the services they require and are receiving and from whom, and how all of these things are projected to change in the foreseeable future are based mainly on *ad hoc* survey data that vary considerably in depth, specificity, validity, reliability, and recency. But they have provided information about some important aspects of the relevant phenomena.

Characteristics of the Elderly Population

Americans are living longer. Improvements in maternal and child health, immunization of children, better nutritional programs, changes in life-style, better understanding of the environment and physiology, along with improved diagnostic and therapeutic interventions, have brought about substantial improvements in mortality rates over the life span, and this trend appears likely to continue.

In 1987 the Bureau of the Census reported that there were 29.8 million Americans aged sixty-five or older. By 2020 this number is projected to grow to 51.4 million—about 20 percent of the total population.[2] Among the elderly population, the fastest growing groups are the very old—those seventy-five to eighty-five and especially those over eighty-five, among whom the prevalence of frailty (some degree of functional disability) is greatest. The over-eighty-five group has tripled in size since 1960 and is expected to double in the next twenty years.[3] More than half of those over eighty-five require some assistance from others, either with activities of daily living (ADLs), such as bathing, dressing, eating, and toileting, or with instrumental activities of daily living (IADLs), such as cooking, cleaning, shopping, and paying bills. Only 13 percent of those in the sixty-five to sixty-nine age range require such help.[4]

The national data on the frail elderly who live in the community come from the National Long-Term-Care Surveys conducted in 1982 and 1984 by the Bureau of the Census for the Department of Health and Human Services. Data on elderly who reside in nursing homes come from the National Nursing Home Survey conducted by the National Center for Health Statistics in 1985, which reported that 1.3 million elderly were in nursing home beds that year. Based on the data from these two surveys, the total number of frail elderly who were dependent on others for assistance with ADLs and/or IADLs was estimated to be between 6.2 and 6.5 million persons in 1985, 4.9 to 5.2 million of whom lived in the community.[5] That is, about four times as many frail elders requiring some long-term-care services reside in the community as live in nursing homes. Most of the care they receive is nonmedical and is provided informally by family or friends. The 1982 National Long-Term-Care Survey found that 74 percent of those receiving care at home received all their care from informal caregivers, 21 percent used both informal and formal care, and 5 percent relied on formal care exclusively. A recent study of some 10,000 frail persons known by agencies of the Robert Wood Johnson's "Interfaith Volunteer Caregivers Program" found that 68 percent of this frail population had no contact with formal social agencies.[6] In the Massachusetts study described in Chapter 2 by John Morris et al., the findings showed that elderly who reside in the community received about four hours of informal care for every hour of care obtained from formal providers.

The number of dependent elderly is projected to more than double by 2020. Whether the same fraction will be able to rely on informal support in the future is unclear, but it is unlikely for at least two reasons. First, the proportion of young and middle-aged women working outside the home has been steadily increasing. For women aged forty-five to fifty-four, this figure is expected to be 70 percent by 1995; for women thirty-five to forty-four, it is projected to be 83 percent in the same year.[7] Second, the proportion of elderly living alone also is increasing. In 1960 the number was 18.6 percent; in 1984 it was 30.6 percent and it is still increasing.[8]

Recent Bureau of Census data (1986) report that the annual income of the elderly population (including those who live alone) is distributed as follows: 13.8 percent have over $35,000; 19.3 percent have $20,000–$34,999; 30.7 percent have $10,000–$19,999; and 36.2 percent have less than $10,000. Among the very old, however, incomes are much lower: For those eighty-five and older, almost three-fourths of the women and about half of the men had incomes under $5,000.[9]

More than 90 percent of elderly persons live in ordinary houses or apartments, including public housing for the elderly and age-segregated residential "retirement" communities (such as Leisure World and Sun City) that were designed for independent elderly. About 5 percent (1.4 million) are in nursing home beds. Roughly one million live in three categories of specialized housing for the elderly: 300,000 in congregate housing, 350,000–700,000 in both licensed and unlicensed residential care facilities, and 200,000 in continuing care retirement communities. An unknown number live in miscellaneous residential settings such as hotels, boardinghouses, and housing.

There are no recent data that show both the characteristics of the residential settings (that is, their suitability for providing long-term care to frail residents) and the characteristics of the residents living in them. In 1978, the last time a survey was done that obtained such information, it was found that 17 percent of residents who had mobility problems lived in housing that did not meet minimal standards for plumbing, kitchen equipment, lighting, and so on.[10]

Coping with Aging in Place Today

For the vast majority of older people, their ability to continue living in their own homes or apartments depends on a number of circumstances: whether they have a spouse or family members who can help them to shop, do laundry, prepare meals, and, if they need it, to bathe and dress; whether they have sufficient income to purchase formal in-home assistance to supplement or substitute for informal care; and whether it is even possible to obtain satisfactory in-home care in their community.

Some states and communities have expanded their capacity to provide in-home and community-based services to facilitate aging in place for the 90 to 92 percent of the frail elderly living in the community. But the requirement for such services is growing faster than the capacity to meet it. There appear to be several reasons for the lag. First, the extent and nature of the requirements for supportive and personal care services in a community is not easily quantified, and, with few exceptions, there are no systematic efforts to collect appropriate data regularly. Second, there is no financing mechanism, other than individual out-of-pocket payment, to pay for the necessary services. The in-home service providers have organized to respond to the requirements of publicly financed programs, mainly Medicare, which pays for a narrowly defined set of home health care services. Without either private or public long-term-care insurance covering a spectrum of in-home services, this set of circumstances is not likely to change very much.

Still, there are successful examples in many parts of the country of locally initiated efforts to organize and operate programs to support frail elders in their own homes. James Sykes describes a few inspiring examples in Chapter 3. They include public housing for the elderly in which successful service programs were introduced through the unusual cooperation of local government agencies, which normally have difficulty in communicating with one another. With over 500,000 elderly living in public housing, these are examples that merit replication by many of the 3,000 local public housing agencies throughout the country. Sykes also calls attention to "naturally occurring retirement communities" — apartment buildings or neighborhoods with high proportions of elderly residents who moved in either as young people or after they retired or were widowed. There are many such communities in the country. They constitute both an opportunity and a challenge to devise ways to help the residents continue to age in place.

A generation ago, before the phenomena of aging in place were understood, the idea emerged of building two different types of "retirement" homes: detached houses or garden apartments set in age-segregated communities, such as Leisure World or Sun City, that were designed to attract the completely independent, well elderly; and facilities that provided safe, comfortable apartments with some supportive services such as a community dining room, housekeeping, twenty-four-hour watch service, transportation, and social programs. Congregate housing facilities, as the latter type came to be called, were conceived as secure, pleasant environments for the well or slightly frail but independent elderly for whom living in their own homes or apartments without some supportive services had become either too difficult or uncomfortable. Some of the early facilities of this type were built by private, nonprofit organizations (mostly church-related), but major growth of congregate housing did not take place until the HUD programs were authorized in the early 1970s.

The HUD concept of aging was static. In the HUD-subsidized projects, residents were required to be "independent," and if they were no longer able to perform ADLs without assistance they were expected to transfer out of the facility, usually to a nursing home. Inevitably, in a relatively few years, aging in place became a major concern of housing project managers everywhere. Many began to improvise responses either by developing personal care units (or services) in their facilities or by constructing a separate personal care facility nearby. Originally, HUD strongly opposed these changes, but its position appears to be softening, at least informally. Most administrators are now convinced that congregate housing without the capacity to provide personal care to those who later become frail makes little sense.

The demand for congregate housing appears to remain strong in many parts of the country, although there is evidence of overbuilding in some localities, particularly for high-cost projects. Rentals in new facilities, however, are all at market rates. And although the HUD Section 202 program for subsidized housing for low and moderate income elderly is still functioning, HUD space and design restrictions have made it impossible for new facilities to include such essential features as meal programs, let alone space for the other amenities and personal care services needed by aging residents. For the past eight years, HUD has been trying to eliminate the Section 202 program, but Congress has insisted that it be continued, albeit at a modest level.

The Congregate Housing Services Program is a demonstration program initiated a few years ago by Congress (over HUD's objections) to add services to help frail residents in elderly housing. Funds for sixty-four projects — about half in public housing and half in Section 202 facilities — were provided to add services such as meal programs. There seems to be little doubt that the program greatly improved the quality of life of the residents. In St. Paul, Minnesota, for example, it enabled a 202 facility to fill forty-five vacant units with residents who were transferred from nursing homes.[11]

Between 350,000 and 700,000 frail elderly people live in residential care facilities, which are called by different names in different states: board and care facilities, adult homes, rest homes, adult foster care homes, adult congregate living facilities, domiciliary care facilities, and so on. These types of facilities were the antecedents of the modern nursing home.[12] In 1987, there were about 41,000 licensed residential care facilities with 563,000 beds,[13] some 65 percent of which were occupied by frail elderly. (The other beds are used by developmentally disabled, mentally ill, and mentally retarded younger persons.) It is estimated that there are at least an equal number of unlicensed beds. Residential care facilities provide meals, personal care (for example, assistance with bathing, dressing, and grooming), laundry, and protective oversight to residents. The facilities vary greatly in size and ambiance: some are very pleasant and offer a warm, family-like atmosphere. Others are bleak and institutional. Many residents live on Supplemental Security Income (SSI) with state supplemental grants.[14] State licensure policies vary widely. It is clear that residential care facilities have emerged in response to real needs. Many of the small facilities are owned and operated by single women. They have been described as "poor people taking care of poor people." Although they are an important category of residential environment for the elderly, very little is known about them. Robert Newcomer and Leslie Grant, in Chapter 5, review what is known about residential care facilities and discuss the policy issues they pose.

Another category of specialized residential facility for the elderly is the continuing care retirement community (CCRC), some of which formerly were called life care communities. This type of facility provides assured access to a full range of long-term-care services: apartments, meal service, personal care, and nursing home care. A substantial fraction of the existing facilities operate a self-insurance program in which costs for all the care — including nursing home care — are borne by the residents through payment of a substantial admission fee and a monthly fee that covers rent and services. The characteristics of CCRCs and the issues they pose are discussed by Sylvia Sherwood et al. in Chapter 6. Access to this type of facility is available only to the relatively affluent elderly, though some efforts are being made to design new CCRCs for persons with moderate incomes (as low as $16,000–$18,000 per year).

The Public Policy Environment

Promoting aging in place requires appropriate and coordinated policies and priorities from several traditional policy domains: health, housing, social services, welfare, taxes, and zoning. As pointed out by Jon Pynoos in Chapter 7, each of these policy domains has separate statutory authorities, and each is served by a bureaucracy at each level of government with its own subculture, priorities, value preferences, and *modus operandi*. They are separated by regulatory and procedural Chinese walls that are patrolled by legislative committees in Congress and the state legislatures. The result is a maze with many blind alleys and discontinuities. At least eighty programs have some bearing on the issues of aging in place (see Table 7-1), but most have different eligibility requirements, are administered by different bureaucracies, and are difficult or impossible to coordinate. This set of circumstances applies to the organization and delivery of long-term care and housing services as well as to their financing.

But the issue is much more than one of program coordination. It concerns the goals of public policy—what we wish as a nation for those who need assistance to remain in their chosen residence. In 1989, federal policy goals did not include the facilitating of aging in place, or major support for long-term care of the elderly except for Medicaid coverage in nursing homes.

In HUD elderly housing programs, tenants must be independent. This means that elderly tenants who become frail and require personal care services they cannot either obtain through public programs or pay for themselves must be moved out—usually to a nursing home.

In the case of the Medicaid program, the Health Care Financing Administration (HCFA) has been reluctant to grant Section 2176 waivers for home care: these waivers supported only 59,000 people in 1986.[15] In any case, the waivers support only those persons who are otherwise eligible for admission to a nursing home. HCFA is concerned about growth of the Medicaid program and is afraid that the Medicaid budget will go up more rapidly if waivers are granted too readily.

The Title XX (Social Services Block Grant) program and Title III of the Older Americans Act have very limited funding. Although the available funds can be used to support aging in place—and do so in many communities—a relatively small fraction of the dependent elderly living in the community are receiving care through these programs.[16] The Older Americans Act Amendments of 1987 explicitly authorize funds for a broad array of nonmedical in-home services for the dependent elderly. But the amounts appropriated are a very small fraction of the amount needed.

The central issue is clearly a societal attitude and priority question: If elected officials become convinced that a policy of facilitating aging in place is something the electorate really wants and is willing to pay for, the design of such a policy framework will take place. Some states have already begun to move in that direction, and with clear evidence of success.[17]

WHO SHOULD PAY FOR LONG-TERM CARE

There is a growing consensus that some system for financing long-term-care services in both residential and institutional environments is both necessary and inevitable, but there is no clear consensus as to whether it should be a universal social insurance program like Medicare, perhaps with a sliding scale of income-related co-payments and deductibles, or whether primary reliance should be on private long-term-care insurance with public funding for the poor. Long-term care is an insurable risk since only a fraction of the elderly require it. But the publicly funded costs are certain to be high and to increase because of the rapid growth projected for the very old and frail population in the next thirty years.

FINANCING SPECIALIZED HOUSING
FOR THE ELDERLY

Although this issue has not received the analytic attention accorded to the financing of long-term-care services, it merits serious attention. The demand for such housing, particularly for service-enriched congregate housing and assisted living facilities, is strong and is certain to grow. But at market rate rentals, it is accessible only to the more affluent elderly. At present there are no programs to stimulate construction of these types of housing for the low- and moderate-income elderly. An aging in place policy requires that this issue be addressed.

ROLES OF FOR-PROFIT AND
NOT-FOR-PROFIT PROVIDERS

Most congregate housing and CCRCs are operated by non-profit organizations, and most of the residential care facilities are operated by proprietary, or for-profit, organizations. Private developers in increasing numbers have been developing CCRCs, congregate housing, and assisted living facilities. Moreover, as the need for case management services has expanded, proprietary case management services have started to appear in many communities.

The home health care industry is largely proprietary and oriented to those who can pay. It is likely that as home care demand grows, many proprietary home health care firms will tailor their services to meet it.

The proprietary organizations have certain attributes that are important. They can command capital in whatever amounts are needed if there is a prospect for reasonable returns to investors. They are also sensitive to market demand, which means they will make special efforts to determine what consumers want and then design programs to satisfy them. Of course, they can only serve customers who can pay market rates. For-profit organizations may also have attributes that are less attractive from a public policy standpoint: In many cases they do not have any special roots in the community, and proprietary enterprises are likely to change ownership and management more frequently than nonprofit organizations. Moreover, concern for maximizing net profits can lead some unethical owner-managers to operate in ways that are hardly in the public interest.

Not-for-profit organizations have a traditional and socially important role in this field. First, they are rooted in their communities, and, if properly organized, have boards that are representative of the communities they serve. Second, they are committed for the long term, and since community service rather than profit is their aim, they are unlikely to change ownership in the abrupt way that characterizes for-profit operations. Third, they are usually rooted in religious communities and draw upon them for volunteers, who can greatly enrich the lives of the residents of the facilities. On the other hand, they seldom can move as quickly or obtain necessary capital as readily as for-profit organizations. Many nonprofit organizations serve mainly middle- and upper-income elderly; others feel strongly that they have a moral obligation to serve clients of low and moderate income who may have to be subsidized through private philanthropy.

In drawing up new policies for financing both long-term-care services and elderly housing, it is important to provide incentives and safeguards to encourage the vigorous participation of both sectors in developing housing and services for the elderly.

REGULATION

Regulation of the services and facilities associated with aging in place programs is primarily a state responsibility. As these programs grow, and as the numbers of specialized facilities for the elderly increase, the pressure to expand regulation to protect the consumers is certain to mount. Well-conceived and properly administered regulation is needed. But poorly designed and insensitively administered regulation can cause unintended harm to consumers, as well as unnecessary costs and powerful disincentives to providers.

One of the biggest risks is that the regulators will impose an institution-like ambiance—analogous to that found in nursing homes—to assure that "quality of care" standards are met. This is almost certain to occur if state health departments are responsible for licensure of residential facilities. But the real goal should be quality of *life,* not quality of *care.* (Quality of care is only one of several factors affecting quality of life.) The ambiance sought should be residential, not institutional.

CCRCs merit special attention, because a major issue is protection from the substantial entrance fee that residents must pay to join such communities. For many residents, the entrance fee represents a major portion of their life savings. Since a number of these projects have failed, regulation to protect CCRC residents is important. The American Association of Homes for the Aging, which represents the majority of currently operating CCRCs, has developed a model state regulatory statute that represents what it considers to be necessary and desirable regulation that should be instituted by all states. (Currently, not all states regulate CCRCs.)

Looking Ahead: Some Underlying Issues

As Brian Hofland points out in Chapter 9, implicit sets of societal attitudes and values toward the elderly are important but invisible influences on policy and program design. As conceptualized by Moody some years ago,[18] there are four implicit societal models of aging that are positioned along a value spectrum ranging from materialistic to idealistic/holistic. The four models are rejection, social services (paternalism), participation, and self-actualization.

The rejection model, no longer fashionable, places very low value on old age since the elderly are viewed as noncontributing members of society. Old people are a problem to be handled with minimum expenditure of society's resources. In Hofland's words,

"Given the negative perspective of this first model, there can be no rationale for supporting frail and dependent older people in the community." Although no longer fashionable, it is by no means absent from our policy assumptions. Does not HUD's consistently negative position toward congregate housing and the congregate housing services program derive from this model?

The second model, social services, has dominated our policies and programs for more than fifty years. It is implicitly imprinted, along with technical knowledge and skills, in the professional education of social service and health professionals. The basic assumption about the value of old age in the first model is not really challenged, but the social service model assumes that society has a moral obligation to meet the needs of those who cannot provide for themselves. But old people are not really viewed as important, valued members of society. They are clients with needs for social services, the nature and setting for which are to be determined by those who know best: the professionals. Under this value model, in Hofland's words, "Old people, perceived as something less than total human beings, are not seriously engaged in activities and projects that are respected and valued by the entire community. They contribute to the community's well-being as consumers rather than as producers, and through leisure rather than through work."

Model III, participation, has a very different view: It assumes that old people, to the extent that their health and functional abilities permit, remain important members of society capable of continued personal growth and meaningful contributions to society. Personal autonomy and choice, central issues affecting quality of life for people of all ages, is perceived as particularly crucial for older people. As Hofland says, "Housing for old people in Model III involves an 'accommodating environment'[19] in the best and truest sense of that term. . . . Supportive services are implemented in partnership and with the consent of old people." As a basis for development of aging in place policy, Model III clearly merits widespread adoption in the policy-making and professional communities, as well as in society as a whole.

Model IV, self-actualization, goes further than Model III in that it assumes that old age brings special possibilities of spiritual growth. This clearly transcends the values of modern society and is suggested as a possible future development without the immediate operational implications of Model III.

These implicit value sets should be made explicit in the course of the forthcoming public policy debates on long-term care, housing, and aging in place.

DESIGNING LIVING ENVIRONMENTS

In the years ahead many new residential facilities for the elderly will be constructed and many older facilities remodeled. Are there special design features that should be incorporated in these facilities that affect quality of life for the residents? Leon Pastalan, in Chapter 10, presents a persuasive case for the affirmative based on the research to date. If we accept the Model III value assumptions, it is important that these design concepts be understood and applied by developers and regulatory authorities. According to Pastalan, we have learned a great deal about designing safe and supportive environments that take account of the normal functional deficits that occur in aging populations, and that enhance the independence and autonomy of the residents.

EXPANDING THE RESERVOIR OF KNOWLEDGE

There is a relatively slender knowledge base on which to rest the design of a set of social policies and programs to foster aging in place. Important gaps exist in three categories of knowledge: (1) statistical information about elderly people, their changing needs, and their residential environments and how they are changing; (2) basic knowledge about the social and psychological phenomena of the elderly population and the effects of various environmental variables on their behavior, health and life satisfaction; and (3) applied research knowledge concerning ways to improve the design and management of facilities and programs, the organization of services, and the training and motivation of staff so as to achieve high quality of life for residents.

In Chapter 11 M. Powell Lawton addresses the first two categories. The failure of the federal and state governments to collect and disseminate even the most basic statistics necessary to track what is going on is a striking illustration of both the implicit value sets that obtain and the failure to recognize the significance of the phenomena of aging in place. Suggested questions for research, mainly in category three, are contained throughout the book. Chapter 2 illustrates the kind of longitudinal study that can contribute importantly to the kinds of knowledge needed for policy and program planning.

Funds for all three categories of research will have to come mainly from public sources, with some modest contributions, perhaps, from private foundations. Sound evaluation of demonstration projects is critical, but tricky. As in all research, asking the right questions is crucial. Much evaluation research in the past has been of questionable value, because either the wrong questions were asked or key questions were not asked.

DISSEMINATING NEW KNOWLEDGE AND ATTITUDES

Education and training are the keys to changing values, attitudes, and behavior. The academic centers' traditional roles of research and disseminating the results of research in their educational programs, and the use of training seminars organized by the various provider and professional associations, remain the primary vehicles for affecting the attitudes and behavior of all the key parties, including policymakers, regulators, developers, professionals, and caregivers.

Consumer organizations, particularly the AARP, perhaps with the aid of private foundations, also have an important responsibility to educate the general public on the policy issues, the underlying values, and the differences between desirable and undesirable programs.

Conclusion

American society, with its deeply rooted faith in pluralism and its complex polity and system of governance, is faced with a major challenge: to devise an adequate response to a major national problem—facilitating aging in place for the frail elderly. The nature and quantitative dimensions of the problem are not fully understood, and the courses of action are difficult to design because they cut across so many entrenched policy domains. The challenge is to design policies that permit innovations in organization and delivery of services at the local level, that provide incentives to both the nonprofit and for-profit sectors to expand capacity to meet the growing needs, and to develop a system of financing, both public and private, that will meet the needs in ways that society as a whole will find equitable, morally attractive, and politically acceptable. Although the authors of the chapters that follow provide no blueprints, they offer some interesting and important insights and directional arrows for the evolution of sound public policy.

Notes

1. Sung by Clari, the Maid of Milan, in the opera, *Home, Sweet Home,* composed by John Howard Payne in 1823.

2. U.S. General Accounting Office (GAO), "Long-Term Care for the Elderly: Issues of Need, Access, and Cost." Report to the Chairman, Subcommittee on Health and Long-Term Care, Select Committee on Aging, House of Representatives. November 1988, p. 8.

3. U.S. Department of Health and Human Services. Report to Congress by Task Force on Long-Term-Care Policies. Washington, D.C., September 1987, pp. 66, 67.

4. Ibid., p. 8.

5. Ibid., p. 12.

6. The Third Age Center, Fordham University. "Religious Congregations and the Informal Supports of the Frail Elderly." Final report (unpublished). New York, May 1988.

7. U.S. Department of Labor, Bureau of Labor Statistics. "Employment Projections for 1995." *Bulletin 2197,* March 1984, p. 3.

8. U.S. GAO, p. 18.

9. See Chapter 4 for Gordon Streib's discussion of these data and for the listing of sources.

10. See Chapter 1 for its discussion of the findings of the 1978 housing survey.

11. This information was supplied by Elaine Anderson, administrator of the Congregate Housing Services Project in St. Paul.

12. Vladeck, Bruce C. *Unloving Care.* New York: Basic Books, 1980.

13. National Association of Residential Care Facilities. *1987 Directory of Residential Care Facilities.* Richmond, Va.: NARCF, 1987, p. 5.

14. A recent survey in New Jersey of more than 6,000 residents in board and care homes found that 45 percent were on SSI. Cited in U.S. GAO, p. 23.

15. Data are from a survey conducted by the National Governors' Association in mid-1987. Cited in U.S. GAO, p. 27.

16. U.S. GAO, p. 27.

17. Justice, D. et al. *State Long-Term-Care Reform: Development of Community Care Systems in Six States.* Washington, D.C.: National Governors' Association, April 1988.

18. Moody, H.R. "Philosophical Presuppositions of Education for Old Age." *Educational Gerontology,* 1:1–16, 1976.

19. Lawton, M.P. et al. "The Lifespan of Housing Environments for the Aging." *The Gerontologist,* 20:56–64, 1980.

PART ONE

Dimensions of the Problem

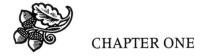

CHAPTER ONE

The Frail Elderly in the Community: An Overview of Characteristics

SANDRA NEWMAN

The debate over the deficiencies in the long-term-care system underscores one essential point: the institutional bias of current policies. This non-neutrality in public policy and financing is implicated in various ills of the current system: the inappropriate use of nursing homes by the frail elderly who need assistance but not at the level or intensity provided by nursing homes, the absence of a residential continuum that would allow the impaired elderly to receive appropriate care, and the lack of support and assistance to the aged in their own homes.

Many proposals for changing long-term-care policy focus on ways to neutralize this bias in current policy. A primary theme is the need for greater choice among services and service settings. Considerable evidence has been accumulated on the implications of an aging population for the need and demand for community-based long-term care, the economics of institutional versus noninstitutional care, and the quality-of-life differences between nursing homes and community living.[1] But there is still uncertainty about such fundamentals as the kinds of elderly persons living in the community who are in need of care, the settings in which they live and in which many of the community-based services would be delivered, and the mix of services they need. Such information is a necessary ingredient for understanding the flaws in the current

3

system and evaluating potential remedies. These dimensions of long-term care have been difficult to characterize largely because the information needed on a range of attributes — sociodemographics, health, housing, social support — was simply not available in any database until the National Long-Term-Care Surveys (NLTCS) were conducted in 1982 and 1984.[2]

We have used the NLTCS data to examine important characteristics of the elderly long-term-care population living in the community, roughly 27 million persons in 1986.[3] First we provide a brief overview of the long-term-care landscape: What characteristics make someone a part of the long-term-care population? What services does this population need? Where do these individuals live? And what is the projected growth of this population over the next several decades? We then turn to a more in-depth examination of the frail elderly living in the community based on special tabulations from the NLTCS. The final section offers some general suggestions for future research useful to the development of community-based long-term-care policy.

The Long-Term-Care Landscape

CHARACTERISTICS AND SERVICE NEEDS OF THE ELDERLY LONG-TERM-CARE POPULATION

There is general agreement that it is the need for long-term assistance in carrying out the normal activities of daily living rather than a particular medical diagnosis that makes someone a part of the long-term-care population.[4] These activities include personal care (eating, toileting, transferring, bathing, dressing), mobility assistance inside the house or outside, and home management (preparing meals, cleaning, shopping). The 1982 NLTCS indicates that roughly 19 percent of the elderly (those aged sixty-five and over) have at least one of these needs for assistance.[5]

It is also generally accepted that these characteristics translate into assistance needs that are largely nonmedical and cover a broad range of health-related, social, and personal needs. But there is far less agreement on such matters as the most appropriate or necessary services or the most appropriate target population for government assistance.[6] In part, these differences in view stem from the fact that the long-term-care population consists of numerous subgroups with different needs for assistance. For example, service needs may vary with different underlying conditions: The primary need of those with mental illness is likely to be monitoring and supervision; for those with physical impairments it may be personal assistance with activities of daily living.[7] Those who retain cognitive functioning — nearly 75 percent of the community-resident elderly — seem better able to cope with functional limitations.[8]

Differences in the informal care network also have been used to distinguish long-term-care subgroups. Two individuals with identical limitations in their capacity for self-care may require different amounts of formal assistance (from either the private or public sectors) "depending on the availability and capacity of their informal caregiving network of family and friends."[9] Recent research emphasizes that simply distinguishing people by their living arrangements (for example, whether they live alone or with others) or by the presence of a social support network does not indicate whether a viable source of informal long-term-care assistance is available. Thus, the fact that more than 70 percent of the elderly long-term-care population live with at least one other person, or even that roughly 89 percent of them can identify a friend or relative who provides some assistance, is not sufficient grounds for assuming that formal care (purchased or subsidized) is unnecessary.[10] What is missing is information on the burden that caregiving represents and the circumstances that enable family and friends to provide care.[11]

Finally, where the frail elderly live also shapes the nature of their demand for long-term care. Characteristics of the residential setting can determine whether outside providers must be relied upon for necessary services. For example, frail individuals who live in barrier-free environments may have less need for personal mobility assistance; those in service-rich settings may never need community-based care.

But for the large majority of the frail elderly who do not live in such supportive housing environments, the question may be more fundamental: whether in-home long-term-care services can be delivered at all. There is limited empirical evidence suggesting that residential characteristics, including physical dwelling attributes, density or concentration of those with needs for assistance, and neighborhood conditions, can affect the ease or feasibility of delivering long-term-care services.[12] According to an analysis of the 1978 National American Housing Survey (AHS), roughly 17 percent of the mobility-impaired elderly live in housing units that do not meet minimal housing standards similar to those used by the U.S. Department of Housing and Urban Development; 6 percent have either incomplete kitchen facilities or unusable kitchen equipment; and more than 4 percent lack complete plumbing.[13] Deficiencies in such essentials may severely restrict the effective delivery of home care services.

WHERE THE ELDERLY LIVE

Despite the effects of the residential environment on the demand for long-term care, there is no reliable information on how many elderly persons live in the various types of residential settings or how the frail elderly are distributed among them. The 1985 National Nursing Home Survey, however, provides much specific information on nursing home residents. Thus, we know that about 1,350,000 elderly persons currently reside in nursing homes. The 27,000,000 noninstitutionalized elderly live mainly in ordinary apartments or houses,[14] but perhaps 1,000,000 of them live in one of three broad categories of specialized housing for the elderly that provide varying amounts of supportive and/or personal care services:

- *Congregate housing:* about 400,000–500,000 elderly live in both subsidized and unsubsidized congregate housing.[15]
- *Residential care facilities* (known by names such as board and care facilities, adult homes, domiciliary care facilities, adult foster homes, and so on): about 350,000–700,000 elderly are living in both licensed and unlicensed facilities of this type.[16]
- *Continuing care retirement communities:* about 200,000 elderly live in these facilities and the numbers are growing.[17]

There are no standard definitions or service packages provided by all facilities in each of these categories. (See Chapters 3 through 5.)

If the findings of the 1982 NLTCS remain valid today, some 5,130,000 of the noninstitutionalized elderly require some amount of supportive and/or personal care on a long-term basis.[18] Even if most of the 1,000,000 who live in specialized housing for the elderly require some long-term care—and many in congregate housing do not—it appears that less than 20 percent of the frail elderly requiring some supportive services have elected to move to residential environments that supply at least some of those services. It is also worth noting that about four times as many frail elderly live in residential settings as live in nursing homes.

PROJECTIONS

Demographic projections of the elderly population, particularly the segment that is likely to need long-term care, indicate that demand for supportive residential settings will increase. Although the exact estimates vary, depending on the assumptions underlying each projection series, all point to major increases. A 1984 report by Manton and Liu projects a 26 percent increase in the population sixty-five and older between 1985 and 2000, and an 83 percent increase between 1985 and 2020.[19] The greatest growth will occur among the very old: Manton and Liu report a doubling of the population eighty-five and older between 1985 and 2020 compared to somewhat more than a 50 percent increase of those seventy-five to eighty-four over the same time period. Another analyst, Karen Davis, reports that in 1980 11 percent of the population was sixty-five and over, but by 2030, this proportion will grow to 19 percent.[20] One set of Census Bureau estimates puts the 2030 elderly population at an even larger figure: 21 percent.[21]

Davis highlights the projected growth in two subgroups who are at great risk of needing long-term-care assistance: older women, particularly those who are widowed or single, and elderly individuals with functional limitations. Women eighty-five and older are expected to increase by 81 percent between 1980 and 2000 and to triple by 2030. The number of women seventy-five and older who are widowed or single is projected to increase from 4.1 million in 1980 to 6.4 million at the turn of the century—a 56 percent increase. Among the elderly in general, those with personal mobility limitations are projected to increase by more than 40 percent (roughly 1.9 million to 2.7 million) over the same twenty-year period; those with more severe limitations, requiring assistance in bathing, for example, will also increase by more than 40 percent (.85 million to 1.21 million).[22]

Manton and Liu's projections focus only on the elderly population with some need for assistance in daily activities. In contrast to Davis, they report the projected prevalence of the population sixty-five and older with either activity of daily living (ADL) limitations or those with instrumental activity of daily living (IADL) limitations exclusively.[23] Their findings are even more dramatic than those of Davis, as shown in Table 1-1. The rates of growth for both IADL and ADL/IADL groups will increase over the six decades between 1980 and 2040. The number of those having only IADL limitations will double in size by 2020 and will almost triple in size by 2040. For the population with at least one ADL limitation, projected increases are even more marked.

As with all projections, some underlying factors are more certain than others. The projections of both the functionally impaired elderly and the elderly population in general result from the aging of the post-World War II baby boomers, a nearly immutable fact. But the projections also assume no major changes in mortality or significant technological or biomedical advances, or even shifts in health behavior that could either affect the incidence of functional limitations or at least mediate their consequences. Despite uncertainty about these important factors, the most likely scenario is a substantial increase in the elderly long-term-care population. And although the demand for supportive residential settings will grow as a result, as will the supply of such settings, the very large majority of the frail elderly will continue to live in their homes and apartments. The next section of this chapter therefore focuses on this

Table 1-1. Projected Rates of Increase in the Elderly
Population, by Functional Limitations

Between 1980 and:	IADL Only	At Least One ADL
2000	50.0% (1.5 million)	60.2% (3.2 million)
2020	105.8% (2.2 million)	122.4% (5.1 million)
2040	189.5% (4.2 million)	221.8% (10.2 million)

Source: Adapted from Manton, K., and K. Liu. "The Future Growth of the Long-Term-Care Population: Projections Based on the 1977 National Nursing Home Survey and the 1982 Long-Term-Care Survey." Paper presented at the Third National Leadership Conference on Long-Term Care, Duke University Center of Demographic Studies, Durham, NC, 1984.

sizable group, with particular emphasis on service needs and possible impediments to meeting them.

The Frail Elderly in the Community

As noted at the outset, the 1982 NLTCS provides a rich source of data for examining multiple attributes of the frail elderly population in the community. The survey was administered to a nationally representative sample of 5,580 chronically impaired individuals sixty-five and older.[24] The data were adjusted by statistical weights that account for differential nonresponse among subgroups in the population.

Although the NLTCS contains more information about the frail elderly's housing environment than any other long-term-care dataset, this information alone is inadequate to assess the residential setting as a possible service setting. Therefore, we have augmented the NLTCS data with five housing indicators from another database, the 1978 National American Housing Survey (AHS): dwelling unit size, ease of access, maintenance problems, structural deficiencies, and affordability. We appended these indicators to the NLTCS by predicting their values in a matched AHS subsample and then imputing these predicted values to the NLTCS.[25] The 1978 AHS was chosen as the donor file because, in that one year, it included a unique supplemental block of questions on health and functional status of each household member along with a rich core of information on housing attributes and background characteristics of household members.[26]

Although the broad parameters of the long-term-care population were laid out earlier, many classification schemes can capture the more specific characteristics of this population. For the present analysis, three such finer categorizations apply: (1) whether the individual has need for IADL assistance only, or whether assistance is needed with one to two ADLs, three to four ADLs, or five to six ADLS;[27] (2) whether the individual needs assistance with each of the six ADLs (transferring, mobility, dressing, bathing, toileting, eating), and the summary class representing whether assistance is needed with any ADL; and (3) whether the individual has cognitive problems, defined in two ways: falling below the mean score for the full NLTCS sample on the Short Portable Mental Status Quiz, or having a proxy reporter for the survey because the sample member is senile or mentally retarded. Table 1-2 lists, for each classification scheme, the fraction of the NLTCS sample and of the elderly population at large represented by each category.

These three classifications have the advantage of identifying the particular functional impairments of the elderly population. But they are imprecise proxies for identifying the population of greatest interest: those at risk of institutionalization. Much research supports the finding that individuals along the full impairment continuum, ranging from moderate to completely bedridden, live in nursing homes or in the community.[28] Therefore, looking only at those with impairments excludes a significant group that is actually at equal or greater risk. To capture this group, we have included a fourth categorization of the frail elderly, namely, those who are definitely at risk of institutionalization. By linking the 1982 and 1984 NLTCS, we can identify this group directly by determining which 1982

Table 1-2. Prevalence Rates of Elderly in Various Long-Term-Care Classifications

Classifications	1982 NLTCS Sample	1982 Population 65 and Older
1. IADL only	44%	6.0%
1–2 ADLs	33	4.5
3–4 ADLs	12	1.7
5–6 ADLs	11	1.6
2. Any ADL*	45	7.9
Transfer	19	3.3
Mobility	22	3.8
Dressing	18	3.8
Bathing	37	6.4
Toileting	13	2.3
Eating	6	1.1
3. Cognitively impaired	27	4.8

Source: 1985 NLTCS.
Notes: Many estimates are approximate because of missing data. All rates are based on unweighted data. The percentages in the first data column are based on a special tabulation of the 1982 NLTCS data. The second data column shows the ratio of the weighted number of cases in each ADL category (in the NLTCS) to the total U.S. population aged 65 and older in 1982.
*Refers to the 1982 NLTCS sample members who had need for assistance with one of the listed activities of daily living for at least three months (actual or expected).

sample members actually became institutionalized by 1984.[29] Roughly 8 percent of the 1982 NLTCS sample fall into this at-risk group and represent roughly 1 percent of the total population. Because this fourth classification allows us to look at the characteristics of individuals prior to their actual institutionalization, we consider it the best measure of the most vulnerable elderly, and we rely on it throughout this discussion.[30]

Table 1-3 compares the functional impairments and availability of assistance for this pre-institutional group, referred to as those "at risk," with the remainder of the 1982 NLTCS sample members known to be frail (in the sense that they need at least some long-term IADL or ADL assistance) but who did not enter institutions within the two-year period covered by the surveys. Each of the measures of level of functioning reveal the substantially greater dependence of the at-risk group. But this group was not without sources of assistance to cope with these incapacities; as the final entry in the table indicates, almost all those who ultimately became institutionalized had either informal (unpaid) or formal (paid) "helpers" available to them for at least some period of time prior to institutionalization. What these data do not reveal is whether the at-risk group remained stably supported throughout the period prior to their institutionalization or whether their support system broke down and, if so, why. Given the greater disability among the at-risk elderly, one reasonable hypothesis is that at some point, the burden of informal caregiving becomes too great, and even the purchase of a range of formally delivered services becomes unfeasible.

At-risk elderly are likely candidates for institutionalization because of severe functional limitations, but they also appear to be vulnerable demographically and socioeconomically. Table 1-4 compares some basic characteristics of this at-risk group with those of two other groups: the frail elderly who are not at risk as we have defined this state, and a representative sample of the community-resident elderly.[31] The at-risk population is older and more likely to be living alone, widowed or not married, female, and poor than either of the other two populations. The rates of most characteristics decrease rather dramatically as one moves across the column entries from left to right (that is, from the most vulnerable to the least vulnerable populations). Although the greater prevalence of these characteristics among the at-risk population confirms the conventional

Table 1-3. Functional Status of At-Risk and
Other Frail Elderly (weighted percents)

	At Risk	Frail, Not At Risk
ADL		
Any ADL	59.3%	43.7%
Transferring	26.7	18.2
Mobility	31.1	21.1
Dressing	30.1	20.8
Bathing	50.9	35.3
Toileting	22.0	12.5
Eating	9.5	6.0
IADL		
Any IADL	90.6	73.0
Food preparation	55.5	34.5
Medicating	43.0	25.9
COGNITIVE PROBLEMS (SPMSQ score)		
0	17.5	27.0
1	15.5	24.0
2	11.2	16.4
3	9.7	9.4
4	4.1	5.4
5	5.2	3.3
6	2.2	1.5
7	1.9	1.0
8	.2	.4
9	.6	.2
10	31.9	11.4
Mean SPMSQ score	4.6	2.6
AVAILABILITY OF SUPPORT		
Any unpaid helpers	91.1	88.2
Any paid helpers	38.3	23.6

Notes: ADL needs represent sample members' reports of the need for another person's assistance whether or not the assistance is actually received and whether or not they need, or use, mechanical aids or equipment. N = 4153.

"At risk" refers to persons 65 years or older in 1982 who were institutionalized by 1984. Stays in nursing homes or hospitals of less than 90 days were excluded except when the individual died in the institution. Total unweighted case count was 457.

"Frail, not at risk" refers to those who reported, in 1982, an ADL or IADL need that had either lasted for at least three months or was expected to last that long, but who, by 1984, had not been in a nursing home or hospital for more than three months. N = 5123.

SPMSQ refers to the Short Portable Mental Status Quiz. The numbers listed are the number of *wrong* answers. The mean to the total 1982 NLTCS is about 3.

image of the most vulnerable groups, this conclusion is not as strongly supported when classifying the long-term-care population by its functional limitations.

The findings for race confirm the tendency reported in previous research for blacks to have lower relative rates of institutionalization compared to whites. Blacks comprise a larger share of the frail population that does not become institutionalized than of the group that ultimately enters an institution: 13.2 percent versus 6.2 percent. This pattern is reversed for whites.[32]

Taken together, the data in Tables 1-4 and 1-5 strongly indicate that those at greatest risk of becoming institutionalized differ fairly dramatically from those who are also frail but not at risk. These differences cover a range of attributes, including functional impairments and availability of assistance as well as demographic and socioeconomic characteristics. But they also suggest that using any one subset of these attributes alone as a proxy for those most likely to become institutionalized is quite imprecise; the combination of vulnerability factors rather than any single factor produces an institutional outcome.

In contrast to these sets of distinguishing features for the most at-risk population, housing characteristics are much less useful. The data in Table 1-6 support this conclusion, showing the distributions of various housing and related characteristics for those who ultimately entered institutions, other frail elderly who did not become institutionalized, and a representative sample of the community-resident elderly.[33] Earlier, it was argued that the housing environment could conceivably affect the risk of institutionalization if, for example, it presented significant obstacles to access to services or the delivery of services in the home. But the data indicate that the at-risk elderly are no more likely to live in nonmetropolitan areas where the supply of services may be unavailable, inadequate, or inconvenient. Nor are they more likely to be still paying off a mortgage, which could represent a major drain on resources that might be used to pay for long-term-care services.

One explanation for this lack of differentiation in housing characteristics is the well-known tendency for the elderly to remain in their long-term residences, a phenomenon often referred to as "aging in place." If the at-risk group were no more likely to move

Table 1-4. Demographic Characteristics of the Elderly (weighted percents)

Demographics	At Risk	Frail, Not At Risk	Total*
SEX			
Male	28.8%	35.4%	41.9%
Female	71.2	64.6	58.1
Total	100.0	100.0	100.0
AGE			
65–69	7.9	21.7	34.0
70–74	10.5	22.1	28.1
75–79	21.2	21.0	19.1
80–84	27.6	17.1	11.5
85 +	32.8	18.1	6.9
Total	100.0	100.0	100.0
MEAN AGE	81 years old	77 years old	74 years old
RACE			
White	93.2	85.4	89.9
Black	6.2	13.2	8.2
Other	.6	1.4	1.9
Total	100.0	100.0	100.0
MARITAL STATUS			
Married	28.5	43.4	55.9
Widowed	58.7	46.9	33.7
Divorced	3.9	3.8	4.2
Separated	.5	1.2	1.2
Never married	8.4	4.7	5.1
Total	100.0	100.0	100.0
NUMBER OF ADULTS IN HOUSEHOLD			
1 person	39.0	31.9	30.3
2 persons	39.3	48.2	55.7
3 + persons	21.7	19.9	13.9
Total	100.0	100.0	100.0
INCOME			
< $5,000	25.7	22.6	13.9
5,000–9,999	34.2	38.2	28.1
10,000–19,999	22.8	26.6	32.1
20,000 +	17.3	12.6	25.9
Total	100.0	100.0	100.0

*"Total" is defined as a cross-section of individuals 65 or older living in the community. Total unweighted case count was 17,802.

Table 1-5. Housing Characteristics of the Elderly (weighted percents)

Housing Characteristics	At Risk	Frail, Not At Risk	Total
TENURE			
Own	63.9%	70.5%	76.8%
Rent	32.6	25.7	21.0
No cash rent*	5.5	3.8	2.2
Total	100.0	100.0	100.0
TYPE OF STRUCTURE			
Single family	70.0	74.9	77.6
Apartment	23.3	19.3	16.9
Mobile home	6.7	5.8	5.5
Total	100.0	100.0	100.0
SIZE OF DWELLING			
<6 rooms	66.8	66.8	61.0
6 rooms or more	33.2	33.2	39.0
Total	100.0	100.0	100.0
NUMBER OF STORIES			
<4	95.3	95.0	94.4
4 or more	4.7	5.0	5.6
Total	100.0	100.0	100.0
LOCATION			
Inside SMSA	55.7	53.5	63.2
Outside SMSA	44.3	46.5	36.8
Total	100.0	100.0	100.0
HOUSING COSTS			
Owners:			
Free and clear	79.0	79.7	80.0
Mortgage debt	21.0	20.3	20.0
Total	100.0	100.0	100.0
Renters: monthly costs			
<$100	37.5	40.7	26.7
100–149	12.1	15.3	14.4
150–249	20.9	20.7	22.8
250 or more	29.5	23.3	36.0
Total	100.0	100.0	100.0
HOUSE VALUE			
(Owners only)			
<$20,000	18.2	21.8	8.3
20,000–34,999	21.5	21.3	17.1
35,000–49,999	21.0	22.8	22.8
50,000 or more	39.3	34.1	51.8
Total	100.0	100.0	100.0
LIVING IN SPECIAL RESIDENCE	12.5	7.8	NA

*No cash renters are included in monthly rent distribution. Rent refers to *contract* rent.

Table 1-6. Housing Problems of the Elderly (weighted percents)

	At Risk	Frail, Not At Risk	Total
HOUSING PROBLEMS			
Physical deficiencies			
Structural	11.6%	14.8%	12.4%
Maintenance	1.8	5.3	1.3
Dwelling use problem: toilet not convenient to bedroom	10.9	14.4	NA
Absence of special dwelling modification that would be helpful	32.9	31.8	NA
Affordability			
Renters:			
housing costs >30% income	42.7	36.0	32.9
housing costs >50% income	26.3	14.9	14.1
Owners:			
housing costs >30% income	21.8	23.8	26.3
housing costs >50% income	5.2	7.2	16.2
NEIGHBORHOOD PROBLEMS			
Neighborhood crime	17.7	18.9	7.9
No convenient grocery	30.1	31.7	13.2
No convenient pharmacy	39.9	43.1	13.2

compared to the other elderly, there would be no reason to expect the attributes of their housing to be different.

Although this interpretation is plausible, there is one piece of evidence that those at risk are somewhat more likely to have adjusted their housing circumstances by moving—though it is not known whether the move preceded or followed the onset of their health-related risk factors. As shown in the last entry in Table 1-5, 60 percent more of the at-risk elderly report that they live in a special residence for older, retired, or disabled persons than do other frail elderly (12.5 percent versus 7.8 percent, respectively).[34] Even taking likely response errors into account, the difference in prevalence rates is probably sizable.

These differences in the data—the first showing consistency in most housing characteristics and the second showing a greater proportion of the at-risk elderly living in special residences—are more compatible than they initially appear. A closer review of each entry in Table 1-5 reveals similarities in most attributes that are unlikely to differ substantially between special residences and other residences, for example, location, size of dwelling, or house value. But two characteristics that are more likely to differ do vary in the expected direction: tenure and structure type. To the extent that most special residences are rented apartments, the somewhat higher rates of renting and of apartment living among the most at risk are reasonable. The somewhat higher rents among this population are also understandable, since many of these special residences are relatively new and many also include some services in their rental fees.

Despite the significant number of the most at risk who appear to have moved to a special residence for the elderly, the large majority are likely to have remained in place. And while the basic characteristics of their dwellings may be largely similar to those at less or no risk, the presence of housing and neighborhood problems may not. There are a number of reasons why the environments of the at-risk elderly might be more deficient. For example, their higher rates of functional impairments and of living alone render them less able to make housing adjustments by either moving or repairing the dwelling. These housing deficiencies, in turn, may increase the vulnerability of this group by limiting the feasibility of long-term care in the home. Thus, the characteristics of the at-risk population may be both the cause and the effect of deficiencies in their residential environments.

Table 1-6 provides data on four sets of housing problems: physical deficiencies, inconveniently located toilets, absence of special dwelling adaptations that would be useful, and excessive expenditures on housing costs. It also includes three neighborhood problems: crime, inconvenient grocery stores, and inconvenient drug stores. Overall, these data do not lend support to the environmental vulnerability hypothesis described above. The most at-risk elderly are actually somewhat less likely to live in dwellings with structural or maintenance defects or in houses with inconveniently located lavatories than those not at risk. These three patterns taken together are once again consistent with the previous finding that a significant number of the at-risk group have apparently moved into special residences which are newer, in better condition, and well designed, albeit more expensive.

No major differences exist in the prevalence of neighborhood problems between the frail at risk and the frail but not at risk. There are, however, very large differences in reported neighborhood problems between the NLTCS sample as a whole and the representative sample of the elderly in the AHS: Reports of neighborhood crime problems are more than twice as great in the NLTCS as in the AHS (17.7 percent versus 7.9 percent), as are reports of inconvenient stores (30.1 percent versus 13.2 percent). These comparisons must be interpreted cautiously because differences could be attributable to measurement error. But if even a portion of the difference is real, then the data suggest that the frail elderly, generally defined, are more likely to live in less hospitable neighborhoods than the elderly as a whole. Nevertheless, there is no evidence that these neighborhood deficiencies are more prevalent among the most at risk of the frail elderly.

Although dwelling unit problems are not more prevalent among the frail elderly who become institutionalized, the most functionally impaired group tends to have a high rate of housing problems. This finding is consistent with empirical research described earlier. Of particular interest is the very high rate of reports indicating the absence of dwelling modifications that would be helpful; for example, more than 40 percent of those with three or more ADLs responded this way. Physical deficiencies and inconvenient toilet location are also more prevalent among the very impaired than among the most at risk of institutionalization. Those with cognitive impairments have particularly high rates of deficiencies — nearly twice as high as the most at-risk group (21 percent versus 11.6 percent). Whether these deficiencies ultimately motivate a residential move by some subset of these individuals is unknown.

These data on the functionally impaired suggest two respecifications of the environmental vulnerability hypothesis. First, although the most at-risk elderly do not have high relative rates of housing problems, the most functionally disabled do. Thus, the notion that functional incapacity may prevent housing adjustments, which is a restatement of the first part of the hypothesis, appears to be borne out. But second, because the most at risk do not seem to suffer disproportionately from housing problems, it is unlikely that the housing environment represents a major obstacle to their receipt of community-based long-term care. Their lower rates of physical dwelling problems seem related in part to previous housing adjustments, since more than 12 percent reported that they lived in a special residence. Whether this move was undertaken in the early years of older age, at the onset of disability or in more advanced stages, or in response to other significant life events such as widowhood is unknown.

It is not clear how to interpret the relatively low rate of housing problems among those who ultimately are institutionalized. This finding suggests two alternative hypotheses: first, that the housing environment has no effect on institutional risk; or second, that although housing conditions may not prevent institutionalization altogether, they may delay it significantly. Some recent results suggest that a small number of environmental features do play a significant role in institutional risk by affecting the efficacy of formal, paid care, although the nature of this role varies for different housing elements.[35] Adequate space in the dwelling unit, for example, results in formal care that lessens the impaired person's institutional risk. Homeownership reduces the elderly person's risk of institutionalization at least in part because it leads to the use of formal support. These preliminary findings lend support to the second hypothesis. But they also underscore the complexity of the relationship among the characteristics of the elderly individual, the environment, and institutional risk. A more complete understanding of this relationship awaits further study.

Conclusion

As pressures for reform of the nation's long-term-care system mount, the need for accurate information on the target populations has become particularly acute. Since a major goal of reform is to expand choices in long-term care services and settings beyond nursing homes, it is crucial to understand who in the community is at great risk of institutionalization, what characteristics put them at high risk, and which of these risk factors can be dealt with in a community setting.

This chapter represents an initial attempt to explore these issues. Using data from the National Long-Term-Care Surveys and the National American Housing Survey, it has been possible to examine a wide variety of attributes of frail elderly individuals who were shortly to enter nursing homes. Although the tabulations support some commonly held images of the most at risk, such as their high rates of functional disability, very old average age, and high prevalence of living alone, two do not. First, despite their high rates of living alone, nearly all of these individuals appeared to have active sources of informal or formal support. Thus, the presence of support is not sufficient to prevent institutionalization. Second, the most at risk do not appear to be especially vulnerable environmentally as measured by attributes of their housing and neighborhood environments. This suggests that characteristics of the at-risk population are neither cause nor effect of residential deficiencies. But these two results must be treated with caution. Reporting the availability of some source of support says nothing about the capacity, burden, or quality of caregiving; there may be a point at which caregiving in the home is no longer feasible. The absence of housing problems may be related to housing adjustments made earlier to get needed care, and residing in such a housing unit may have delayed eventual institutionalization. There is also limited evidence from other research that at least some housing characteristics may have an indirect effect on institutional risk by facilitating formal service delivery in the home. Simple distributions such as those relied on in this chapter cannot detect such complex relationships.

In fact, the inappropriateness of simple conceptualizations for studying the at-risk elderly is a major theme of this report. Identifying the characteristics of this population provides one clear example: Although the most at risk do tend to be severely functionally impaired, a definition that relies strictly on impairments is seriously flawed, since a combination of factors rather than any single one puts an elderly person at great risk. The long-term-care policy debate would be well served by research on a number of these complexities. Four areas suggested for study are (1) how the characteristics of caregiving (for example, burden, quality) and of caregivers (for example, true capacity) affect risk; (2) the nature of the transition to high-risk status; (3) the nature, timing, and effects of residential moves by those who ultimately constitute the at-risk group; and (4) how the supply of supportive housing environments affects residential moves by the frail elderly and, in turn, mediates the risk of moving to a nursing home.

Notes

1. Feder, J., and W. Scanlon. "The long-term-care market place: An overview." *Journal of the Healthcare Financial Management Association,* January 1984.

   Newman, S. "The aging of America: Implications for the future of the welfare state." *Policy Currents* 2, 1. Baltimore: The Johns Hopkins University Institute for Policy Studies, 1988.

   Berkeley Planning Associates. "Evaluation of Coordinated Community-Oriented Long-Term Care Demonstration Projects." Final Report, Contract 500-80-0073. Berkeley, California, 1985.

   Heumann, L., et al. "A Cost Comparison of Congregate Housing and Long-Term Care Facilities in the Midwest." Urbana, Ill.: Housing Research and Development Program, University of Illinois, 1985.

2. Bureau of the Census for the Department of Health and Human Services, Office of the Assistant Secretary for Planning and Evaluation (ASPE) and the Health Care Financing Administration (HCFA). "National Long-Term-Care Surveys," 1982 and 1984. See also Mochan, C. "1982 Long-Term-Care Survey." Internal memorandum to Ronald Dopkowski, Chief, Special Surveys Branch, Demographic Surveys Division. Washington, D.C.: Bureau of the Census, 1983.

3. Sirrocco, A. "Nursing and related care homes as reported from the 1986 inventory of long-term-care places." In *Advance Data,* No. 147, Vital and Health Statistics of the National Center for Health Statistics, 1988.

4. Katz, S., et al. "Progress in development of the index of ADL." *The Gerontologist,* 1, 1:75–99, 1970.

   Feder and Scanlon. "Long-term-care market place."

   Technical Work Group on Private Financing of Long-Term Care for the Elderly. "Report to the Secretary on Private Financing of Long-Term Care for the Elderly." Washington, D.C.: HCFA, pp. 391–414, 1986.

   Macken, C. "A profile of functionally impaired elderly persons living in the community." *Health Care Financing Review,* 6, 3:33–49, 1986.

   Doty, P., et al. "An overview of long-term care." *Health Care Financing Review,* 6, 3:69–78, 1985.

5. As described later, the NLTCS sampled Medicare beneficiaries 65 and older. Note that this rate is nearly twice as high as that reported by Feller (1983) using the National Health Interview Survey. This difference appears to be caused by the NLTCS' inclusion of needs for assistance that are *expected* to last for three months in addition to those that have already existed for three months. See Macken, Note 4, for a discussion of this discrepancy.

6. Berkeley Planning Associates. "Demonstration Projects." Newman, S., and R.

Struyk "An alternative targeting strategy for housing assistance." *The Gerontologist,* 24, 6:584-592, 1984.

7. Feder and Scanlon. "Long-term-care market place."

8. Macken. "Profile."

9. Technical Work Group. "Private Financing."

10. Estimates based on tabulations of the 1982 NLTCS.

11. Feder and Scanlon. "Long-term-care market place." Doty, P. "Family care of the elderly: The role of public policy." *The Milbank Quarterly,* 64, 1:34–75, 1986.

12. Lawton, M.P., et al. "The lifespan of housing environments for the aging." *The Gerontologist,* 20:56–64, 1980.

    Noelker, L. "The impact of environmental problems on caring for impaired elders in a home setting." Paper presented at the 35th Annual Meeting of the Gerontological Society of America, 1982.

    Newman, S. "Housing and long-term care: The suitability of the elderly's housing to the provision of in-home services." *The Gerontologist,* 25, 1:35–40, 1985.

13. The 1978 AHS included a special health and housing modification supplement. Newman. "Housing."

14. Sirrocco. "Nursing."

15. The Senate Special Committee on Aging reported that as of 1984 the following amounts of congregate housing for the elderly had been built under U.S. Department of Housing and Urban Development Programs:

Section 202	200,000 units
Section 236	56,000 units
Section 221 d(3)	26,000 units
Section 221 d(4)	104,000 units
Total	386,000 units

Although later data are not available, both Sections 202 and 221 d(3) have been actively supporting construction of additional congregate housing since 1984. Based on authorizations and appropriations since that time, it is estimated that through Fiscal Year 1989 at least 75,000 additional units have been built or were under construction under these two programs. In addition to HUD-assisted projects, an unknown (but probably significant) amount of congregate housing has been built by private sponsors and some states.

16. The National Association of Residential Care Facilities, Richmond, Va., conducted a survey of state licensure agencies in 1988. Their unpublished report shows that there were 41,196 licensed facilities with 513,550 beds. In a 1984 telephone survey conducted by the Institute for Health and Aging, University of California, San Francisco, it was found that about 65 percent of the beds in

licensed facilities were occupied by frail elders. The balance of the beds were used for the developmentally disabled, mentally retarded, mentally ill, and so on. The U.S. General Accounting Office estimates that there are at least as many unlicensed beds as licensed beds. See Chapter 4 for a more complete discussion of these data.

17. Data furnished by the staff of the Continuing Care Accreditation Commission, American Association of Homes for the Aging, who maintain a data base on CCRCs.

18. This represents 19 percent of 27,000,000.

19. Manton, K., and K. Liu. "The future growth of the long-term care population: Projections based on the 1977 National Nursing Home Survey and the 1982 Long-Term Care Survey." Paper presented at the Third National Leadership Conference on Long-Term Care, Durham, N.C., Duke University Center of Demographic Studies, 1984.

20. Davis, K. "Health implications of aging in America." Paper presented at the Office of Technology Assessment Conference, the Impact of Technology on Aging in America, Baltimore, Johns Hopkins University, 1983.

    Davis, K. "Financing health care for the elderly in the U.S.: Current policy debate and future directions." Paper presented at the Commonwealth Fund Forum, Improving the Health of the Elderly: Best Prospects from Five English-Speaking Countries, Baltimore, Johns Hopkins University, 1983.

21. Technical Work Group. "Private Financing."

22. The projection period for the bathing limitation population is 1977 to 2000.

23. The former group includes the subsets having personal mobility problems and need for bathing assistance reported by Davis, plus several other limitations (for example, eating, transferring, and toileting).

24. The sampling frame was a list of 36,000 names from the Health Insurance Master File (that is, Medicare beneficiaries). "Chronically impaired" is defined as having, or expecting to have, a problem for three months or longer with any ADL (such as eating, getting in or out of chairs, mobility inside, mobility outside, dressing, bathing, getting to or using the toilet, and incontinence of bladder or bowel), or IADL (preparing meals, doing laundry, light housework, grocery shopping, managing money, taking medicine, or making phone calls). Screening was done either in person or by phone. Although 6,393 cases were screened into the sample, 508 were determined to be "false positives" (for example, when the ADL or IADL need no longer existed at the point of the interview), and another 203 cases were no longer available for interviewing at the time of the actual survey (mainly due to death). We dropped the false positive cases from our analysis file, yielding an initial analysis sample of 5,580 (U.S. Department of Health and Human Services. Undated memorandum on 1982 National Long-Term-Care Survey Data; Manton, K., and K. Liu. "The 1982 and 1984 National Long-Term-Care Surveys: Their structures and analytic

uses." Paper presented at National Conference on Long-Term-Care Data Bases, May 21–22, 1987).

25. The detailed description of these procedures is reported in Newman, et al. "Overwhelming odds: Caregiving and the risk of institutionalization." Unpublished paper, Washington, D.C.: The Urban Institute, 1987.

26. The four-year time difference between the two surveys should represent a problem only if there were systematic changes in the housing characteristics of the at-risk elderly population. Given the low mobility of the elderly and the slowness at which the housing stock changes, we doubt that the time difference affects any nonfinancial attributes. In contrast, financial characteristics are known to have fluctuated over this period but, fortunately, can be adjusted through standard procedures (see Newman, et al. "Overwhelming odds").

27. This categorization was used by Manton and Liu, "Future growth."

28. Brody, E., et al. "The family caring unit: A major consideration in the long-term-care support system." *The Gerontologist,* 18:556–61, 1978.

   McCoy, J., and B. Edwards. "Contextual and sociodemographic antecedents of institutionalization among aged welfare recipients." *Medical Care,* XIX, 9:907–21, 1981.

   Doty, P. "Family care."

   Wan, T. "Evaluation research in long-term care." *Research on Aging,* 8, 4:559–85, 1986.

29. We limited this group to those who had been institutionalized for at least 90 days to eliminate short-term stays (except where the individual dies in the institution). The 1984 response rate among the 5,580 members of the 1982 sample was 97 percent.

30. Tabulations based on each of the other classifications are available from the author.

31. The latter is drawn form the 1983 National American Housing Survey (AHS). Because the AHS is based on a sample of housing units, it was converted to a person-level file for this analysis.

32. Blacks are also substantially overrepresented among those with cognitive impairments.

33. The same conclusion obtains for the three functional limitation subgroups defined earlier.

34. The specific question asked was: "Is this place part of a building or community intended for older, retired, or disabled persons?"

35. Newman, S., et al. "Overwhelming odds."

CHAPTER TWO

Aging in Place:
A Longitudinal Example

JOHN N. MORRIS,   CLAIRE E. GUTKIN,
HIRSCH S. RUCHLIN,   AND
SYLVIA SHERWOOD

"*Aging in place*" is a relatively new phrase. It refers to the changes in functional status and residential circumstances of cohorts of older people over time, and the extent to which various types of residential environments permit elders to grow old in familiar surroundings. To date, however, even simple descriptive data of this sort for cohorts of older people are scarce. This absence of data may have contributed to the presumed failure of many community intervention programs designed to keep frail elders from moving to nursing homes.

For years, federal long-term-care policies have centered around programs to keep frail elders from entering nursing homes. The motivation was to slow the growth of the Medicaid budget, about 40 percent of which pays for nursing home care of the elderly.[1] The most ambitious of these experimental efforts was the National Long-Term Care Channeling Demonstration,[2] which facilitated access to community-based services for elders impaired in activities of daily living (ADL). This demonstration removed financial and regulatory barriers, served a self-selected client population, and delivered services through a case-management control system. The results were disappointing. Similar findings from earlier demonstrations[3] underline the need to increase our knowledge of the changes over time in the functional capabilities of cohorts of elders residing in the community.

High risk elders have proved difficult to identify.[4] Although many elders have functional and health deficiencies, in the study discussed in this chapter we found few who had serious unmet needs, and fewer still who entered nursing homes. The majority of elders who actively sought care in the community were successful in their quest. When institutional placements occurred, they often were transitory. Large numbers of impaired elders continued to live in the community for long periods of time.[5]

The study in this chapter suggests a way to develop important information about the experiences of a cohort of elders as it ages in the community. The study examined a sample of elderly people living in the community in the state of Massachusetts.[6] They all were aging in place in a variety of residential settings and they drew upon whatever supportive services were available. The aging in place perspective was not restricted by public policy concerns with cost reductions, the need to justify the role of the public sector in caring for elders in the community, or by limiting the study only to a subset of highly impaired elders.[7]

The data show that placements in a nursing home are rare and that informal care is available to most elders living in the community. We looked at the extent to which informal and formal care systems respond to the needs of the elderly and measured the consistency in service levels over a four-year period for a representative cohort of elders.

We relied on descriptive information for a representative sample of 2,898 elders. The members of the cohort were 62 years of age and older when first interviewed in 1982, and 66 years of age or older at the end of the four-year follow-up period in 1986. Baseline characteristics and service use estimates for the first of the four follow-up years apply to all elders in the cohort; year two and subsequent estimates are limited to cohort members who were alive during the remainder of the follow-up period. Our analyses thus center on the experience of a cohort of elders, tracking it at distinct points in time.

Although the findings are limited to elders from one state, they may be indicative of what is occurring in some other industrial states, particularly those with programs that foster in-home care for frail elders.

Findings are disaggregated by type of residential setting: private homes, apartments in facilities for the elderly, and private apartments. Private homes include free-standing homes, condominiums, and mobile homes, whether the elder owns the dwelling or whether he or she is the head of the household; private apartments include privately owned two-unit to multiunit dwellings (as well as residential hotels) where the elder, or someone on behalf of the elder, pays rent as a condition of residency.

The issues discussed in this chapter include the distribution of types of elders in the different residential settings; entry into a nursing home; return to the community following entry into a nursing home; change in community residence; support services received; unmet need status; and functional status. The presentation is primarily descriptive, although explanatory hypotheses are suggested.

We believe that findings of this type are useful in laying a foundation for new long-term-care paradigms.[8]

Living Environments

Over three-quarters (78 percent) of the representative sample of Massachusetts elders residing in the community lived in private homes at the time of the initial (baseline) survey. The next most prevalent setting was private apartments (16.2 percent), followed by housing for the elderly (5.8 percent).

Sociodemographic descriptors of the sample are reported in Table 2-1. The oldest cohort resides in housing for the elderly, a quarter of whom are over 80 years old. The age profiles for the two remaining housing groups are fairly comparable. Slightly less than half were 62 to 69 years of age, and 20 percent or less were age eighty or above. Over 70 percent of elders in elderly housing and private apartment settings were female, but only 55.3 percent of those living in private homes were female. Eighty-five percent of the residents in elderly housing were not married at baseline, but only 63.4 percent living in private apartments and 42.2 percent of those living in private homes were unmarried. Similarly, two-thirds of those living in elderly housing reported that they lived alone. Following the marital status pattern, the distributions of those living alone in the private apartment and private home settings were 43.8 percent and 23.2 percent, respectively.

Table 2-1. Sociodemographic Characteristics

Characteristic	Total Cohort	Residential Setting at Baseline		
		Private Home	Elderly Housing	Private Apartment
AGE				
62–69	46.0%	47.7%	26.7%	44.9%
70–74	19.4	19.9	22.9	16.0
75–79	17.4	16.4	25.3	19.3
80–84	10.2	9.8	11.7	10.9
85 +	7.0	6.2	13.4	8.9
SEX				
Male	41.0	44.7	26.2	28.6
Female	59.0	55.3	73.8	71.4
MARRIED				
Yes	51.9	57.8	15.0	36.6
No	48.1	42.2	85.0	63.4
LIVES ALONE	29.1	23.2	66.1	43.8
HOUSEHOLD INCOME				
Less than $5,000	13.6	10.4	23.8	25.5
$5,000–$9,999	54.4	53.3	64.8	55.8
$10,000–$19,999	21.2	24.1	6.2	12.7
$20,000 +	10.8	12.2	5.2	6.0
(Total Sample N = 2,898)				

(Total Sample N = 2,898)
Source: Data from longitudinal study done by the Department of Social Gerontological Research, Hebrew Rehabilitation Center for the Aged, Boston, Massachusetts, 1982–1986. "Identification of Persons at Risk of Institutional Placement." John Morris, principal investigator, Sylvia Sherwood, co-principal investigator.

In addition to being older, more predominantly female, less likely to be currently married, and less likely to live with someone, residents of elderly housing were poorer than their counterparts in the other two housing settings. Almost a quarter (23.8 percent) reported an annual household income below $5,000, and only 11.4 percent reported an income level above $10,000. Elders living in private apartments ranked second lowest in income. While 25.5 percent of this group also reported an annual household income below $5,000, 18.7 percent reported income in excess of $10,000.

Those residing in private homes were the most affluent — only one in ten reported income below $5,000, whereas 36.3 percent reported income above $10,000.

Placement over Time

Two important findings emerge from the data in Table 2-2, which reports the residential status of the sample of elders 24 and 48 months after the initial interviews. First, the vast majority of elders were still alive and living in the community — 92.9 percent at the two-year follow-up, and 83.2 percent at the four-year follow-up. If we look only at those who were alive in these periods, 98.6 percent were in the community at the end of 24 months, and 97.5 percent at the end of 48 months.

The second major finding concerns admissions to nursing homes. Only 3.4 percent of the original cohort were in a nursing home during the initial 24-month period, and 8 percent during the 48-month period. Of those alive at the end of each of these periods, only 1.4 percent were in a nursing home at the end of 24 months, and 2.5 percent at the end of forty-eight months. Thus, for many elders, nursing home placements are either transitory or occur at the end of one's life.

Among institutionalized elders who were alive at the end of 24 and 48 months, the number who returned to the community was similar to the number who remained in nursing homes: At 24 months, 1.3 percent of the original cohort were in a nursing home and 0.9 percent had been in a nursing home at some point during the 24-month period but had returned to the community by the end of

Table 2-2. Residential Status at Designated Follow-up Points

Residential Status	Total Cohort	Residential Setting at Baseline		
		Private Home	Elderly Housing	Private Apartment
STATUS AT 24 MONTHS*				
Overview				
In community	92.9%	93.4%	87.0%	92.2%
In nursing home	1.3	1.1	1.9	2.1
Dead	5.8	5.5	11.1	5.7
Ever in nursing home				
Total	3.4	3.0	7.0	4.6
(Now in)	(1.3)	(1.1)	(1.9)	(2.1)
(Was, now in community)	(0.9)	(0.9)	(2.6)	(0.6)
(Was, now dead)	(1.2)	(1.0)	(2.5)	(1.9)
Residency for those alive at 24 months				
In community	98.6	98.8	97.9	97.8
In nursing home	1.4	1.2	2.1	2.2
STATUS AT 48 MONTHS				
Overview				
In community	83.2	84.4	79.0	79.6
In nursing home	2.1	1.8	2.0	4.0
Dead	14.6	13.9	19.0	16.4
Ever in nursing home				
Total	8.0	7.3	10.6	11.3
(Now in)	(2.1)	(1.8)	(2.0)	(4.0)
(Was, now in community)	(2.5)	(2.4)	(2.7)	(3.2)
(Was, now dead)	(3.4)	(3.1)	(5.9)	(4.1)
Residency for those alive at 48 months				
In community	97.5	97.9	97.5	95.2
In nursing home	2.5	2.1	2.5	4.8

*At 24 months, 96 cases were lost to follow-up due to refusal to respond or study's inability to locate; at 48 months, 195 cases were lost for these reasons.

the period. Two years later, at 48 months, the pattern was even stronger, 2.1 percent were in a nursing home at the end of month 48, and 2.5 percent had returned from a nursing home to the community.

Of those who died, the risk of institutional placement was considerably higher than the overall averages might suggest — one in five over the initial two-year period, and one in four over the four-year period. By the end of month 24, of those who had entered a nursing home 35 percent had died, 38 percent were still in a nursing home, and 27 percent had resumed community residency. In 48 months, 43 percent of those who had entered a nursing home had died, 26 percent were still in a nursing home, and 31 percent had returned to the community.

The use of nursing homes differs only slightly among residents living in different settings. At the end of month 24, while 1 percent of elders from private homes were in nursing homes, 2 percent of elders from the two apartment settings were in nursing homes. By the end of month 48, residents of both private homes and housing for the elderly shared a lower likelihood of nursing home placement (2.1 percent to 2.5 percent) than residents in private apartments (4.8 percent).

The likelihood of ever having resided in a nursing home during the four-year period is highest for elders in the two apartment settings (about 11 percent) and lowest for those in private housing (7.3 percent).

Of the elders who entered a nursing home during the 48 months and who were alive at the end of that period, those in private homes and housing for the elderly (at baseline) had a 57 percent chance of returning to the community. For the elders who had moved to a nursing home from a private apartment, the rate of discharge from a nursing home back to the community was somewhat lower — 44 percent by the end of month 48.

Of those who died during this period, institutional placement rates were lowest for residents in the private home subgroup (22 percent), compared to those in private apartments (25 percent) and those in housing for the elderly (31 percent).

Cohort death rates were 5.8 percent in the initial 24-month period, and 9.3 percent in the second 24-month period for those alive in month 25. This increase is attributable to both an aging cohort and the fact that in the second period (between 24 and 48 months) a substantial number of the original sample of elders had been institutionalized. When identified (at baseline) in 1982, all sample members lived in the community. At the beginning of the second two-year period, 1.4 percent of elders resided in nursing homes. Over four years, we can see the importance of this change in the makeup of the cohort: 42.5 percent of those who were ever in a nursing home had died, although only 12.2 percent of those who had never been in a nursing home had died.

Through 24 months, the death rate was highest for those living in elderly housing — 11.1 percent. This was almost double the rate for elders in the other two settings. By the fourth follow-up year, the cumulative death rate was still highest for those who had resided in elderly housing at baseline (19.0 percent). This difference, however, was due entirely to the differential death rate in the initial 24-month period. During the period from month 25 through month 48, the elderly housing subgroup who were alive at month 25 had an 8.9 percent death rate, a rate identical to that of elders in private housing (8.9 percent) and less than that of elders in private apartments (12.0 percent).

Shifts in residential setting since baseline are summarized in Table 2-3, representing the baseline and follow-up sites of residence. Of those living in private homes at baseline, 91.5 percent were still

Table 2-3. Shifts in Residential Setting

Residential Setting at Designated Follow-up Period	Residential Setting at Baseline		
	Private Home	Elderly Housing	Private Apartment
24 MONTHS (N = 2615)			
Private home	91.5$	1.4%	10.0%
Elderly housing	1.2	79.7	4.5
Private apartment	6.1	16.7	83.3
Nursing home	1.2	2.2	2.2
48 MONTHS (N = 2216)			
Private home	89.5	3.1	18.3
Elderly housing	2.1	63.7	6.5
Private apartment	6.3	30.7	70.4
Nursing home	2.1	2.5	4.8

living in private homes at 24 months, and 89.5 percent at the 48-month follow-up. Only 1.2 percent were in a nursing home at 24 months and 2.1 percent at 48 months. About 6 percent of this cohort were in private apartments at each of the follow-up intervals and 1% and 2%, respectively, were in elderly housing.

Comparable but somewhat lower levels of residential stability characterized elders in private apartments and elderly housing. Among those living in private apartments, movement was largely into private homes — 10 percent through months 24 and 18.3 percent through month 48. Movement to a private home was most often accompanied by residency with others: At month 48, 53 percent lived with a spouse, 21 percent lived with a child, 9 percent lived with some other relative, and only 17 percent lived alone. A much lower rate of movement to private homes is noted for those in elderly housing at baseline — 1.4 percent through month 24, and 3.1 percent through month 48. If a tenant in elderly housing moved, the community alternative was almost always a private apartment, and the majority lived alone following the move: At month 48, of those who entered a private apartment, 56 percent lived alone, 16 percent resided with a spouse, and 28 percent resided with a child.

Of those in elderly housing and private apartments, 2.2 percent were in nursing homes at the end of month 24. By the end of month 48, 2.5 percent of elderly housing tenants and 4.8 percent of those in private apartments were in nursing homes.

Changes in Functional Status

The functional status estimates presented in this chapter rely on an expanded version of the HRCA Vulnerability Index.[9] The HRCA Index differentiates elders into two groups: the functionally independent and the functionally impaired. Impairment is defined as requiring support in at least two areas of daily activities such as meal preparation, housework, taking out the rubbish, dressing, and climbing stairs. In this chapter the impaired are further disaggregated into those with activity of daily living (ADL) and those with instrumental activity of daily living (IADL) dependencies. ADL-dependent elders require support with personal care activities, particularly dressing, and with medication management. IADL-dependent elders do not have ADL deficiencies, but do have problems in preparing meals independently, removing rubbish, or completing light housework activities. Based on this expanded version of the HRCA Vulnerability Index, at baseline 77.8 percent of elders were functionally independent, 17.2 percent had IADL deficits, and 5 percent had ADL deficits (Table 2-4). Those living in private homes were most likely to be functionally independent, but those living in housing for the elderly were most likely to have IADL and ADL deficits.

Although some individuals changed in functional status, there was little change in the proportion of elders remaining in the cohort who were functionally independent and nonindependent during the forty-eight-month study period. At each of the three data collection points, 78 percent of the cohort members were found to be functionally independent.

At baseline, elders in private homes were most independent, while those in elderly housing were the most dependent. At the same time, only elderly housing tenants, in line with their higher death rate in the initial twenty-four-month period (see Table 2-2),

Table 2-4. Functional Status Distributions at Three Points in Time

		Residential Setting		
	Total Cohort	Private Home	Elderly Housing	Private Apartment
FUNCTIONAL STATUS AT BASELINE				
Independent	77.8$	80.5%	59.4%	71.5%
IADL problem	17.2	14.8	32.7	23.3
ADL problem	5.0	4.7	7.9	5.2
FUNCTIONAL STATUS 24 MONTHS LATER				
Independent	78.7	80.0	71.7	74.8
IADL problem	13.3	12.4	19.8	15.4
ADL problem	8.0	7.6	8.5	9.8
FUNCTIONAL STATUS 48 MONTHS LATER				
Independent	77.7	79.0	67.5	75.3
IADL problem	12.1	11.7	18.5	11.7
ADL problem	10.2	9.3	14.0	13.0

(Total cohort N = 2898; at 24 months N = 2615; at 48 months N = 2216)

experienced an appreciable shift in the distribution of impaired elders over time. This resulted in a net increase in the proportion who were independent for the residual cohort at 24 months compared with the total cohort at baseline.

Aging in place over the four-year period was not accompanied by a rapid loss of functional independence for surviving sample members. At the same time, concentrating only on the estimate for those with the most severe functional problems, there is a tendency in all housing settings for the proportion with ADL deficits to increase over time.

Selected sociodemographic characteristics of those with IADL/ADL deficits at baseline are reported in Table 2-5. Among those under 75, 16 percent had one or more deficits. This figure rises to 24 percent among the 75 to 79 age group, and to 44.1 percent among those 80 and older. In the first two age groups (under 75 and 75 to 79), a higher proportion of those living in elderly housing had one or more deficits than those living in private homes (37.1 percent versus 13.9 percent). The same pattern holds true for those age 75 to 79. For both of those age categories, those living in private apartments occupy a midpoint position—a greater proportion had IADL/ADL deficits than their counterparts living in private homes, but their rate was less than that of those living in elderly housing. However, for age 80 and above, the percentage with IADL/ADL deficits was fairly comparable in all three housing settings.

Fourteen percent of those who were married and 30.5 percent of those not married had one or more functional deficits. Sixteen percent of males and 26.3 of females had such deficits. For both of these sociodemographic characteristics, deficit rates were generally highest for those in elderly housing and lowest for those living in private homes. Comparable patterns are noted for elders living alone or living with others.

Changes in functional status over time are shown in Table 2-6. Close to 85 percent of elders alive at each follow-up period who were functionally independent at baseline remained functionally independent at follow-up. A large proportion of the survivors, close to half in five of the six cells in the table, displayed an improvement in functional status over the follow-up periods, but 15 percent or fewer became less functionally independent over time.

Among those who were IADL-dependent at baseline, less than 19 percent were more dependent at 24 months and less than 25

Table 2-5. Relationship of Functional Status to Selected Demographic Characteristics

Percent Who Have One or More IADL/ADL Deficits

Designated Background Characteristic	Total Cohort	Residential Setting at Baseline		
		Private Home	Elderly Housing	Private Apartment
Less than 75	16.0%	13.9%	37.1%	21.0%
75–79 years of age	24.0	19.9	43.0	33.2
80+ years of age	44.1	42.9	45.6	48.1
Married	14.5	12.8	28.9	25.0
Not married	30.5	28.6	43.1	30.6
Male	16.4	13.1	23.2	37.8
Female	26.3	24.8	46.5	24.5
Live alone	25.4	22.7	37.4	25.2
Live with others	20.8	18.5	48.5	31.6

(Total cohort N = 2898)

Table 2-6. Change in Functional Status

| | | Residential Setting at Baseline | | |
	Total Cohort	Private Home	Elderly Housing	Private Apartment
PROPORTION OF INDEPENDENT ELDERS AT BASELINE WHO REMAINED INDEPENDENT				
At 24 months	82.8%	87.7%	84.9%	89.0%
At 48 months	85.9	86.0	90.6	84.0
PROPORTION WHO BECAME MORE INDEPENDENT (EXCLUDING THE INDEPENDENT AT BASELINE FROM DENOMINATOR)				
At 24 months	45.9	46.5	50.7	41.4
At 48 months	45.4	45.2	33.9	53.2
PROPORTION WHO BECAME MORE DEPENDENT (EXCLUDING THE ADL-DEPENDENT AT BASELINE FROM DENOMINATOR)				
At 24 months	13.1	13.3	13.9	12.1
At 48 months	15.4	15.2	11.9	17.4
PROPORTION OF IADL-DEPENDENT AT BASELINE WHO BECAME MORE DEPENDENT				
At 24 months	17.6	18.9	10.7	16.5
At 48 months	23.5	24.6	16.2	24.2
PROPORTION OF ADL-DEPENDENT AT BASELINE WHO BECAME LESS DEPENDENT				
At 24 months	25.8	27.3	34.0	16.5
At 48 months	42.1	43.8	35.8	35.2

(At 24 months N = 2615; at 48 months N = 2216)

percent were more dependent at 48 months. Large proportions of those who were ADL-dependent became less dependent, as shown in the last two rows of data in Table 2-6 — 26 percent through two years and 42 percent through four years.

Access to Support Resources

Data on the annual amounts of supportive services received by the sample of elders was estimated for homemaking, chores, meals, personal care, medication management, shopping, and transportation. Table 2-7 shows that home-based care is a pervasive feature in the lives of elders as they age in the community. Between 72 percent and 79 percent of elders in the three residential settings received informal care, levels that are considerably higher than the 22 percent of elders shown to have IADL and/or ADL deficits in Table 2-4. Informal supports were almost always present if elders had reduced functional capacities; 91.2 percent and 95.8 percent, respectively, had IADL and ADL deficits. Even for those without functional deficits, however, informal care was the norm — with almost three-quarters of these elders receiving some type of assistance by family and/or friends. (Reciprocal helping behaviors between functionally independent spouses was not included in the definition.)

On average, recipients of informal care were assisted with two or more activities — 2.6 for those who were functionally independent, 3.6 for those with IADL impairments, and 4.9 for those with ADL impairments. In the twelve-month period following assessment of those elders who received informal care, the majority were assisted with shopping (ranging from 73 percent for the independent to 93 percent for the ADL-impaired) and transportation (ranging from 55 percent to 76 percent). Among these recipients of informal care, assistance with meals and housework was received by one-quarter of functionally independent elders, a little less than half of IADL-impaired elders, and about three-quarters of ADL-impaired elders. Informal assistance with personal care was generally limited to those who exhibited ADL impairments, and was received by 4 percent of independent elders receiving informal care, 11 percent of the IADL-impaired, and 64 percent of the ADL-impaired.

Table 2-7. Distribution of Elders Receiving Care from Others (averaged over four study years)

Total Cohort or Functional Subgroup	Total Group	Residential Setting at Baseline		
		Private Home	Elderly Housing	Private Apartment
Average annual % who received informal care				
Total Cohort	77.6	77.8	71.9	79.2
Independent	73.5	74.3	61.0	74.1
IADL-dependent	91.2	91.8	85.8	90.0
ADL-dependent	95.8	96.8	92.1	92.5
Average annual % who received formal care in the community				
Total Cohort	40.0	37.4	66.4	43.9
Independent	35.0	31.7	59.3	41.9
IADL-dependent	54.0	54.3	78.4	43.7
ADL-dependent	52.5	47.4	75.7	68.9
Average annual number of areas in which recipients of informal care were assisted				
Total Cohort	2.9	2.9	2.6	2.9
Independent	2.6	2.6	2.2	2.6
IADL-dependent	3.6	3.7	3.1	3.4
ADL-dependent	4.9	5.2	3.4	4.8
Average annual number of areas in which recipients of formal care in the community were assisted				
Total Cohort	1.8	1.7	2.4	2.1
Independent	1.6	1.5	1.8	1.7
IADL-dependent	2.3	2.1	2.7	2.9
ADL-dependent	2.9	2.6	3.3	3.3

Significantly fewer elders made use of formal support services in the community — about 40 percent overall, ranging from 35 percent of those who were functionally independent to 54 percent of those with IADL and/or ADL deficits. To some extent, the use of formal services by those who were functionally independent represents a private market or life-style choice by elders and their families. At the same time, it also reflects the fact that some of those who were independent at baseline experience transitory or permanent changes in need status during the intervening time period (see Table 2-6). For example, of those who were independent at both baseline and at the two-year follow-up, about 33 percent made use of formal services; of those who became IADL-dependent, about 44 percent used formal services; and of those who moved from independent to ADL-dependent, about 53 percent used formal services.

On average, recipients of formal care in the community were assisted with 1.8 activities, ranging from 1.6 activities for those who were functionally independent to 2.3 and 2.9, respectively, for those with IADL and ADL impairments. In the twelve-month period following assessment, there was no service area in which a majority of elders receiving help obtained that help from a formal source. The two most prevalent areas of support were meals and transportation, in which 38 percent and 33 percent, respectively, of the recipients of formal care were assisted. Little difference in receipt patterns across the functional subgroups was noted. In addition to these two services, 17 percent of functionally independent recipients of formal care received help with housework and personal care, whereas less than 10 percent received help with shopping and medication management. For IADL- and ADL-impaired recipients of formal care, approximately 40 percent received formal help with housework and transportation, and 25 percent of the IADL-impaired and 47 percent of the ADL-impaired received help with personal care. Finally, formal assistance with medication management was largely localized to those who were ADL-impaired: It averaged 3 percent of the independent, 12 percent of the IADL-impaired, and 35 percent of the ADL-impaired.

Differences exist in the usage estimates in the three housing settings. Although 74 percent of independent elders in private homes and private apartments received informal care, only 61 percent of independent elders in housing for the elderly received such care. Elderly housing tenants who are functionally independent appear to be less able to rely on friends and relatives for support in the everyday activities of life. This housing-associated difference in access to informal care was not observed for elders with ADL impairments; for those elders, the difference was not in the receipt of care but rather in a reduction in the number of areas in which informal care was provided.

Interresidential patterns of access to formal community services are more complex. Tenants residing in housing for the elderly were most likely to access formal support systems. For those who were functionally independent, 59 percent received formal care, but for those who were functionally impaired, slightly over 75 percent received formal care.

For elders in private homes and apartments, use of formal care was less than that observed in elderly housing, except for those in private apartments who had ADL deficits. In the latter case, the rates were about the same. In addition, for ADL-dependent elders in both apartment settings (elderly and private), although not displayed in table 2-7, the percentage using home-based formal care decreased over time, from 87.4 percent to 66.4 percent over the four-year interval for tenants in elderly housing, and from 74.8 percent to 63.0 percent for tenants in private apartments. Although we have not explored the reasons for these shifts, we note that this decreasing utilization pattern begins to bring these elders into closer proximity with the considerably lower usage experience of ADL-dependent elders residing in private homes. In addition, as indicated in Table 2-2, a higher proportion of tenants in the two apartment subgroups spent time in a nursing home (thereby reducing their need for home-based formal care).

Of those living in private homes, formal usage levels mirror the values for the total sample. In contrast to those in apartments, ADL-dependent elders living in private homes were considerably less likely to make use of formal support services in the home. Elders in private homes were much more likely to reside with a spouse (see Table 2-1), and this undoubtedly played a large part in this unique helping pattern. Such people may simply be less likely to require supports beyond those provided by family. When elderly individuals in private homes have a need for ADL support, it is more likely to be provided informally. In addition, for the subgroups of elders in private homes who were functionally independent or had IADL deficits, the percent using home-based formal care increased over time—rising from 19.1 percent in the first year to 32.4 percent in the fourth year for those who were functionally independent, and from 46.2 percent to 62.1 percent for those who had IADL deficits.

In assessing the use of formal services in Massachusetts it is important to consider the extent to which the state's widespread case-managed home care system is involved in the care provision process. Massachusetts uses state funds to provide homemaking, chore, transportation, and other home-based services to approximately 4 percent of elders in the state. This pattern represents a relatively unique commitment by a state to providing community-based long-term-care services. Our data suggest that significant numbers of impaired elders, particularly those in apartment settings (private apartments and elderly housing), benefit from this program. Approximately 70 percent of ADL-dependent elders and 50 percent of IADL-dependent elders received formal services in their homes. For functionally impaired elders residing in private homes, approximately 44 percent of ADL-dependent and 23 percent of IADL-dependent received formal in-home services. At the other extreme, for functionally independent users (some of whom will have deteriorated over time) of formal services, home care participation was at a much lower level—5 percent for those in private homes, 7 percent for those in private apartments, and 14 percent for those in elderly housing.

Services Used

Table 2-8 contains estimates of the annual hours of informal and formal care, based on average utilization values, provided to sample residents during four one-year periods. Also included are systematic trends representing either increasing or decreasing levels of care. The initial, and in many ways most important finding, was the absence of significant shifts over this four-year period in informal and formal utilization levels for the total group of elders in the cohort. On average, community elders who were alive in any study year received 101 hours of informal care and 26 hours of formal care—representing 4 hours of informal care for every hour of formal care. These findings suggest a system in equilibrium. They are consistent with our earlier finding of longitudinal stability in the estimated proportion of functionally independent elders (see Table 2-4). They also fit within a model of oscillating capabilities: Some elders

Table 2-8. Average Annual Hours of Informal and Formal Care (average of four one-year periods)

	Total Group	Residential Setting at Baseline		
		Private Home	Elderly Housing	Private Apartment
		Average Annual Hours of Informal Care		
TOTAL SAMPLE AVERAGE OF FOUR ONE-YEAR-PERIODS	100.9	104.1	54.7	100.1
AVERAGE FOR ELDERS IN DIFFERENT FUNCTIONAL CATEGORIES AT BASELINE				
Independent	80.4*	84.0*	41.7*	72.5
IADL-dependent	149.4	164.9	71.5	137.2
ADL-dependent	264.4*	278.3*	136.9*	280.5*
		Average Annual Hours of Formal Care		
TOTAL SAMPLE AVERAGE OF FOUR ONE-YEAR PERIODS	26.1	22.2*	53.1*	35.9*
AVERAGE FOR ELDERS IN DIFFERENT FUNCTIONAL CATEGORIES AT BASELINE				
Independent	19.3*	18.2*	29.3*	22.7*
IADL-dependent	48.6	37.5	74.4	73.1*
ADL-dependent	67.3*	57.7*	136.7	66.5*

*There was a steady increase in the annual hours of care from year 1 to year 4.

die and some deteriorate, but others improve, and the net effect of these changes for a given cohort is longitudinal stability in estimated risk levels and utilization profiles.

At the same time, interresidential differences existed in informal utilization levels. Informal care was least intensive for tenants in housing for the elderly, averaging 55 hours per year or about one-half the average for elders in private homes and private apartments. These interresidential differences were consistent over time, and there was no indication that informal support levels were changing for the cohort as a whole, nor that elders in one setting were more or less likely to experience shifts in the intensity of informal care available to them. As would be expected, informal supports increased with disability status, with tenants in elderly housing receiving the lowest level of care at each level of disability. Highest informal care levels were found for elders with ADL deficits who lived in private apartments and private homes: They averaged 280 hours of care per year, or a little more than three-quarters of an hour per day. In addition, for elders who were independent at baseline, we observed an increase in informal support levels over time. This occurred because this group became slightly more functionally dependent—increasing from an average of 73.8 hours of care in the first year to 85.6 hours in the fourth year.

For functionally independent tenants in housing for the elderly, the annual averages rose from 34.8 hours in the first year to 47.6 hours in the fourth year; for functionally independent elders in private apartments, there was no systematic pattern of increasing informal hours of care over time.

Finally, for elders who were functionally (ADL) impaired at baseline, a different pattern of longitudinal shifts in average cohort utilization values occurred. For the high-level users who resided in private homes and private apartments, utilization went down over time—from 345.5 hours to 252.3 hours in the four-year period for those in private homes, and from 313.8 hours to 223.5 hours for those in private apartments. To some extent these changes reflect the death or institutional placement of the most disabled of these cases. In addition, some experienced improvement, that is, they became more functionally independent. For ADL-dependent elders in housing for the elderly at baseline, the pattern over time is much different. The average hours of care in the first follow-up year for this cohort was only about 40 percent of the level observed for ADL-dependent elders in the other two settings. More importantly, their average hours of care increased over time, rising from 134.7 hours (on average) in year one to 151.8 hours in year four. By year four, their average hours of informal care had increased to about 63 percent of the level observed for ADL-dependent elders in the other two settings. It appears that informal supporters are less responsive if the elder resides in an elderly housing site, although there is some indication (at least for those who are functionally independent or have ADL deficits, although not for those with IADL deficits) that the level of these supports can increase over time.

Formal care levels also differed by residential setting. Unlike the preceding findings, formal care is most intensive for tenants in housing for the elderly—averaging fifty-three hours per year, or about equal to the level of informal care received by these tenants. This level of care is twice that for elders in private homes and one and one-half times the level for elders in private apartments. As would be expected, formal support levels increase with disability status, averaging 19 hours per year for those who are functionally independent, 49 hours for those with IADL deficits, and 67 hours for those with ADL deficits.

Three remaining findings are worthy of special note. First, universally lower levels of formal care were observed for elders in private homes who do not have ADL deficiencies. Second, the average level of formal care for ADL-dependent adults who continue to live decreased over time, from an average of 77.2 hours in the first year to 56.4 hours in the fourth year. Third, ADL-dependent elders in housing for the elderly have average utilization levels that far exceed those of ADL-dependent elders in other residential settings.

Unmet Needs

The unmet-need estimates in Table 2-9 summarize subjective judgments of whether additional support is required with home-making, chores, meals, personal care, medication management, shopping, and transportation. To be scored as having an unmet need, a respondent must report the need for additional support in a service area in which he or she has had some level of functional

Table 2-9. Percentage of Elders with Unmet Needs
(averaged over three rounds of interviews)

Total Cohort or Functional Subgroup	Average Annual Percentage Who Report Unmet Needs			
	Total Group	Residential Setting at Baseline		
		Private Home	Elderly Housing	Private Apartment
Total cohort	5.0	3.8	9.2	6.0
Independent	2.7	2.3	6.5	3.5
IADL-dependent	13.7	14.5	12.4	11.7
ADL-dependent	17.1	17.6	14.1	17.2

restriction (no matter how minor). As indicated in the table, unmet needs in Massachusetts were not a pervasive factor in the lives of most elders—only 5 percent of elders reported unmet needs. Although not shown in the table, the needs reported were seldom viewed by the respondents to be of major significance. In addition, very few elders required additional support in more than two areas, and most who required such supports had a need in only one area.

Unmet-need levels were higher for elders with IADL and ADL deficits—13.7 percent and 17.1 percent respectively. But even here, approximately five out of every six impaired elders believed that they were receiving sufficient support services. Finally, although there is some fluctuation across residential settings, the basic shape of the distributions and relative levels of unmet need were not dramatically different.

Conclusion

Very little published information exists on the types of changes to be expected as elders age in the community. This study provides data that suggest the importance of conducting this kind of research throughout the country. The population of elders in the community is diverse, and it is this diversity that must be studied. Elders live in different types of residential settings, and although the importance of adequate housing for maintaining elders in the community has been pointed out by some researchers,[10] it has not received as much attention as have, for example, the large number of community-based case-management programs evaluated under federal sponsorship. For long-term-care professionals housing has been of secondary interest, often characterized as simply the opposite of institutional residency without further differentiation. By focusing on the concept of aging in place we can begin to remedy this oversight. We therefore examined longitudinal data for subgroup cohorts of elders in three distinct types of housing, and provided descriptive information on residential mobility, death, functional status, institutional placement, and service utilization.

The data have made it possible to highlight a series of factors essential to planning long-term-care services for the frail elderly in this country. We have found that residential mobility patterns differ for elders who live in the three types of settings studied. Institutional placements were relatively rare, and many who entered a nursing home subsequently returned to the community. Informal support was found to be available to most elders; helping patterns begin prior to functional decline, escalate with increasing disability, and achieve different levels of intensity in the three types of housing. Formal care also was a factor in the lives of large numbers of elders living in the community. Moreover, the use of some formal care did not require that the elder be impaired. Its spread for those in apartments was related to the presence of a statewide program of case-managed home care services.

In presenting these data, we hope to highlight the need for new service paradigms. There is much to be gained by finding out what is happening in the community and providing descriptive information that can be used for more effective organization of services. We recognize that, despite the fact that the data cover four years, the lessons to be learned are limited to information from a single time period (1982 to 1986) and from a single state (Massachusetts). We believe it would be useful to both states and the federal government to replicate this type of study in many other places in the country; a single national survey will not provide the information needed for realistic planning on the local or statewide level. Local factors of particular importance are residential density, the distribution of minority and disadvantaged populations, the rate of in- and out-migration, the extent of state or local support for community-based service systems, and local variations in the access or use of third-party insurance. Because long-term care is so related to systems of informal care as well as to local variations in community and institutional service availability, we recommend that replications be completed for populations in different states with the overall effort coordinated at the national level.

Notes

1. U.S. Department of Health and Human Services. "Health United States, 1987." DHHS Publication No. (PHS) 88-1232, Table 113, 1987.

2. U.S. Department of Health and Human Services. "National long-term care channeling demonstration." March 1987.

3. Brown, T.E., Jr., D.K. Blackman, R.M. Learner, M.B. Witherspoon, and L. Saber. "South Carolina Community Long-Term Care Project: A report of findings under HCFA Project Grant No. 11-P-97493/4 to South Carolina State Health and Human Services Finance Commission." 1985.

   Capitman, J., B. Haskins, and J. Bernstein. "Case management approaches in coordinated community-oriented long-term-care demonstrations." *The Gerontologist,* 26:398–404, 1985.

   Weissert, W.G. "Seven reasons why it is so difficult to make community-based long-term care cost-effective." *Health Services Research,* 20:423–33, 1985.

   U.S. General Accounting Office. "The elderly should benefit from expanded home health care but increasing these services will not insure cost reductions." GAO/IPE-83-1. Gaithersburg, Md.: U.S. General Accounting Office, 1982.

   Hicks, B., H. Raisz, J. Segal, and N. Doherty. "The triage experiment in coordinated care for the family." *American Journal of Public Health,* 71:991–1002, 1982.

   Skellie, F.A., G.M. Mobley, and R.E. Coan. "Cost-effectiveness of community-based long-term care: Current findings of Georgia's alternative health services project." *American Journal of Public Health,* 72:353–58, 1982.

   Holahan, J., and M. Stessen. "Long-term care demonstration projects: A review of recent demonstrations." Working paper 1227-2, Urban Institute, Washington, D.C., 1981.

   Hammond, J. "Home health care cost effectiveness: An overview of the literature." *Public Health Reports,* 94:305–11, 1979.

4. "High risk" is the term applied to those who are most likely to require nursing home care.

5. Weissert, W.G. "Seven reasons."

Morris, J.N., S. Sherwood, and C.E. Gutkin. "Inst-Risk II—An approach to forecasting relative risk of future institutional placement." *Health Services Research*, in press.

Morris, J.N., C.E. Gutkin, H.S. Ruchlin, and S. Sherwood. "Housing and case-managed home care programs and subsequent institutional utilization." *The Gerontologist*, 27:788–96, 1987.

6. Supported by grant #87ASPE183A from DHHS, Assistant Secretary for Planning and Evaluation (ASPE).

7. Christianson, J.B. "The effect of channeling on informal caregiving." *Health Services Research* 23:99–117, 1988. Kemper, P., R. A. Applebaum, and M. Harrigan. "Community care demonstrations: What have we learned?" *Health Care Financing Review*, 9:87–110, 1987.

8. Weissert, W.G. "Seven reasons."

Morris, J.N., C.E. Gutkin, H.S. Ruchlin, and S. Sherwood. "Long-term care community services: Risk groups and level of care." In preparation.

Lawton, M.P. "Housing for the elderly in the mid-1980s." In G. Lesnoff-Caravaglia (Ed.), *Handbook of Applied Gerontology*. New York: Human Sciences Service Press, 1987.

Newman, S.J. "Demographic influences on the future housing demand of the elderly." In R. J. Newcomer, M. P. Lawton, and T. O. Byerts (Eds.), New York: Van Nostrand Reinhold Company, 1986.

Brody, E. "Service options in congregate housing." In R.D. Chellis, J.F. Seagle, and B.M. Seagle, (Eds.), *Congregate Housing for Older People*. Lexington, Mass.: Lexington Books, 1982.

9. Morris, J.N., S. Sherwood, and V. Mor. "An assessment tool for use in identifying functionally vulnerable persons in the community." *The Gerontologist*, 24:373–79, 1984.

10. Sherwood, S., and J.N. Morris. "The Pennsylvania domiciliary care experiment: Impact on quality of life." *American Journal of Public Health*, 73, 1983, and in L. H. Aiken and B. H. Kehrer (Eds.), *Evaluation Studies Review Annual*. Beverly Hills, Calif.: Sage Publications.

Sherwood, S., J.N. Morris, C.C. Sherwood, S. Morris, E. Bernstein, and E.S. Gornstein. Final report of the evaluation of congregate housing services program, in connection with HUD contract #HC-5373, 1985.

Sherwood, S., D.S. Greer, J.N. Morris, V. Mor, and Associates. *An Alternative in Long-Term Care: The Highland Heights Story*. Cambridge, Mass.: Ballinger Press, 1981.

Sherwood, S., C.E. Gutkin, T.G. Lewis, Sr., and C.C. Sherwood. "Housing alternatives for an aging society." In *Legislative Agenda for an Aging Society: 1988 and Beyond*. Proceedings of a Congressional Forum by the Select Committee on Aging, House of Representatives and the Special Committee on Aging, United

States Senate, November 1987. Washington, D.C.: U.S. Government Printing Office, 1988 pp. 105–44.

Byerts, T.O., S.C. Howell, and L.A. Pastalan (Eds.). *Environmental Context of Aging.* New York: Garland STPM Press, 1979.

Newcomer, R.J., M.P. Lawton, and T.O. Byerts (Eds.). *Housing an Aging Society: Issues, Alternatives and Policy.* New York: Van Nostrand Reinhold Company, 1986.

PART TWO

Current Residential Realities

CHAPTER THREE

Living Independently with Neighbors Who Care: Strategies to Facilitate Aging in Place

JAMES T. SYKES

*W*here people live is central to the quality of their lives. Over time, the significance of "home" increases as older people face the loss of other symbols of independence and connections to the mainstream of life. Nearly every study affirms the conventional wisdom that older people strongly prefer to age in place, to grow old within familiar territory that has provided a context for their lives, whether they live in single family dwellings, elderly housing complexes, or naturally occurring retirement communities.

How the marketplace provides shelter for an aging society and what government does to develop, coordinate, and finance support systems for those most vulnerable will affect the quality of life for millions of older Americans.

The past two decades have seen dramatic shifts in the demography and health status of older persons, and these trends are continuing. There are millions more older people, their health is considerably better, and their preferences are diverse. However, for many, advanced age brings frailty and the need for supportive living environments. Society now faces an immense challenge to provide sufficient affordable housing that suits the preferences and meets the changing needs of older Americans.

53

As the number of very old persons increases rapidly, the need for imaginative responses in shelter and services becomes urgent. Society may choose to pay a relatively small sum to modify apartments and increase services, or to pay substantially more later when elders move into nursing homes, spend their resources, and become dependent upon Medicaid.

Fortunately, there are groups and individuals creating new living arrangements, designing appropriate housing, organizing services, and experimenting with programs responsive to older people's needs. We're beginning to see the results of social experimentation, innovative programs, and community responses to the aging in place phenomenon.[1]

The combination of new ideas in living arrangements and society's willingness to increase support to people living in community augers well for the future of elderly housing. However, before too much is made of progress to date, the balance sheet must account for the loss of quality housing stock,[2] particularly in rural America.[3] Government programs have failed to keep pace with the great need for affordable housing with supportive services—especially for elderly people near or below the poverty line.

Demographic facts provide ample evidence of the aging of our society and underline the extent to which the blessings of long life are diminished by the incidence of chronic illness. The poor and very old with little or no family support, principally women, are in double jeopardy. Efforts to make Medicare and Medicaid more comprehensive and accessible need to be integrated with reforms in the housing policy arena. Housing is a critical component of a long-term-care system for those suffering from infirmities associated with long life, who—with a little help—can continue to live semi-independently within the community.

This chapter describes how a few local communities have successfully accommodated residents who have grown increasingly dependent. In addition, the efforts of three states to implement a positive strategy for dealing with the needs of aging individuals suggest that the cutting edge of housing policy may well be in state capitals rather than in Washington. A brief section on naturally occurring retirement communities (NORCs) describes how individuals are aging in place fairly successfully without the support of organized services. NORCs demonstrate that a majority of older people age in places where they have important ties to the community.

The chapter concludes with a discussion of the key role housing plays in the long-term-care system and provides a list of important issues about which too little is known and that merit serious attention by the research community.

Community Examples

Throughout the nation communities are developing innovative elderly housing ideas in response to local needs. Housing for the elderly is not a new enterprise, but the need is becoming more urgent as the population ages. The service needs of the very old exceed the capabilities of available facilities. The cases cited here illustrate solutions that may apply in many places. They include government and nongovernment programs, initiated both privately and publicly, in small towns and large. Common to each is a high level of integration between housing and supportive services essential to an individual's well-being.

SUN PRAIRIE, WISCONSIN

Sun Prairie, a small community not far from the state capital in Madison, applied for public housing at about the same time communities all over the nation began to look to the federal government to finance public housing.[4] Like hundreds of other towns, Sun Prairie did not make HUD's approved list: There were too many proposals and too little money. Undiscouraged, leaders of the city's senior center, the Colonial Club, urged a local corporation to develop elderly housing under provisions of another HUD program. The application was in the pipeline when the Nixon administration announced a moratorium on all federally assisted housing. Sun Prairie's elders saw their promising project rejected before it left the planning board.

However, corporate officers of The Wisconsin Cheeseman, a closely held private corporation, decided to develop housing to meet the well-documented needs of the community's elders. Thus began Colonial Acres, a housing development that now includes 154 corporate-owned units, 94 Section 202/8 units, and two group homes with accommodations for 16 people. The housing units were built on land adjacent to the senior center, an attractive facility built and donated by The Cheeseman. The campus was designed to provide various levels of housing for persons with changing needs.

Beginning with ninety-eight independent living, garden-type apartments, the corporate owners asked the senior center staff to identify those most in need of moving into the housing — whether for health, social, or economic reasons. Through efficient construction and management, the corporation was able to set rents below market rates. A corporate grant to a local church provided support to those who needed help with their rent. Campus residents and older persons around the area received a wide variety of services including transportation, subsidized meals, counseling, adult day care, information and referral, and, equally important, an opportunity to participate in an active program.[5]

The apartments were designed to accommodate independent elderly persons who wanted to be close to the senior center's programs, services, and people. In the Sun Prairie community, Colonial Acres is viewed not as an elderly ghetto, but as a pleasant neighborhood surrounding an attractive senior center. This image holds even as the average age of residents rises and the number of individuals requiring assistance increases.

When it became evident that additional housing was needed and that such housing should include meals, housekeeping, and personal assistance, the Colonial Club applied to HUD for a direct federal loan (Section 202) to build a congregate housing facility. The application was approved, and a ninety-four unit congregate housing facility was added to the campus. A part-time geriatric nurse practitioner was hired whose skills and knowledge added substantially to the center's capacity to serve aging residents.

The Colonial Acres story is a success story for many reasons, but it stands out because it provides housing for both poor and well-off persons, for healthy, vigorous individuals as well as those in need of supportive services. That a private corporation has developed and financed housing in cooperation with a senior center is an idea worthy of replication.[6]

DURHAM, NORTH CAROLINA

Before the first resident moved into Oldham Towers, a high-rise housing facility for about a hundred elderly poor, the Coordinating

Council for Senior Citizens of Durham offered to help the Housing Authority plan for the residents' future.[7] The council, a private, nonprofit agency responsible for aging programs and services, urged the Housing Authority to provide space for a senior center within the facility. The council offered to finance the additional space and provide vital services for residents and older people living in the area. The authority agreed, and a center program, already begun in a nearby church, moved into space in the facility — avoiding the usual turf problems that occur between residents and "outsiders."

Ten years later, the authority developed a second high rise, the Henderson Housing Center, which provides 179 apartments in another part of town. With ten years of positive experience and financial support from a Community Development Block Grant and federal revenue sharing, the authority quickly agreed to provide community space for a senior center offering health and personal care services. The Coordinating Council administers the center and provides special services, including transportation, health promotion, counseling, and a clinic for residents and area seniors.

The success of over twenty years of integrating services and programs at Oldham Towers and ten productive years at the Henderson Housing Center is acknowledged by the Housing Authority and the Coordinating Council for Senior Citizens. Residents and other elders in Durham, a city of about 160,000 people with 20,000 persons over sixty, benefit from this cooperative effort. The development of a clinic for elders has met an important need, especially as many residents of public housing have grown very old.

According to the executive director of the Coordinating Council, the services integrated into the elderly housing facilities make it possible for about 8 percent of the residents to continue to live relatively independently despite severe functional losses. Although research comparing costs of delivering services in the community to costs of institutionalization does not always affirm substantial cost-savings for the former, leaders in the Durham aging network have no doubt that the personal and social benefits of their system far outweigh any potentially higher costs. The Coordinating Council avoids potential problems in Durham by ensuring that services are arranged and delivered without costly overlap. The Housing Authority recognizes the value of these services and trades space and utility costs for vital services for residents.

The value of a working relationship between housing officials and service agencies is obvious in Durham.

ST. PAUL, MINNESOTA

The Public Housing Agency of the City of St. Paul and the Wilder Foundation have long recognized the vital relationship between housing and services — especially for residents who become frail.[8] Ramsey County has allocated resources to individuals at risk of institutionalization and, because of the cooperation between the Housing Agency and the Wilder Foundation, many frail persons are able to stay where they prefer, in their apartments.

The Wilder Foundation has developed and administered an adult day health program in one public housing facility. That program has been so successful that it was extended from a day program to a twenty-four-hour service — the Assisted Living Program. The Housing Agency provides space and staff and the Wilder Foundation covers operational costs. This collaboration between a private foundation and the Housing Agency enables frail residents to age in a place that provides far more than shelter.

In addition, the Housing Agency received a congregate housing services program grant from HUD for residents with special needs. When the three organizations realized there were residents who needed additional services, the Wilder Foundation took the lead to develop an assisted living program to provide these services.

The Wilder Foundation assures that residents' needs are met through its own in-house programs and through collaboration with other community agencies. Due to the success of these efforts, the foundation has decided not to expand its nursing home capacity. "We believe that the older people of St. Paul, including those in Wilder Foundation housing, prefer to retain their independence with limited services rather than move into a nursing home. Our energies and resources are being devoted to expanding the range of alternatives for older people, especially when they face personal and health-related losses," reports an official of the foundation.

In St. Paul, frail residents of public and private organized housing for the elderly receive the benefits of cooperation and collaboration between local government and the private not-for-profit sector. Each has done what it is best suited to do: The Housing Agency has interpreted its functions broadly to do far more than provide housing to eligible individuals; county government has adopted a policy to shift money from nursing home payments to cover the cost of home care, including assisted living services; and the Wilder Foundation has invested private funds to experiment with program design and service delivery. Appreciative elders are the primary beneficiaries of well-designed supportive services, but their families and the community share the benefits.

SUMMARY

There's nothing extraordinary about any of these examples, but each suggests elements essential to providing successful housing for older people. In each instance there was careful planning, from sophisticated surveys and analyses in St. Paul to informal information gathering in Sun Prairie, Wisconsin.

Planners recognized that people aging in place need more than just an attractive apartment, and that their needs differ widely. Close attention was given to coordinating services within housing programs and among community agencies serving older adults. Most importantly, these projects serve aging residents and use taxpayers' dollars efficiently.

State Initiatives

Medicaid forced states to subsidize the housing costs of the "medically indigent" frail elderly to whom they provided long-term care in nursing homes. Finding their budgets buckling under the pressure of rapidly escalating Medicaid costs, state governments undertook policy initiatives to reduce costs. But costs continued to rise.

Some states recognized that they could curb costs by developing a housing strategy and encouraging the development of community-based services to keep people in their homes as long as possible. Three states in particular — Massachusetts, New Jersey, and Illinois — have developed effective programs that address the need for housing alternatives with supportive services.

MASSACHUSETTS

Massachusetts is notable for its continuing efforts to study what ought to be done for its elders and how to meet those needs. In 1978 the state developed plans for programs that would help older residents maintain their independence by coordinating services for those most in need. A 1985 study of housing options for the elderly,[9] prepared by the state's housing finance agency, identified strategies to help frail residents age in place and also to develop more housing designed for these special populations. Under the state program, coordinators at each housing site manage services provided to eligible residents. They interview residents to assess needs and connect them with community services.

Through a home care program financed by general purpose revenues as well as Medicare and Medicaid resources, residents of congregate housing facilities receive priority status for home care services. In addition, the state encourages housing development for impaired elders who, with shelter and services, can remain independent.

A guidebook, *Independence through Interdependence: Congregate Living for Older People,* expresses the state's philosophy and commitment to housing alternatives for people in need. And the *Congregate Housing Directory,* published by the Executive Office of Elder Affairs, provides information on more than 150 facilities and programs that integrate shelter and services for the state's elders.[10]

Massachusetts has initiated a variety of programs in response to the studies. Each initiative, based on sound principles, is a workable, sustainable program supported by the state and coordinated at the local level. Other states will benefit from studying Massachusetts's programs.

NEW JERSEY

In New Jersey, the legislature found that "housing requirements of the growing population of senior citizens are significantly different from the rest of the population" and that "a need exists to fill the gap in the housing continuum between independent living and institutionalization."[11]

The legislature acknowledged that a large percentage of the elderly population cannot pay for essential services. To ensure that older persons receive needed services in their apartment settings, the state adopted a congregate housing services program designed to provide a "supportive environment for persons of low income or suffering economic hardships."

Targeted to not more than 25 percent of a facility's resident population, the program provides assessment, congregate meals, housekeeping, and personal services, and other specific support services. It links at-risk residents with community health services.

New Jersey's Office of Housing and Community Development also has initiated a program, in cooperation with the Warren County Housing Authority, to place elder cottages for low-income individuals who need support close to caring families. The cottages can be inexpensively built and easily removed as needs change. Section 8 rent subsidies were made available to the low-income tenants. County ownership of the structures ensures that the facilities serve only those eligible for the program. These elder cottages, or "granny flats," or "Echo housing" offer housing alternatives that permit individuals to continue to live independently, and with informal support right next door.

Although most state programs now divert at-risk residents from nursing home placements, New Jersey's programs benefit many more than the at-risk population.

ILLINOIS

An Illinois study has investigated the need for supportive services in elderly housing and found that the state is facing tremendous near-term pressure for additional housing.[12] It suggests that the state should support efforts to convert existing housing into congregate facilities for those who, without such support, face nursing home placement. Conducted by the University of Illinois, the research establishes the importance of examining ways to meet future needs in the least restrictive, least expensive manner possible.

Illinois's situation resembles that of most states: A large number of subsidized apartments are occupied by individuals who have become quite frail. They are beginning to have difficulty with certain tasks necessary for self-sufficiency. They need nutritious, well-balanced meals, but find "cooking for one" difficult, grocery shopping nearly impossible. They appreciate help keeping their apartments clean and their clothes laundered. Taken separately, these tasks are not so onerous, but together they become too much for many residents.

The study suggests that the Illinois Housing Development Agency, Public Aid, and the Office on Aging cooperate to develop services for elders at-risk of institutionalization and to encourage sponsors to design programs supporting residents in their preferred setting: their apartments or homes.

The researchers concluded that "only a policy that *extends* independent subsidized housing to allow frail tenants to age-in-place can assure appropriate retention and postpone transfer to a time when dependent care is truly needed."

SUMMARY

The impetus for change may be the push of increasing demands and costs or the pull of wanting to create the best possible environments for elders. In either case, states are seriously looking at the fiscal and personal consequences of relying entirely on nursing homes to meet the long-term-care needs of a growing population of frail elderly. Waiting for the federal government to develop a national policy that meets this large and growing need does not appear to be realistic. States have initiated a variety of programs designed, in part, to strengthen community-based services, encourage development of informal support networks, and curtail past practices biased toward institutionalization.[13] However, states are discovering that expected savings from keeping individuals out of nursing homes are not nearly enough to finance housing for the thousands of at-risk persons who, without an alternative, will end up—inappropriately—in a nursing home.

There are demonstrably effective programs to study and replicate. What is needed is a firm commitment to allocate sufficient resources for individuals to remain in their homes and receive the services they require. Fortunately, for every individual over eighty who needs the support of extensive services, there is another individual who continues to maintain herself, often with family help, in the community. Millions of elders have housing that generally meets their needs. A look at how the vast majority of older people live without special services or purpose-built elderly housing may be instructive.

Naturally Occurring Retirement Communities

Over 90 percent of older people continue to live in their homes or apartments in neighborhoods familiar to them. How and why do residents in these settings continue to flourish without organized services and specially designed environments?

Naturally evolving retirement communities—apartment complexes occupied by individuals of diverse ages, usually located in desirable neighborhoods—can be found throughout the nation. After ten, twenty, even thirty years, these apartment buildings continue to provide attractive housing for residents who have grown older. The residents, primarily widows, prefer to live where they have lived independently for years, among friends in the same neighborhood.

University of Wisconsin researcher Michael Hunt has chosen the term "naturally occurring retirement community" (NORC) to describe apartment buildings neither designed nor particularly intended for older adults but which have more than half their residents over age sixty-five.[14] The term may describe either a single building or a housing complex. A NORC, he says, can be an older part of town "where residents have aged and others have been attracted to the point that the neighborhood houses a preponderance of older people."

In Hunt's initial study of three NORCs—apartment complexes with 238, 89, and 80 residents respectively, located in three different neighborhoods of Madison, Wisconsin—he found that 80 percent of the residents were widows living alone. Thirty percent moved in prior to their sixtieth birthdays and 50 percent made the move between 60 and 75 years of age. Sixty percent of the residents have lived in their apartments for more than ten years. Nearly all moved from single-family dwellings in a nearby neighborhood into the building which, over time, became a NORC.

In nearly every community, naturally occurring retirement facilities offer security and stability to aging residents. Those interviewed by Hunt indicated they would move only if rent increased dramatically or they required more health care. Hunt's findings confirm what is well known: Older people prefer to stay where they are despite the loss of a spouse. Residents like their independence, their neighborhood, the feeling of security, and the ambiance of their residence.

Moreover, it appears obvious that such residences offer not only a tie to one's roots, attractive housing, and affordable rent, but also an opportunity for community-based agencies or organizations to deliver services to residents who need and want assistance. An owner with a large number of very old residents may consider introducing limited services even though, as Hunt points out, the very nature of a NORC is that formal services are not provided. The NORC, he reports, demonstrates that "attractive housing for older people is attractive to younger people as well," even though the reverse may not be true. "Housing should be designed and planned with the needs of older people in mind in order to provide attractive housing for all," Hunt concludes.

Hunt's research has broad implications for an aging society. Although thoughtfully designed, well-located, service-rich environments are needed for a rapidly increasing population of vulncrable older people, there are thousands of residential settings that continue to provide an attractive alternative not only to nursing homes, but also to purpose-built elderly housing.

Owners, in cooperation with local service providers, may arrange services for individuals who want to retain a strong sense of independence despite growing loss of function. The nature of the apartment complex may change as the majority of residents become frail, but the idea of maintaining an image of independent living within the neighborhood has great appeal to many elders. The dynamics of a NORC suggest that purpose-built elderly housing complexes should be designed and developed in a way that avoids the image of "elderly housing" yet selectively provides essential services to vulnerable elders.

Frail, Yet Almost Independent

One's home and its immediate environment have a profound effect on the activities of daily living and the quality of one's life.[15] Elderly housing projects built in the 1970s and early 1980s have experienced a large increase in the mean age of their residents. Moreover, the population moving into elderly housing today is considerably older than was typical a decade ago. A major challenge facing owners and managers of such housing is how to provide the necessary services that will enable frail residents to continue living in the same facility.

Where there are a large number of older people congregated in one project or neighborhood, the potential efficiency of providing services increases. The challenge is to develop supportive services and a financing scheme to pay for them without destroying the image of independent housing. Experiments in the development of community-based housing with services warrant analysis and replication.

In Wisconsin, the state's Community Options Program (COP) enables frail individuals to receive services in their homes and communities. This program, using Medicaid waivers, signals a significant shift from a policy that provided skilled nursing *and* housing (in a nursing home) to one that undergirds a community-based support system. It ensures that institutionalization is a last resort for individuals in need of support.[16]

COP provides for assessment of a person's physical condition and social circumstances. If there's a way to enable elders to remain in their homes, COP will fund community-based services up to the cost of nursing home placement. For some individuals, modifications in the home will suffice. For others, special living arrangements will increase the likelihood of remaining in the community.

Individuals residing in subsidized and unsubsidized elderly housing comprise a group for which services can effectively be provided. As residents who moved into elderly housing ten or more years ago grow older, sponsors and managers face the difficulty of deciding at what point residents require more support than the housing complex can provide. Usually, by adding rather simple services management may extend the period in which residents can remain in their apartments.

Sponsors of elderly housing should decide early whether to apply rigid rules of independent living to residents or to add services and adapt spaces within the apartment complex to accommodate individuals who require assistance.[17] Although there is something to be said for retaining an ambiance of independence and preventing independent housing from appearing like a nursing home, there are compelling reasons to adapt housing and introduce programs that enable residents to continue living, with support, in familiar settings. When such modifications are made, many frail residents may avoid premature or unnecessary transfer to nursing homes.

Sponsors of such housing, with support from agencies serving older people, can fill a gap in the community-based long-term-care system and ensure that residents continue to enjoy the benefits of living where they choose.

Even with a service-rich environment, some residents will need to move to a nursing home. Nonetheless, it is a worthy goal to delay that move as long as practicable for as many residents as possible.

While there is increasing pressure on sponsors of elderly housing to add services for at-risk residents, there are inexpensive steps they may take to assist at-risk residents. For example, programs designed to train managers of elderly housing to identify emerging problems and make appropriate referrals may provide an important defense for the frail resident. The University of Wisconsin–Madison Vice-Chancellor for Health Sciences, with support from the Wisconsin Housing and Economic Development Authority, has embarked on a program to provide vital information to housing managers about the principal health problems that undermine residents' ability to live independently.[18]

Managers have received training and materials on such problems as incontinence, alcohol and drug abuse, depression, Alzheimer's disease, mental health problems, and sensory and mobility losses. They have attended summer institutes on the aging process that provide valuable material about the biology and biophysiology of aging, the aging brain, and chronic illnesses. They have been helped to identify problems and make appropriate referrals. These efforts, developed in collaboration with the Wisconsin Bureau on Aging, the Veterans Administration Hospital, and the University's Institute on Aging, have received considerable commendation for helping housing managers to become effective care managers in a community-based long-term-care system.

Another development in the housing field directly affecting the community's capacity to support frail residents is the hiring of nurses with geriatric training to provide assessment, consultation, and support for residents. A number of universities now offer graduate training leading to a geriatric nurse practitioner (GNP) certificate. With this training graduate nurses become key members of the team working to enable frail residents to maintain their independence despite chronic diseases and disabilities.

A team of professionals and managers working together with residents and their families can determine whether and when residents may have to move. Proper assessment of residents' potential for independent living and the community's capacity for providing supportive services enable residents to receive the services they require in the setting of their choice.

Although it is not easy, adding services to residential settings designed for independent living is one way to give frail elderly the opportunity to remain in place and receive the help they need. Every community should provide a range of options so that elders may choose an attractive housing environment appropriate to their needs.

A Research Agenda

The challenges created by an aging society are of great magnitude. Research directed at lengthening the period of good health and providing years of disability-free, self-directing life needs to be creative, collaborative, well conceived, and adequately funded. Although advances in the biomedical arena have been substantial, environmental factors for an aging society are underconceptualized and underexamined. Research is needed on the social as well as the physiological aspects of aging. The following areas merit attention by the research community.

HOUSING OPTIONS

If succeeding generations of older people are to be able to choose among housing alternatives, the total number of units must increase and the variety of housing options must expand considerably. We have evidence that such approaches as congregate housing, group homes, accessory apartments, and independent living units provide satisfactory living arrangements for an increasing number of aging persons. However, we should investigate new models, new sponsors, and issues such as location, management, and scale to find workable solutions to older persons' housing problems and attractive alternatives to satisfy their preferences.

Sponsorship. Investigators should identify incentives that encourage sponsors to develop new housing and to preserve and modify existing housing for older people. We need studies to identify as many types of projects and sponsors as possible and to develop directories of projects by geographic area and types of sponsorship, with sufficient information to answer certain questions: For whom was the housing developed, at what cost, in what location, with what problems, and what successes?

Home equity conversion. Recent national legislation provides for demonstration projects by HUD to show how home equity can be converted into cash for the nation's aging population. The fact that millions of older Americans have considerable equity in their homes indicates that with appropriate consumer safeguards, many of these elders will be able to maintain their homes, purchase supportive services, and add certain amenities important to their sense of well-being. Instruments for converting equity into cash need to be skillfully developed to protect the homeowner and carefully marketed to those whom such a program would benefit. Careful evaluation of home equity programs is an important research priority.

Design of elderly housing. What is the optimum number of units in elderly housing that will offer homelike ambiance and facilitate unobtrusive but efficient delivery of services? This is a difficult question for developers and policymakers. We need environments that are attractive to older residents, who may prefer smaller scale developments, but we also want to ensure the delivery of cost-effective services. Research may uncover ways to preserve homelike qualities and provide vital services.

Conventional wisdom suggests that we do, indeed, need to create substantially more housing and diverse forms of housing that meet changing needs of aging people. However, we need to examine carefully what happens to individuals when they can no longer live independently. It is not enough to design attractive buildings or to hire sensitive managers, although we surely need both. As a society, we must also find ways to deal with the myths and the realities of aging that enable residents to maintain their dignity when they move into housing that suggests dependency. This is a most important issue facing those engaged in developing housing, building social support systems, and devising policies that encourage independence.

What can we learn from successful NORCs that can be applied to purpose-built housing for the elderly? Are there styles of architecture and management that contribute to a mainstream image and yet provide needed services and supportive design? We need to learn more about location and the relative merits of concentrated housing and scattered site development.

How can we retain or create "homelike" qualities in elderly housing yet achieve economies of scale and meet an increasing need for housing? We have learned that high-rises can offer homelike qualities and small homes can seem like institutions, depending on different factors and expectations. We must initiate behavioral and environmental investigations to help us identify and preserve homelike characteristics while substantially expanding the number of units.

TRANSITION ISSUES

Given the importance of realistic expectations, what can we learn about a person's decision to move to elderly housing that will make the transition from one kind of housing to another as free of trauma as possible? How can people adjust to more institution-like settings without losing their sense of independence? If the idea of creating alternatives is to work effectively, then we must study transitions within a system of alternatives to understand what happens before, during, and after such moves. What do these moves mean to the individual?

INTEGRATION OF SERVICES WITH SHELTER

This chapter has underscored the importance of providing attractive housing for residents who need services in order to live somewhat independently. Examples of successful programs have been cited, indicating that with planning, coordination, and sensitivity, housing can be enriched without becoming too institutional. The goal of most housing sponsors and managers is to integrate services into the housing scene so effectively that residents will have the best of two worlds: independent living and essential services. The letterhead of the Colonial View Apartments in Sun Prairie reads: "Living independently with neighbors who care." The lesson is clear. Many residents could not reside there without the help of neighbors, services, and staff. Yet the ideal of independent living is reaffirmed each day.

To what extent can services be introduced into NORCs without unduly disturbing the positive image of those developments? The attractiveness of NORCs has a great deal to do with the fact that they are *not* "elderly housing." As individual tenants need help, they can contract with local agencies. A group with similar needs may want to negotiate a package of services at a reasonable cost. We need to learn how to introduce services in an unobtrusive manner while preserving those qualities that make NORCs attractive.

In integrating services with shelter, we need to study a number of important, specific questions.

Mix of frail and independent residents. What balance between frail and hardy residents is needed to provide services and keep a facility from taking on the image of housing for dependent persons? This question has been asked for many years and remains unanswered, partly because it has not been studied seriously. At what point does independent housing lose its image of being for "normal" older people? Is there a formula to calculate this? For example, if some fraction — perhaps 30 to 40 percent — of the residents are quite impaired, will a facility be perceived by residents and outsiders to resemble a nursing home?

Fostering dependence. Does a service-rich environment "cause" individuals to become more dependent? This fear, stated or not, arises in discussions about adding services to independent housing. Another view suggests that older people, like people of all ages, want to be able to choose services and amenities without someone else deciding what is good for them. We badly need research into this subject so that well-intentioned sponsors of elderly housing do not needlessly assume unfortunate consequences to adding services nor contribute, on the other hand, to the very problem the services are intended to ameliorate.

Selecting and training housing managers. How do we select and train housing managers to ensure appropriate values, attitudes, and competence? Managers are the key to creating environments in which residents feel good about themselves and their homes. It is certainly clear that residents have aged dramatically over the past decade and that new residents are moving in with greater needs. It is also apparent that elderly housing is a vital part of a community-based, long-term-care system and that housing managers are increasingly playing care-manager roles. Research is needed to identify managerial qualities that add to or detract from a good housing environment. With this research, those who select and train managers will be able to do so with greater understanding and confidence.

Admission and termination policies. What guidelines are needed for admitting, continuing, and terminating residents in "independent" housing? Every month a typical housing manager has to decide whether a person with chronic illnesses should be admitted, whether a frail resident can return after hospitalization to the facility, and when a resident must be asked to leave. All too often, the manager has few guidelines and little support. Most independent housing is only for those fully able to care for themselves; inevitably, the resident's first need is rather simple to meet. Needs increase slowly and the number of residents needing help also increases slowly. Managers facing these problems need the benefit of thoughtful research and the support of owners and sponsors.

The prescient work of Powell Lawton[19] provides researchers with a foundation for examining different aspects of the broad questions: Where and how will older persons live, what will add to their sense of well-being, and what will undermine that value? The questions raised here are merely "openers." The research community, in close collaboration with housing managers, owners, sponsors, and policymakers, needs to set a broad research agenda so that policies and decisions that affect the quality of life for millions of older people will have the benefit of rigorous and practical research. Our goal must be to create environments and design support programs that will enable residents to continue to live independently with neighbors who care, to retain their dignity, and to receive, as a right, the attention and services they need.

Conclusion

Where an older person lives is a crucial element in a community-based, long-term-care system. Each element in the system needs development: adding and modifying housing units, strengthening formal and informal supports, and delivering services as needed and where preferred—in the home. For the system to work well, those dependent on it must retain their sense of dignity and self-respect while receiving care.

No single strategy ensures that those growing old and frail will be able to remain in their homes or apartments. In fact, a wide variety of programs and services must complement the informal network of individual self-care and family support. Formal programs such as congregate and home-delivered meals, transportation, housekeeping, personal assistance, adult day care, and respite programs are essential.

Intensive community planning and a variety of resources are required to develop such systems. Wherever older people congregate—in elderly housing, neighborhoods with a concentration of very old people, or in small group homes—is an appropriate setting for a "shelter with services" strategy.

There are many lessons to be learned from NORCs. For relatively healthy residents, the apartments in which they have lived for a long time provide qualities they cherish. Owners of NORCs are well aware that they have a resident population that is stable, pleasant, and ideal in many ways. They will want to find ways to keep these residents, even though their needs increase, *and* maintain the ambiance of attractive apartments for independent elders. Therefore, developers and owners of elderly housing should carefully examine the qualities that make NORCs attractive places to live—not only for the well but also for people with increasing disabilities and needs.

NORCs provide a key to how we can effectively integrate frail with fully independent residents. It seems clear to those studying NORCs that these communities escape the stigma of subsidized and congregate housing by being part of the community and not requiring residents to admit either poverty or disability.

Housing, whether intentionally built for the elderly or naturally occurring along Main Street, whether in small villages or huge cities, cottages or high-rises, is at the very center of the long-term-care system. The wisdom of using available resources such as homes, supportive families, and community services becomes increasingly clear to policymakers, especially as they discover relationships between where older people live and their need for support over the long term. But the way our society's elders are to be housed and served is far too important to leave solely to government policy, marketplace realities, or chance. The eldest members of our society are entitled not only to security and shelter, but also to lives as full as their desires and health permit. To do so, communities must create well-designed, well-staffed housing programs using the vision and expertise of a variety of organizations.

Needed most is the willingness to act. Tomorrow's generation of vulnerable elders deserves the benefits of our thoughtful planning and commitment to creating environments in which people can flourish despite their disabilities. We have the knowledge, the models, and the resources. We need a catalyst, people of vision, enlightened policies, and the determination to act.

Notes

1. See the NCOA publication "Housing and living arrangements for the elderly: A selected bibliography," edited by H. Boston, 1985, for a fairly comprehensive listing of books, articles, and reports available to 1984.

2. Clay, P. "At risk of loss: The endangered future of low-income rental housing resources." Neighborhood Reinvestment Corporation, Washington, D.C., 1987.

3. Nathanson, I. "Housing needs of the rural elderly and handicapped." U.S. Dept. of Housing and Urban Development, 1980.

4. Information for this vignette comes from the author's twenty years of direct involvement with all aspects of the Sun Prairie developments.

5. Sykes, J. "A community-based long-term-care system: The Sun Prairie experience." Unpublished Grand Rounds presentation, Middleton Memorial Veterans Hospital, Madison, Wis., March 1985.

6. Sykes, J. "Needs of older people met by the Colonial Club's campus." *Perspective,* 15, NCOA, 1986.

7. This information is from the executive director of the Coordinating Council for Senior Citizens of Durham, N.C., 1987.

8. This vignette is based on conversations with officials of the Public Housing Authority of St. Paul and the Wilder Foundation, 1987. The 1986 Annual Report of the Amherst H. Wilder Foundation, entitled "Eighty Years of Serving the Greater St. Paul Community," contains an interesting description of the foundation's response to community needs.

9. Tiven, M. and B. Ryther. *State Initiatives in Elderly Housing.* Council of State Housing Agencies and the National Association of State Units on Aging, Washington, D.C., 1986.

10. Elements of the Massachusetts program were described to the author by the deputy director of the state's Executive Office of Elder Affairs. See also "Massachusetts Community Care and Housing Services," a report issued by the Executive Office of Elder Affairs in 1987.

11. Parkoff, B. "Adding services to existing buildings." In *State Initiatives in Elderly Housing.*

12. Heumann, L. "The retention and transfer of frail elderly living in independent housing." Report prepared for the Illinois Housing Development Authority,

Department of Public Aid and Department of Aging, by the Housing Research and Development Program, University of Illinois at Urbana-Champaign, 1985.

13. Tiven and Ryther, "State Initiatives."

14. Hunt, M. and G. Gunter-Hunt. "Naturally occurring retirement communities." *Journal of Housing for the Elderly*, 3, 1985. See also L. Pastalan, et al., *Retirement Communities: An American Original*. New York: Haworth Press, 1984.

15. See, for example, S. Howell, "The Meaning of Place in Old Age," in G.D. Rowles and R.J. Ohta, editors, *Aging and Milieu: Environmental perspectives on Growing Old*. New York: Academic Press, 1983.

16. "An evaluation of the Community Options Program," Wisconsin Legislative Audit Bureau, 1987. See also J. Spahn, "The Community Options Program: A public choice for personal choice in long-term support," Lafollette Institute of Public Affairs, University of Wisconsin-Madison, 1987.

17. M.P. Lawton, M. Greenbaum, and B. Leibowitz. "The lifespan of housing environments for the aging." *The Gerontologist*, 20, 1:1980. For a thoughtful analysis of the conceptual underpinnings of aging in place, see also M. P. Lawton, *Planning and Managing Housing for the Elderly*. New York: Wiley-Interscience, 1975.

18. See J. Sykes (Ed.), *Health Issues for Housing Managers*, a series of primers developed by the Center for Health Sciences, with a grant from the Wisconsin Housing and Economic Development Authority.

19. Lawton, et al. "Lifespan."

CHAPTER FOUR

Congregate Housing: People, Places, Policies

GORDEN F. STREIB

The expanding population of those over 75, and particularly of those over 85, highlights the importance of special residential environments for the elderly that include some supportive services. Congregate housing is one of the options developed by public agencies and private organizations to meet the needs of large numbers of older people unable – or unwilling – to continue living in ordinary apartments or single family homes.

There is no precise definition of congregate housing for the elderly. In most cases, however, it refers to a multiunit apartment building in which the apartments all have bathrooms and kitchens or kitchenettes, and where the management provides some supportive services, such as a dining room where residents can obtain at least one main meal a day, optional housekeeping, transportation, and twenty-four-hour watch service. Usually there is common space for residents to engage in social, educational, and other group activities, and often the management arranges for other services – such as health monitoring, or a beauty parlor – that are desired by residents.

Congregate housing differs from residential care facilities (see Chapter 5) in that the management of a congregate housing facility normally does not provide personal care (that is, assistance with activities of daily living such as bathing or dressing) or any kind

75

of health-related services to the residents. It may, however, arrange for those services to be offered (by other organizations or individuals) in the building. In general, congregate housing facilities do not admit residents who require personal care.

Unfortunately, the definitional distinctions between congregate housing and residential care homes or facilities (which are labelled personal care, board and care, domiciliary care, adult foster homes, group homes, and so on) are sometimes blurred. Florida, for example, combines congregate housing, residential care facilities, and continuing care retirement communities into one licensure category called "Adult Congregate Living Facilities." It is difficult to make sense of a definition that includes both an 8-bed personal care facility and a 200-unit congregate housing facility. In the latter every apartment has a kitchen and private bath, and the management does not provide personal care to the residents. On admission, at least, residents must be relatively independent, able to function adequately with the limited amount of supportive services provided. The personal care facility residents, on the average, are much more disabled. They receive three meals a day as well as personal care. Many have semiprivate bedrooms and rarely a private bath. By including such disparate facilities in the same definition, it becomes difficult to say anything meaningful about the category: The residents, services, staffing requirements, economics, and public policy issues all are quite different.

Part of the confusion stems from an early discussion of congregate housing in a 1975 report of the United States Senate's Special Committee on Aging.[1] It states that congregate housing is "a residential environment which includes services such as meals, housekeeping, *health, personal hygiene,* and transportation, which are required to assist *impaired,* but not ill, elderly tenants to maintain or return to a semi-independent life style and avoid institutionalization as they grow older" (emphasis added).[2] This definition is clearly too broad since very few, if any, congregate housing facilities supply health or personal hygiene services or admit residents who are significantly impaired.

Congregate housing was the term used in the 1970 and 1974 Housing and Urban Development Acts, which described low-rent public housing that provided food and other services. And a recent glossary published by the National Institute on Aging (NIH) defined congregate housing as "apartment houses of group accommodations that *provide health care* and other support services to *functionally impaired* older persons who do not need routine nursing care." (emphasis added)[3] This clearly perpetuates the definitional confusion.

This chapter discusses congregate housing as it is most generally understood and organized—and as explained in the beginning of this chapter. Residential care facilities (facilities that provide personal care to significantly impaired people) are discussed in Chapter 5.

Why do people enter congregate housing? The process of aging for many people involves declining health and a reduced ability to carry on such instrumental activities of daily living as housework, shopping, laundry, and meals preparation. There is also constriction of social networks of friends, family, and neighbors, perhaps worries about neighborhood security, and increased concern about the ability to obtain help in medical emergencies. All of these considerations contribute to an elder's decision to move to a new housing environment with supportive services, such as congregate housing, but the decision may also be influenced by family, friends, or a physician.

Congregate housing has some features that make it unattractive to many people who prefer to remain in their own apartment or house. In a congregate facility they may have to mingle with people whom they do not like. There is likely to be some loss of privacy, and there is mandatory scheduling of some life activities such as meals, which may not always mesh with a resident's personal desires. Thus, the decision to move to a congregate facility is often made reluctantly.

Federal Support of Congregate Housing

Although privately developed congregate housing predates federal involvement, the number of such units has been relatively small. It was the initiation of federal support, authorized by the Housing and Urban Development Act of 1970, that stimulated development of congregate housing on a national scale. This housing, which included shared but self-supporting eating facilities, was designed for the elderly and also displaced and handicapped persons. Under four titles in the law—Sections 202, 236, 221(d)(3) and

221(d)(4)—about 300,000 units of congregate housing for the elderly have been built by both nonprofit and for-profit developers.[4] Only Sections 202 (subsidized housing for low-income elderly and disabled) and 221(d)(4) (mortgage insurance for market-rate facilities) are still available.

Before federal statutory authority existed, four demonstration congregate housing developments were initiated in the mid-1960s.[5] The goal was to determine the need for this new approach and its utility in housing low-income elderly who needed some supportive services. At that time, congregate housing was available only to persons with higher incomes in facilities that were privately financed and managed.

The demonstration facilities are located in Toledo and Columbus, Ohio; Alma, Georgia; and Burwell, Nebraska. These projects explored the way in which federal, state, and local government agencies could provide shelter and services to the low-income elderly. The projects varied in size and in the way facilities were provided. The Columbus and Toledo developments, with 246 and 100 units, respectively, were able to include a kitchen and a central dining room because the state contributed land in prime locations. These savings were then applied to the cost of the extra space required in the facilities, particularly for the kitchen and central dining room. In discussing the project the 1975 report of the Senate's Special Committee on Aging states that "none of the tenants need nursing service. Congregate tenants are not thought of as frail. They are seen as elderly persons needing a friendly hand."[6] However, one manager states that all of his tenants living in the congregate facility would be in a nursing home if this type of housing and services did not exist.

What We Know about Congregate Housing

This section summarizes some of the major studies of congregate housing. We have selected reports that cover a period of approximately twenty years. Research was chosen because of its quality and scope, with particular attention given to studies with a longitudinal design. (More recent research has focused on specific issues such as cost comparisons and social networks in congregate housing.) The reports summarized here also illustrate the spectrum of environments that can be designated as congregate housing. Finally, because of the variation in research reports, we have presented the materials as case summaries rather than descriptions broken down by variables into topical issues (such as size of buildings, average age of residents, health function, and change in disability over time).[7]

EARLY RESEARCH: TWENTY-SEVEN SITES

The first comprehensive research reported on the range of congregate housing in the United States and evaluated its impact on the elderly.[8] The report, published in 1978, contained information on (1) development policies, management policies and practices, delivery of services, and design features; (2) residents and applicants at congregate housing facilities; and (3) financial matters.

Twenty-seven congregate housing sites in four regions constituted the sample. The housing projects were stratified into three service levels, three rent levels, and three building sizes (nine each of units of 70 to 125, 126 to 200, and 201 or more). Only a few of the many findings can be presented here. The researchers found that there is a large variety of congregate housing facilities and congregate housing residents. They also emphasize the importance, in serving residents and maintaining continuity, of being flexible in adapting to the constantly aging population.[9]

The survey used a target sample of 25 residents and 10 applicants at each of 19 sites (total sample sizes were 469 and 85, respectively). Applicants were much more reluctant to be interviewed because they felt it might jeopardize their admission to a facility. About one-half of the applicants were 75 years of age or older compared to 72 percent of the residents. Eighty percent of the residents were women. Income data were difficult to obtain due to confusion or refusal. However, income stratification was an interesting factor that revealed striking contrasts. Malozemoff and her colleagues found that "upper income respondents were attracted to facilities which were close to their families, in locations with good climates, which had good quality health programs and housekeeping services. Lower income respondents chose facilities according to their cost, their location in safe neighborhoods, or because there was no other alternative."[10]

It is also interesting that design features were ranked low — fifteenth out of nineteen features listed in terms of importance.[11] On the other hand, residents found on-site medical services important because of their easy accessibility. One of the most striking observations is that the vast majority of respondents evaluated the congregate meal programs positively.

The performance of the management was a difficult subject to assess because respondents used personal criteria. Respondents' housing experiences prior to living in a congregate project influenced their evaluation, and a consistent pattern emerged showing that negative assessments of management's performance increased as the health of residents declined. Residents stated a major need for assistance in maintaining an independent life-style. This underscores the need for flexibility in operation. But the authors stress that as physical capabilities decline, the need for on-site services increases. The availability of services prolongs activity by alleviating problems of access and mobility.

The area of cost analysis was the most difficult to study and the results were the most problematic. Only six of the twenty-seven sites provided detailed data, and three did not provide any information. Twelve sites reported a loss for the study period.

Some conclusions from this early national study are particularly noteworthy. Congregate housing serves many different types of elderly persons. And although a wide range of age groups, physical capabilities, and income levels can be served, this research shows that higher-income elderly receive a very different housing and services package than do the poor. Only upper-income elderly can pay for extensive services. And the budget deficits that were reported existed in the facilities with higher service levels. A large proportion of the owners of the facilities in the study were church-sponsored, nonprofit organizations and were able to operate because deficits were covered by gifts. The authors conclude their study by stating that congregate housing projects providing a medium or high level of services *do* have lower costs of operation than the national average for all nursing homes and that they had significantly lower total costs than skilled nursing facilities.

This early national study serves as a benchmark for later research. Although there were problems in research execution, sampling, applicant refusal, and most importantly, cost data, the study is a valuable source of data and research procedure.

A PIONEERING MODEL AND LONG-TERM RESEARCH

Victoria Plaza in San Antonio, Texas, is a unique public housing project that merits discussion in this chapter for three reasons: (1) It was one of the first service-enriched public housing projects for the elderly; (2) It provided a broad array of needed services and amenities; and (3) It has been studied repeatedly over the years, notably by F.M. Carp.[12] It was different from other elderly public housing projects in San Antonio in several respects. First, it was planned for a limited age group, with an average age of 72 for the first residents. Second, it was the first high-rise public housing project and the tallest apartment building in the area. Third, Victoria Plaza had special features to make it more functional for older residents.

The San Antonio Housing Authority showed considerable foresight by including the county's first senior center as a tenant on the ground floor of the building.[13] The upper eight floors contain 184 private apartments.[14] From the beginning there was a community kitchen for social events and also a large recreation room. Later, a second meeting room was constructed. This space has been used by various agencies (the Department of Public Welfare, the Social Security Administration, and the Housing Authority) who come to provide their services. The ground floor of the building contains offices for building personnel and the Senior Center's director and staff. Next to these offices are a hobby and crafts room, and a library. At the end of this wing is an eight-room clinic used by the Public Health Department. The ground floor's east wing contains a post office, two counseling offices used by the Retired Senior Volunteer Program (RSVP), and the building custodian's apartment. Victoria Plaza is clearly a model public housing project with features that should have been included in later projects.

After the building was occupied for eight years, Carp conducted a follow-up user evaluation study on the effects of improved housing on old people. The tenants were generally well satisfied, primarily due to the good qualities of the physical environment.

The original design did not include meal service. When residents were asked at the end of one year about services they felt were important, 37 percent mentioned a place to buy meals (restaurants were some distance away). However, after eight years, 78 percent stated that provision of meals was the most important need.

Carp also conducted a study of the health benefits of the project and concluded that appropriate housing "may not only improve psychological and social well-being during the later years, but may also extend those years and benefit health status during them."[15]

THE HIGHLAND HEIGHTS EXPERIMENT

The Highland Heights experiment is another example of detailed, longitudinal research on congregate housing.[16] This facility was a medically-oriented, semi-independent housing project located on the grounds of a municipal hospital for the chronically ill in Fall River, Massachusetts. HUD approved the building of a low-income, fourteen-story apartment house with 208 apartments. The building design and other features included health and other community services. The outpatient clinic of the hospital was located in the basement of the HUD project. When the building was ready for occupancy, the government's precise definition of congregate housing had not yet been formulated. Thus, there were problems concerning the design of space for medical facilities, and there was no way of approving space for congregate dining if the apartments had kitchens. And although HUD had a legal mandate to provide housing, it also held a reputation for being concerned primarily with "bricks and mortar" and not with the multiple services that might be required by elderly residents of public housing.

Highland Heights was unique because it had a contract to develop screening techniques for selecting occupants and to develop a program that would help to meet the social service and medical needs identified in the screening process. The project was designed to be a viable alternative to institutionalization. In the beginning the Housing Authority exerted pressure to fill the apartments immediately, so all of the applicants on the waiting list were accepted. Later, higher priority was given to frailer persons and the highest priority was awarded to those who had transferred from an institution.

The second major objective was the development and stimulation of services to deal with the residents' needs. Over a period of seven years the project delivered an array of programs: health and basic support services, counseling and casework, social and recreational activities, volunteer and community activities, nutritional and meal services, and transportation. These multiple services required considerable administrative and community involvement to sustain them.

The patchwork nature of the program is illustrated by the fact that for four years, Highland Heights provided a noon meal service through Meals-on-Wheels five days a week. Finally, the Massachusetts Office of Elder Affairs sponsored a nutrition program, and the meals were prepared in the hospital kitchen.

Research findings validated the major aim of the congregate housing intervention design and showed that service-rich housing is a viable alternative to institutionalization for many people. The researchers stated: "Throughout the five year impact study period, the Highland Heights residents were significantly less likely to become institutionalized and spent less time in a long term care facility as compared with their matched controls."[17]

The data on persons who moved directly from long-term-care facilities to Highland Heights were also very positive. People who had been sick enough to be institutionalized according to Medicaid standards were able to live in supportive public housing. All but one lived for more than one year, and some lived as long as six years in Highland Heights.

A cost-benefit analysis indicated an average saving of almost $3,000 per person over a three-year period.

PHILADELPHIA GERIATRIC CENTER STUDIES

A team of researchers at the Philadelphia Geriatric Center have carried out important studies on the match between the needs of the elderly person and the resources available in his or her environment. They state: "Ideally, congruent matches should provide few services for the independent elderly and many services for the less independent."[18] The matching of the environment and the person alters because both change over time. Lawton, Greenbaum, and Liebowitz have reported on studies of two housing projects (one for a fifteen-year period and the other for twenty years) in which services were added over the years as the health of both the original residents and the new tenants declined.[19] This approach has been called the "accommodating model" of housing, since accommodation is made to increase services as the competence of the tenants declines. These authors contrasted this model with the "constant model," which attempts to control the nature of the original population by three means: (1) stringent admission standards that keep out anyone who has too many health needs; (2) by terminating tenure through monitoring and asking residents to leave if impairment is evident; and (3) by encouraging and fostering independent behavior.

To study what happens over time in congregate housing under different conditions, a follow-up study was conducted at five housing facilities that had opened earlier, in 1966 and 1968.[20] At each of the federally assisted, age-segregated housing projects, one hundred randomly selected tenants were interviewed prior to admission and one year after moving in. Twelve years later, a new representative sample of one hundred residents from each of the housing units was interviewed to obtain a picture of the long-term characteristics of the tenants.

The issue of major interest is the twelve-year change in characteristics of the population. The average age increased from 72.8 to 77.7 years. Marital status changed dramatically: 25.5 percent were married in the original population and 7.9 percent in the follow-up sample. The mean number of living children per tenant also decreased, from 2.1 to 1.6.

Tenant well-being was presented for each housing unit in eight domains, including health, mobility, and morale, and despite some variability between the sites, the residents declined in competence and well-being as they aged. The decline was smallest in the two measures of functional health related to activities of daily living. There was an increase in hospitalization and a decline in mobility during the study period. The researchers note a general decline in the quality of life, which they say is evidenced by the increase in passive activities such as watching television, looking out the window, and sitting and thinking, and a decrease in eleven active activities, such as visiting in one another's apartments, leaving the neighborhood, and going out after dark.

The Balanced Model of Person-Environment Interaction

Ehrlich, Ehrlich and Woehlke address the issue of aging in place in congregate housing in their report of research on the changing needs of the residents of a St. Louis housing project thirteen years after it opened.[21] The study raised the question of whether a constant or an accommodating model of person-environment change was followed as the original cohort of healthy people aged. A constant model provides for only healthy elderly and stipulates that residents must leave when they can no longer maintain their independence. The accommodating model increases service programs gradually to meet the needs of the residents as they age.[22]

The Ehrlich team found that age alone is not a factor in determining function level, needs, or wants. They concluded that neither the constant nor the accommodating model could be considered the "ideal environment." Instead, they support the concept of a balanced environmental model that would "allow for the maintenance of the traditional mobile-well independent environment while still assuring some support if needed. . . . Development of a strong peer-oriented, reciprocal informal network is suggested as a practice method for operationalization of the balanced environmental concept."[23] They believe that there should be limited intrusion of bureaucratic systems but major involvement in a strong peer-oriented, reciprocal, informal helping network. It was found that morale increases when elderly people assist each other in basic supportive tasks.

A Recent Study of Cost Comparisons

A recent study comparing costs of congregate housing and nursing homes in Illinois was conducted by L.F. Heumann and associates.[24] The study was designed to determine if congregate housing provides savings in comparison to long-term-care facilities. Cost comparisons are complex and formidable and the researchers point up the major reasons: (1) The two types of facilities are quite different living environments; (2) Different care alternatives are provided, with one having on-site staff and the other, intermittent and visiting services; and (3) About three-fourths of the persons in nursing homes are too frail to live in congregate housing, yet the costs of their support are difficult to separate from the 20 to 30 percent of residents who might be able to transfer to congregate housing. Earlier studies tend to exaggerate the cost savings because controls were not employed to determine comparable services in the two types of housing.

The Illinois research team selected representative study sites, but the high refusal rate among for-profit facilities resulted in only one such project being included in the study. Refusals among the proprietors occurred primarily because they were not willing to reveal their costs and charges.

Representative study sites were carefully selected and in order to insure comparability, facilities in urban locations and single buildings (not multibuilding campuses) were the research locations. The size of the facilities was controlled, so that the average had 133 residents (the range was from 75 to 225 units), and the median age of residents was 78 years (range 75 to 82).

The Illinois researchers conclude: "A single best comparison would be the range of cost differences created by comparing Level II congregate housing charges with both private pay and private pay/public aid mixed charges for long-term care. This comparison produces a savings per person per year of $1,320 to $2,964 for residents of congregate housing."[25] Or comparing the units on a total facility basis, the savings per year range from $195,360 to $438,672, favoring congregate housing. The saving can be specified more precisely by normalizing capital costs and debt service, by considering the quality of life factors, which are difficult to price, and by reintroducing the conservative assumptions that were part of the selection of the sample. When these issues are taken into account and the savings per year calculated with all capital costs and debt service normalized to 1985 cost levels, the savings per resident per year in congregate housing would range from $4,288 to $5,880 less than the cost of nursing home care. After reviewing the conservative assumptions of the Illinois research team, one agrees with their conclusion: "The cost savings for congregate housing uncovered in this study are both substantial and realistic."[26] In areas with higher nursing home costs, savings would be even greater.

The quality of life factors are difficult to compute in accurate dollar values, but they are important considerations, particularly to the residents of the various kinds of facilities. The nursing homes included in the Illinois research were progressive, but it is nonetheless true that the independence of residents is limited in all nursing homes. Indeed, the worst of these facilities are custodial and do not encourage independent living.

A study of congregate housing in Massachusetts reported that the residents of congregate housing who formerly lived in nursing homes stated overwhelmingly that the move into congregate housing improved their quality of life.[27] Congregate living provided them with greater freedom to come and go, to control their money, and to purchase what they wanted. The service provider reported improvements in health and in attitudes as measured by fewer medications, less depression, increased self-confidence, and so on.

Social Life within a Project

Kaye and Monk have studied the impact of aging on the social life of "enriched housing."[28] The facility in question, which was sponsored by a religious group, housed 1,424 elderly persons. A 25 percent random sample was drawn and 210 tenants were personally interviewed. They had a median age of 77 years and the median length of residence in the project was five years. Fifty percent were widowed, and 79 percent had living children. One-half of the latter were in contact with their children daily (through either phone calls or visits), and 14 percent stated that they never had contact. One focus of the research was the availability of social confidants. Research on confidants was divided into two components: expressive needs (sharing happiness or talking about personal problems) and instrumental needs (helping with chores, shopping assistance, and so on).

Among the significant findings were that the oldest residents (75 and older) are less likely to receive help. As the authors write, "the very cohort of older people who are expected to receive the most help are least likely to receive it from their friends."[29] It is interesting that all respondents felt that they gave more assistance to their neighbors than they received. When respondents were asked to identify the person or organization they would call on first during a *personal emergency*, slightly less than half mentioned a relative, spouse, or housemate, and 19 percent said they would turn to management. There tends to be symmetry in the exchange assistance patterns of respondents and their friends and fellow tenants in the building, but this must be considered in relation to whom a respondent will turn to first in an emergency.

Residents in poor health had less frequent contact with the social network than those who were healthier. The nature of the withdrawal process, however, is not clear from the report. Do the frail residents withdraw from neighbors and relatives, or do other people withdraw from them? Are those in poor health too proud to seek help when they can no longer reciprocate, or do neighbors find it depressing to see their deterioration and tend to withdraw? The researchers do note that unbalanced helping relations may arise when residents deteriorate in health. They suggest that enriched-housing sponsoring agencies consider initiating programs to make those in informal support systems more aware of the needs of the frail elderly. The researchers conclude: "Early intervention in the form of housing policies and programs which promote ongoing opportunities for social exchange and support between older tenants and their significant others both within and outside of the housing development can insure increasingly satisfying lives for the elderly themselves at the same time that the costs accruing to formal service delivery are maintained at reasonable levels."[30]

A State Initiative

A team of researchers in Massachusetts carried out an assessment of congregate housing in the state to determine how it works and whom it serves best. The study is diagnostic because the research on congregate housing is relatively undeveloped, and specific hypotheses could not be proposed at the beginning of the project. The research design identified the varying types of congregate housing facilities. The research team used a contextual research design because a particular project would have varying combinations of building design, developers, management, support, and resident characteristics.

One of the most powerful influences on congregate housing is the community in which it is located. Mollica et al. wrote that "in many critical ways, congregate housing is a local phenomenon. Its localness is reflected in many ways including the organizational interrelationships necessary for its development, management and service provision; in the reputation it is awarded by others in the community—which often affects project and resident self-perceptions; and in the level and way in which resources get channeled to the project. To study congregate housing, then, means to appreciate its community context. This approach also permits the researcher to understand why another setting might inhibit its success."[31]

Congregate Housing Services Program

The Congregate Housing Services Program (CHSP) is a demonstration program in which the Department of Housing and Urban Development linked supportive services with its subsidized housing.[32] The CHSP's basic premise is that community-based supportive services can help frail elderly and handicapped persons avoid institutionalization. The eligible projects are those built and managed by local public housing authorities and those organized under Section 202 of the Housing Act of 1959. Section 202 housing provides direct long-term federal loans to eligible private nonprofit organizations for financing rental housing for the low-income elderly and/or handicapped. CHSP awards funds to housing projects if they are able to show that its services are needed because existing services are inadequate to meet residents' needs. CHSP has several important features:

1. Residents in the buildings must receive two on-site meals seven days a week.
2. Additional nonmedical services such as housekeeping, transportation, and social services may also be provided to fill gaps in the service system.
3. CHSP services are not a substitute for services already provided but must be additional services.
4. Participation in a CHSP building is generally limited to 20 percent of the residents in order to create an atmosphere of independent living.
5. A professional assessment committee (PAC) of volunteers must screen all of the applicants for the services at each project.
6. Residents must make some contribution toward the cost of services.

Evaluation was integral to CHSP, focusing on process, performance, and impact in forty-eight projects. The process evaluation involved analysis of the program start-up, and the performance evaluation concentrated on use of program services by residents. This evaluation also examined how services were targeted and monitored the cost of the program. The impact evaluation analyzed the effects of CHSP on mortality and institutionalization, on functional health and quality of life, and on whether CHSP replaced services supplied informally.

Data from forty-eight sites found the process of implementing CHSP to be successful in the first year of the program. Part of the success was due to the fact that housing managers were able to use community expertise. About 20 percent of the CHSP buildings had no services previously; only a minority had a package of more than two services. The general conclusion was that CHSP was instrumental in increasing the availability of services at their sites. For example, housekeeper/chore and personal care had been provided previously at 38 percent of the sites; after CHSP, 78 percent provided these services.

Performance evaluation measured the degree to which the CHSP model provides services to those who need them — the "vulnerable" persons who need help in at least one Activity of Daily Living (ADL). "Tailoring" was the term used to describe whether CHSP residents received services appropriate to their assessed needs. CHSP projects did target services to the most vulnerable tenants, for 85 percent of them became participants in the program. Ten different services (meals, transportation, shopping, and so on) were included, and the evaluation research found that a majority needing a service at the start of the program received services from at least one source during the research period. A few persons had received service for which there was no apparent need at the time of the survey. But it must be emphasized that CHSP served the vast majority of elderly and handicapped who were identified as needy. The average monthly cost per participant was $204, and meals accounted for 54 percent of these costs.

Impact evaluation was the third component. It focused on whether CHSP replaced services provided by informal caregivers or other providers and whether the program's effects were positive or negative on the functional health and quality of life of the participants.

After fourteen months, there were no statistical differences between the experimental (CHSP) and the control group as to costs and illness. However, this result must be carefully qualified by noting the relatively short time period of study—fourteen months. CHSP did not reduce rates of admission to nursing homes because CHSP residents were in a low-risk category.

The data on quality of life are limited and short-term. Long-term effects may be different. However, the results are generally positive. Detailed information is provided on four topics: functional health, psychological status, tenant satisfaction, and social activities.

In summary, the Congregate Housing Services Program demonstrated many positive aspects. The organization and implementation of the program was effectively carried out and the services were generally on target. The researchers question whether the two-meal-a-day program in itself reduced institutionalization of the residents. Over two-thirds of all formal service time was given to meals. There is a definite possibility that other services might receive more time, and a different mix of services may be more appropriate and more effective. This topic warrants further study and shows the importance of flexibility and tailoring.

Highlights of the Research

The varieties of congregate housing for the elderly described in this chapter are a reflection of the housing situation generally in the United States. Congregate housing covers a number of types, which vary by building structure, sponsorship, services, size, atmosphere, and cost. All of these varying housing environments have as a major objective the assisting of the elderly to age in place. Research on congregate housing shows that most of these forms can be flexible in meeting the changing needs of their residents. Improving the relationship between the person and the environment in late life requires greater adaptability from the people managing the environment than from the older residents themselves. This observation, however, does not imply that the housing environment should foster dependency and passivity. The research on congregate housing indicates that sensitive management and personnel can encourage autonomy and independence.

One conclusion from our review of the literature is that congregate housing must be understood in terms of a life-course orientation that involves more than the psychology and biology of aging. Housing must take into account a person's income and assets and position in the system of stratification in late life. There are three broad strata whose needs for congregate housing vary because of their socioeconomic position: the affluent, served by private developers; the poor, served by government-subsidized programs; and those of middle income, who are ineligible for publicly subsidized congregate housing but cannot afford private, market-priced congregate housing. Many of the middle-income group own their homes and have a strong psychological attachment to them. This can be an impediment to their considering new housing arrangements more congruent with their declining health or ability to function in the activities of daily living, and thus their need for some kind of supportive services.

Another major conclusion from the survey of research is that congregate housing is a cost-effective living environment in comparison to nursing homes. Moreover, congregate living arrangements offer greater freedom and autonomy than is possible in most institutionalized environments.

The review of research also indicates that the potential population for congregate housing is large and growing, representing a challenge and an opportunity for private and public sectors of the society to expand the numbers of facilities available. The studies also demonstrate that the complicated structure of American society with its multiple layers of government demands local initiative and involvement in housing. Because of the "localness" of congregate housing, there is bound to be a veritable patchwork of new facilities and programs as well as local agendas that differ considerably from one community to another. Moreover, these agendas are influenced or constrained by state laws and local ordinances controlling land use and zoning. These may act as an impediment to development of innovative housing solutions.

Research also indicates that the success of congregate housing often depends on "street level bureaucrats."[33] Like other aspects of the aging service industry, congregate housing relies on many untrained, low-paid personnel. These people, who are involved in day-to-day operations, have an important effect on the quality of life in the facility.

The studies of the Congregate Housing Services Program indicate that public housing facilities can be "tailored" to meet the needs of their residents as they age in place.

Housing and Its Social Context

Congregate housing as one type of housing for the elderly must be placed in the general culture of American society. Most older Americans are homeowners. Approximately 80 percent of people over 60 own their homes, and almost two-thirds own them free of mortgage.[34] Seventy percent of these live in single-family houses and 30 percent live in other types of housing, mainly low-rise apartments, condominiums, and mobile homes. Home ownership in American society represents for most older persons a lifetime of thrift. It is their major asset, and thus is the central part of their legacies. For many older Americans, passing something on to their children is a significant social goal and a commitment to family cohesion and solidarity. Home ownership also has important symbolic values for residents. There is a strong attachment to the house as a place where personal and family treasures are kept. It is a repository of memories, for many significant events have occurred there and many important activities have been carried out.

The attachment to place is a recognized characteristic of the elderly, for as an AARP survey reports, 66 percent of the respondents had lived in the same community for twenty-one or more years, and 46 percent had lived in the same house for that period.[35] Thus, moving into congregate housing involves dropping a long-standing commitment to a place with important sentimental and traditional characteristics. It is noteworthy that the national survey sponsored by AARP, "Understanding Senior Housing," reported that the women over 80 years of age are especially unwilling to move.

INCOME DISTRIBUTION

Recent annual income statistics for persons 65 or older (including single persons living alone) show that 13.8 percent have incomes over $35,000; 19.3 percent have $20,000 to $34,999; 30.7 percent have $10,000 to $19,999; and 36.2 percent have under $10,000.[36]

These statistics on income levels point to three general target populations for congregate housing.[37] At the top of the income ladder, 20 to 30 percent of the elderly are able to pay market rates for various kinds of congregate housing. At the bottom of the income ladder, about 35 percent of people have incomes low enough to be eligible for subsidized housing if a needs test were applied. In between these two layers is some 35 to 40 percent of America's elderly, who are not eligible for subsidized housing and in many instances cannot afford the market price for congregate housing. Further, current trends suggest that the family's financial ability to provide support for those in the middle strata is expected to decline.[38] The economic trends for this expanding older population are accentuated in a downward direction because of the very unbalanced sex ratio and the fact that widowhood causes most older women to experience a decline in income.

When discussing the housing of the elderly, it is essential to focus on a subcategory — those 85 and older — and to note their income distribution. Rosenwaike's data show that almost three-fourths of the older women and about one-half of the men had incomes under $5,000.[39] Moreover, the data for the very old men and women who are institutionalized present a starker picture: One-third had no income, and another one-third had incomes of less than $2,000 per year. Approximately 1 percent had incomes of over $15,000.

Recommendations

The research reviewed above suggests that as people age in place our government agencies and private organizations must be flexible in coping with the growing population requiring supportive services. The preceding discussion has also shown that Americans in the field of housing and gerontology are innovative in developing a variety of housing options that are feasible, cost-effective, and satisfying to the residents. The following policy recommendations are offered:

1. The various branches of the federal government must be more flexible in dealing with the complex issues bearing on older persons and their living environments. The Department of Housing and Urban Development has demonstrated, through the Congregate Housing Services Program, that it can mount an effective program that goes beyond its traditional emphasis on building structures. Unfortunately, HUD has repeatedly tried to terminate this program. If HUD does not wish to enlarge this area of its mission, some other branch of the federal government should be vested with this responsibility.

2. Given the federal nature of our government structure, it is essential that state and local governments be involved in the initiation, financing, management, and evaluation of congregate housing.[40] Review of the research literature indicates that projects are successful when they have strong local involvement and support.

3. A major policy issue concerns the amount of financial support the federal government is willing to give to congregate housing.[41] Perhaps new funding mechanisms should be established in which revolving trust funds would operate separately from the annual budgetary and appropriation system of the federal government. The disbursement of these trust funds should be allocated to states that apply according to a matching fund principle. A formula should be developed that takes into account the percentage of a state's population who are eligible functionally and financially for congregate housing.

4. The policymakers who allocate funds should consider the distribution of the older population and the structure of government in the particular states. Small states have an administrative advantage, adaptability in responding to the complex problems of congregate housing. In large states, subdivisions such as health and planning districts might be more suitable administrative units.

5. With the increasing trend toward privatization, the non-profit sector might be increasingly involved in the actual development and operation of congregate housing. The knowledge and expertise of professional organizations like the American Association of Homes for the Aging, the

National Council on Aging, the Gerontological Society of America, and others are natural candidates for such an operation.

6. There is a need for a broad educational program to make Americans aware of the growing social need for congregate housing. The changing demographic structure, the increased involvement of women in the paid labor force, and the mobility of American families all point to the need for more congregate housing. As one of its major goals this educational program should alert Americans to life-course developments. We must alter our belief that the private single-family home is the ultimate form of environment for the elderly.

Because this last suggestion touches a new area related to age policy that may be sensitive and controversial, the observation of Alan Pifer is pertinent: "It is possible that new types of advisory, quasi-judicial, or arbitrative bodies may develop to provide protected environments for the nonpartisan, disinterested exploration of sensitive new issues arising from population aging — issues that would only be exacerbated if subjected too early to the rough and tumble of the traditional process of public policy formation."[42]

Since 1965 the Older Americans Act has been amended many times. However, the ten goals of the act have remained fixed despite changes made by the various Congresses and signed into law by every president. These objectives serve as our watchword on housing for America's elderly and research about their environment. In Title I of the act, objectives three and nine are as follows:

Objective 3: Suitable housing, independently selected, designed and located with reference to special needs and available at costs which older citizens can afford.

Objective 9: Immediate benefits from proven research knowledge which can sustain health and happiness.

This chapter has described some steps taken to meet these fine objectives and examined new and valuable increments to our knowledge. It is now the task of the policymakers to translate this research knowledge into programs that will serve the needs of our older citizens.

Notes

1. Special Committee on Aging, U.S. Senate. *Congregate Housing for Older Adults: Assisted Residential Living Combining Shelter and Services.* 94th Congress, 1st Session, Report No. 94-4778. Washington, D.C.: U.S. Government Printing Office, 1975.

2. Ibid., p. 4.

3. National Institute on Aging. *Age Words: A Glossary on Health and Aging.* Bethesda, Md.: National Institutes of Health, 1986, p. 49.

4. Congressional Budget Office. *Federal Housing Programs Affecting Elderly People.* Report No. 88-576E. Washington, D.C.: Congressional Budget Office, 1988.

5. Special Committee on Aging, "Congregate housing." It should be noted that the author of the working paper for the Special Committee on Aging was Marie McGuire Thompson, Commissioner, U.S. Public Housing Administration, 1961–67. She had previously been director of the San Antonio Housing Authority during the planning, construction, and early evaluation of Victoria Plaza, which is described and analyzed in this chapter.

6. Special Committee on Aging, p. 60.

7. In summarizing a large body of research, some rich and subtle aspects of the research reports had to be left out. The reader should consult the original sources for additional data. Our goal has been to offer an overview of the research on congregate housing and provide a base for discussions of public policy and future research opportunities in housing options for the elderly.

8. Malozemoff, I.K., J.G. Anderson, and L.V. Rosenbaum. *Housing for the Elderly: Evaluation of the Effectiveness of Congregate Residences.* Boulder, Colo.: Westview Press, 1978.

9. Ibid., p. 63.

10. Ibid., p. 108.

11. Malozemoff et al. wrote: "The high degree of satisfaction with the design program at all types of sites also suggested that elderly residents are very adaptable and complacent with regard to the physical environment they live in." However, the importance of building design has been demonstrated convincingly in the comparative study of two public housing projects in a large midwestern city. Peterson, Longino, and Phelps reported in 1979 that Horizon

Heights, which had space for a nutrition site, had a much higher degree of sociability than Metro Towers, a similar-sized building with a large atrium but no common facility for dining. See Peterson, W. H., C. F. Longino, Jr., and L. W. Phelps. *A Study of Security, Health and Social Support Systems, and Adjustment of Residents in Selected Congregate Living and Retirement Settings.* Kansas City, Mo.: Center on Aging Studies, University of Missouri, Kansas City, 1979.

12. Carp, F.M. *A Future for the Aged: Victoria Plaza and Its Residents.* Austin, Tex.: University of Texas Press, 1966.

13. Carp, F.M. "User evaluation of housing for the elderly." *The Gerontologist* 16:102–11, 1976.

14. Carp, F.M. "A senior center in public housing for the elderly." *The Gerontologist* 16:243–48, 1976.

15. Carp, F.M. "Impact of improved living environment on health and life expectancy." *The Gerontologist* 17:247, 1977.

16. Sherwood, S., D.S. Greer, J.N. Morris, V. Mor, and Associates. *An Alternative to Institutionalization: The Highland Heights Experiment.* Cambridge, Mass.: Ballinger Publishing Company, 1981.

17. Besdine, R.W. and S. Sherwood. "Health care needs of elderly in congregate housing." In Robert D. Chellis, et al. (Eds.), *Congregate Housing for Older People.* Lexington, Mass.: Lexington Books, 1982, p. 202.

18. Lawton, M.P., M. Moss, and M. Grimes. "The changing service needs of older tenants in planned housing." *The Gerontologist,* 25:258, 1985.

19. Lawton, M.P., M. Greenbaum, and B. Liebowitz. "The lifespan of housing environments for the aging." *The Gerontologist,* 20:56–64, 1980.

20. Lawton, M.P. *Social and Medical Services in Housing for the Aged.* Rockville, Md.: National Institute of Mental Health, 1980.

    Lawton, M.P., and J. Cohen. "Environment and the well-being of elderly inner city residents." *Environment and Behavior,* 6:194–211, 1974.

    Lawton, M.P., and J. Cohen. "The generality of housing impact on the well-being of older people." *Journal of Gerontology,* 29:194–204, 1974.

21. Ehrlich, P., I. Ehrlich, and P. Woehlke. "Congregate housing for the elderly: Thirteen years later." *The Gerontologist,* 22:399–403, 1982.

22. Lawton, et al., "Lifespan."

23. Ehrlich, et al., "Congregate housing."

24. Heumann, L.F., J.L. Rose, and T.P. Palton. *A Cost Comparison of Congregate Housing and Long-Term-Care Facilities in the Midwest.* Chicago: Illinois Housing Development Authority, 1985.

25. Ibid., p. 52.

26. Ibid., p. 59.

27. Mollica, R., J. Zeisel, et al. *Congregate Housing for Older People: An Effective Alternative* (Final report). Boston: Executive Office for Elder Affairs, 1984.

28. Kaye, L.W., and A. Monk. "Patterns of social network reciprocity in elder congregate housing." Paper presented at the 40th Annual Scientific Meeting of the Gerontological Society of America, Washington, D.C., 1987.

29. Ibid., p. 14.

30. Ibid., p. 22.

31. Mollica, R., Zeisel, J., et al., *Congregate Housing*, p. 18.

32. Kaye, L.W., B.E. Diamond, and A. Monk. "Congregate housing for the elderly: An analysis of program adequacy and effectiveness." Paper presented at the 39th Annual Scientific Meeting of the Gerontological Society of America, Chicago, Illinois.

    Ruchlin, H.S., and J.N. Morris. *Service Cost Analysis* (Performance Issue 3). Boston: Department of Housing and Urban Development, 1984.

    Sherwood, S., N.D. Layzer, J.N. Morris, S. Morris, M. Rosentraub, and C. Sherwood. *Evaluation of the Congregate Housing Services Program* (Performance Report 2). Boston: Hebrew Rehabilitation Center for the Aged, 1984.

33. Lipsky, M. *Street-Level Bureaucracy: Dilemmas of the Individual in Public Services.* New York: Russell Sage, 1980.

34. Consumer Affairs, American Association of Retired Persons. *Understanding Senior Housing.* Washington, D.C.: American Association of Retired Persons, 1987.

35. Ibid.

36. Reported in *The New York Times,* January 24, 1988, based on 1986 Bureau of the Census data. For a discussion of the socioeconomic patterns see G.F. Streib, "Socioeconomic strata," in E.B. Palmore (Ed.), *Handbook on the Aged in the United States,* Westport, Conn.: Greenwood, 1984, pp. 77–92.

37. The stratification issue of "age or need" is discussed in B.L. Neugarten, (Ed.), *Age or Need? Public Policies for the Elderly,* Beverly Hills, Calif.: Sage, 1982. A more recent discussion is contained in B. Neugarten and D.A. Neugarten, "Age in the aging society," *Daedalus,* 115, 31–49, 1986, where they write: "And when all federal programs are considered together — the direct payments, the in-kind transfers, the tax benefits — it is evident that most of the benefits are going to those older people who are in the top third of the income distribution. Further, if these programs continue in their present direction, they will not only maintain the present inequalities, they will create even further disadvantage for those older persons who are poor."

38. Rosenwaike, I. *The Extreme Aged in America: A Portrait of an Expanding Population.* Westport, Conn.: Greenwood Press, 1985, p. 91.

39. Ibid., pp. 84-85.

40. Nachison, J.S. "Congregate housing for the low and moderate income elderly—A needed federal state partnership." *Journal of Housing for the Elderly,* 3:65–80, 1985.

41. Nachison, J.S. "Who pays? The congregate housing question." *Generations,* Summer, 34–37, 1985.

42. Pifer, A. "The public policy response to population aging." *Daedalus,* 115, 1:394, 1986.

CHAPTER FIVE

Residential Care Facilities: Understanding Their Role and Improving Their Effectiveness

ROBERT J. NEWCOMER, LESLIE A. GRANT

Residential care facilities and boarding home living form a major component of the nation's long-term-care delivery system, housing up to one million people.[1] A variety of terms describe this housing: residential care; community care; personal care; domiciliary care; supervisory care; sheltered care; adult foster care; board and care facilities; and family, group, and boarding homes. "Residential care facility" or "RCF" is used in this chapter as a generic label for the subclassifications of licensed facilities. This usage is preferred by the RCF industry and its professional association. The term "boarding home" will refer to unlicensed facilities.[2]

These living arrangements encompass multiple levels of care and have the potential to fill major gaps in the long-term-care continuum. Proponents view the RCF as an integral element in the continuum of long-term care; it bridges an important service gap for people who do not need nursing home care but who find in-home

This chapter updates and expands the background paper "Descriptive Analysis of Board and Care Policy Trends in the 50 States," prepared in 1983 for the U.S. Administration on Aging. We thank Robyn Stone and A.E. Benjamin for their assistance in conceptualizing these issues; Joel Weeden and Shawn Ginther for their assistance in updating the literature review and state innovations; Ida Red, editor; and Norton Twite, senior word processing technician.

101

assistance inadequate or too expensive. Opponents view RCFs as another form of institutionalization — one that is underfunded, poorly regulated, and likely to expose the public to questionable care. They want to tightly limit the levels of care provided in RCFs.

These are not simply academic issues. Anecdotal information from RCF operators suggests that residents have become more impaired in recent years. Perhaps the change in impairment level is due to more stringent screening of nursing home placements or to the limited supply of nursing home beds. Perhaps it reflects the greater number of RCF residents aging in place.

Regardless of the cause, the wide range of care received in RCFs may have its basis in the failings of the overall long-term-care service system, rather than in the RCF concept itself. The presence of ambulation-impaired persons in RCFs with their increased need for services illustrates the issue and the concern. Does the solution to providing appropriate care to such individuals lie in upgrading the staffing, service mix, and environmental standards of RCFs? Is the answer to ban entry or occupancy by persons with mobility handicaps? Is it to change the preadmission screening criteria and financing for nursing home care?

This chapter provides data for making a balanced assessment of RCFs and their role in the continuum of long-term care. We will examine current knowledge of the residential care industry, its clients, and the regulatory and financing structures affecting its operation.

Bed Supply in Residential Care Facilities

The diversity of supportive housing categories causes variable estimates for the number of residential care facilities and their residents both nationally and by state. These facilities are classified by the level of care, size, or population served. At least seven groups are served: the elderly, the mentally ill, the developmentally disabled, the mentally retarded, alcohol and/or drug abusers, the physically handicapped, and children.

Although standardized definitions have not been established among the fifty states, several characteristics distinguish RCFs from nursing homes and other forms of group housing. Residential care refers to the provision by a nonrelative of food, shelter, and some degree of protective oversight and/or personal care that is generally nonmedical in nature.[3] The personal care and oversight responsibilities usually include cleaning the residents' rooms, doing their laundry, helping with transportation and shopping, supervising residents' medication, and assisting them in obtaining medical and social services. Available on a more limited basis is assistance with activities of daily living (for example, eating, bathing, and grooming). Other services are sometimes provided, and these vary with the needs of the client population; for example, the needs of the mentally impaired differ from those of the physically impaired.

There is no national directory of residential care facilities, but estimates of the number of facilities have been developed from time to time. One source of data is a 1982 report issued by the Office of the Inspector General, U.S. Department of Health and Human Services.[4] Several other studies conducted in the early 1980s provide information about the types of clients served. Approximately 90,000 mentally retarded persons are in "private community-based" residences.[5] Just over half (49,000) of this number are mentally retarded adults.[6] Another study in 1981 estimated that between 60,000 and 80,000 mentally ill adults reside in RCFs, with the largest proportion in adult foster care facilities.[7] The National Association of Residential Care Facilities (NARCF) estimates that there are a total of 41,196 residential care facilities and 513,550 beds in the U.S.[8] These estimates generally affirm an Institute for Health & Aging (IHA) telephone survey of state residential program licensing agencies. This survey found that the elderly are the primary users of residential care facilities. Nationally about 65 percent of licensed beds are designated for persons over age 65.[9]

Table 5-1 shows the total number of adult RCF facilities and beds per 1,000 persons in each state, using the NARCF data. The total number of licensed beds varies widely across states and tends to be associated with state size. Totals vary from only 130 beds in North Dakota to almost 120,000 in California. Eighteen states license fewer than one RCF bed per 1,000 persons, whereas ten states have three or more beds per 1,000. Table 5-2 displays the number of facilities by bed capacity using IHA data. Although there are overcounts or incomplete reports for some states, it is nevertheless clear that small facilities with 1 to 8 beds outnumber those with a larger

Table 5-1. Number of Licensed Residential Care Facilities and Beds, 1987

State	Number of Licensed Facilities	Number of Beds	Beds per 1000 Population
Alabama	432	5,386	1.33
Alaska	18	180	0.34
Arizona	277	4,784	1.44
Arkansas	556	2,011*	0.85
California	8,632	119,163	4.42
Colorado	328	3,973	1.22
Connecticut	299	3,500	1.10
Delaware	514	229*	0.36
District of Columbia	354	2,000	3.19
Florida	2,298	57,000	4.88
Georgia	1,208	6,403	1.05
Hawaii	618	3,000	2.82
Idaho	155	2,695	2.69
Illinois	48	550	0.05
Indiana	191	709	0.13
Iowa	129	1,717	0.60
Kansas	567	28,596	11.62
Kentucky	787	10,922	2.93
Louisiana	†	†	†
Maine	533	4,034	3.44
Maryland	440	1,150	0.26
Massachusetts	104	632	0.11
Michigan	4,205	29,240	3.20
Minnesota	600	1,200	0.28
Mississippi	67	1,175	0.45

*Known undercount due to incomplete data.
†Data are not available.

Table 5-1. Number of Licensed Residential Care Facilities and Beds, 1987 (*cont.*)

State	Number of Licensed Facilities	Number of Beds	Beds per 1000 Population
Missouri	1,373	22,621	4.47
Montana	163	409*	0.50
Nebraska	73	3,237	2.03
Nevada	134	1,212	1.26
New Hampshire	802	14,800	14.41
New Jersey	395	6,898	0.91
New Mexico	421	†	†
New York	4,085	44,400	2.50
North Carolina	1,222	18,531	2.93
North Dakota	50	130	0.19
Ohio	2,040	18,874	1.76
Oklahoma	112	2,100	0.64
Oregon	254	4,553	1.69
Pennsylvania	2,137	20,500	1.72
Rhode Island	22	†	†
South Carolina	356	5,242	1.55
South Dakota	148	435	0.61
Tennessee	387	3,955	0.82
Texas	381	9,052	0.54
Utah	70	†	†
Vermont	47	989	1.83
Virginia	397	17,488	3.02
Washington	1,130	14,813	3.32
West Virginia	995	3,634	1.89
Wisconsin	600	9,000	1.88
Wyoming	22	425	0.84
U.S. mean	41,196	513,550	2.21

Source: National Association of Residential Care Facilities, unpublished data, 1988.
*Known undercount due to incomplete data.
†Data are not available.

Table 5-2. Estimated Number of Residential Care Facilities by Facility Size, 1983

State	1–8 Beds	9–24 Beds	25–59 Beds	60–99 Beds	100+ Beds	Unknown	Total
Alabama	62	36	5	3	2	0	108*
Alaska	55	6	6	1	1	0	69
Arizona	129	31	36	6	5	0	207
Arkansas	14	18	0	0	0	45	77*
California	5,509	1,120	389	153	220	0	7,391
Colorado	390	32	5	2	2	15	446
Connecticut	267	92	47	7	1	8	422
Delaware	197	6	5	0	1	0	209
District of Columbia	295	38	12	1	2	9	357*
Florida	3,217	15	12	0	5	1,196	4,445
Georgia	1,374	2	0	0	0	70	1,446†
Hawaii	575	5	7	2	0	0	589
Idaho	43	29	14	6	2	0	94
Illinois	45	33	34	12	5	81	210
Indiana	375	28	0	0	0	0	403
Iowa	140	104	84	31	17	0	376
Kansas	247	13	0	0	0	0	260
Kentucky	514	68	75	34	10	0	701*
Louisiana	154	15	0	0	0	0	169
Maine	462	48	30	2	1	0	543
Maryland	439	36	37	11	4	0	527
Massachusetts	1,818	168	124	21	4	400	2,535
Michigan	2,881	271	74	18	32	639	3,915
Minnesota	0	0	1	0	0	214	215
Mississippi	24	21	1	1	0	0	47

* Incomplete data or undercount.
†Known overcount or possible overcount.

Table 5-2. Estimated Number of Residential Care Facilities by Facility Size, 1983 (cont.)

State	1–8 Beds	9–24 Beds	25–59 Beds	60–99 Beds	100+ Beds	Unknown	Total
Missouri	250	228	84	13	14	255	844†
Montana	199	9	0	0	0	0	208
Nebraska	327	33	17	4	8	2	391*
Nevada	60	11	5	0	3	0	79
New Hampshire	103	31	6	1	1	38	180
New Jersey	936	25	0	0	0	531	1,492*
New Mexico	0	0	0	0	0	182	182
New York	2,366	333	1	0	92	2,770	5,562*
North Carolina	738	160	135	63	14	22	1,132
North Dakota	19	21	17	5	2	0	64
Ohio	0	472	0	0	0	71	543*
Oklahoma	22	42	25	3	1	0	93
Oregon	964	51	1	0	0	171	1,187*
Pennsylvania	1,601	368	177	29	14	0	2,189*
Rhode Island	56	9	1	0	0	35	101
South Carolina	90	121	56	0	0	6	273
South Dakota	192	51	8	0	0	0	251*
Tennessee	0	0	0	0	0	512	512
Texas	9	52	19	18	23	30	151*
Utah	94	13	3	1	3	0	114
Vermont	96	83	18	0	0	5	202†
Virginia	82	72	74	1	25	140	394*
Washington	750	—	—	—	—	—	750†
West Virginia	617	32	24	1	1	0	675
Wisconsin	327	191	36	11	11	0	576
Wyoming	48	0	0	0	0	0	48
Total	29,172	4,643	1,705	461	526	7,447	43,954

Source: IHA, 1984.
* Incomplete data or undercount.
†Known overcount or possible overcount.

bed capacity in two out of every three states. Nationally, these small facilities account for two-thirds of the total number of facilities, and between one-quarter and one-third of all beds.

Who Are the Residents?

Paralleling the piecemeal information about the distribution of RCF beds is the equally fragmented knowledge about RCF residents.[10] Most studies to date have been limited to one or perhaps a handful of purposefully selected states (for example, six to eight). Typically, these investigations have relied on case studies and convenience or haphazard samples of facilities.

Despite the limitations of these studies, a few general patterns in resident characteristics emerge. About 60 percent of persons in RCFs for the aged are women. The populations of facilities for the mentally ill and mentally retarded are almost equally divided between men and women, and these residents tend to be age forty or younger. At least half of the men, regardless of facility type, have never been married. At least three-fourths of the women have been married, but most are widowed or divorced. All RCFs tend to have an underrepresentation of ethnic minorities. Length of residency in RCFs ranges from three to five years for the aged, which is slightly longer than for other resident groups.

Health status and functional ability among the various client groups have not been well quantified. A survey of 27,000 persons in 230 facilities in New Jersey provides one of the best estimates and description of the characteristics of populations served in licensed RCFs and unlicensed boarding homes.[11] Almost half the residents in residential care facilities were found to need some help in their activities of daily living, as did eight percent of those in boarding homes. More importantly, in both groups a high proportion of residents needed some form of mental health service (37 percent of the RCF group and 30 percent of the boarding home group). Similar rates have been reported in other studies.[12]

Paralleling the prevalence of mental illness in RCFs is the use of psychotropic medications and the need for other assistance in care. General findings from these studies indicate that about two-thirds of the residents needing mental health services receive them.

About one-third of the residents in facilities serving the aged or mentally ill have had a recent hospitalization. Among the mentally retarded, the rate is about half this level.

How the needs of RCF residents vary by facility size and by health or functional status has not been studied systematically. However, it is known that mentally ill and mentally retarded residents are more commonly found in small RCFs than are the aged.

Staffing

Depending on the size of the facility, employees in RCFs provide such services as housekeeping, kitchen work, personal care, building maintenance, transportation, and managerial and clerical services. In general, the average ratio of residents to staff is smaller in facilities for the mentally retarded than in RCFs for the aged or the mentally ill. These patterns are affected by funding and state regulations and requirements for care. An examination of regulations governing residential care facilities nationwide found that 70 percent of the regulations require a responsible person to be present at the facility at all times, and 28 percent specify a maximum resident-to-staff ratio.[13] A seven-state study found the lowest resident-to-staff ratios in Massachusetts (2.2 to 1 for facilities serving the elderly and 2.4 to 1 for the mentally ill).[14] The highest resident-to-staff ratios were found in Texas (4.7 to 1 for the elderly and 4.2 to 1 for the mentally ill).

A national study of residential care facilities for the mentally retarded found that staffing ratios vary by the size and type of facility and by the type of ownership.[15] Resident-to-staff ratios tend to be low in small facilities. Ratios tend to be lowest in specialized foster homes (1.9 to 1) and small group residences with fewer than sixteen beds (2.9 to 1) and highest in large public residences with between sixteen and sixty-three beds (8.7 to 1).

Matching RCF Supply and Resident Need

An issue without clear resolution is the ability of existing RCF resources to provide personal care and even medically oriented services to residents. Existing studies do not address this issue well, as most cover one point in time. Two longitudinal studies have examined the benefits of residence in supportive housing. One of these studies involved medically oriented housing for the physically impaired and elderly.[16] Activity programs and noon meals were available in this facility. Homemakers, home health aides, and nurses were available as needed, from community-based agencies. A second study involved the Pennsylvania domiciliary care program.[17] The program consisted of both family-oriented homes providing shelter for up to three clients and somewhat larger facilities for four to thirteen clients. Personal care and protective services were provided in addition to room, board, laundry, and other needed household services. Clients included aged, mentally ill, and retarded persons.

Findings from these studies demonstrate that both medically oriented congregate housing and case-managed, foster family housing can have a positive effect on the quality of life of the residents and reduce transfers to nursing homes. The state of Oregon under a Section 2176 waiver of Medicaid regulations has reportedly had similar success in diverting about 2,300 people from nursing homes to RCFs.[18]

But a less optimistic conclusion also is drawn by the same study. Using data from the 1985 National Nursing Home Survey[19] and the seven-state RCF resident and staffing levels study by Dittmar and associates,[20] Feder and associates examine the extent to which RCF care is or might be used as a substitute for nursing home care. A basic assumption tested in their analysis is that the primary nursing home candidates for lower levels of care are those who require little personal care — at most, assistance in bathing and dressing — or no personal care at all. Such individuals are estimated to account for about 35 percent of the U.S. nursing home population.[21] According to Feder and associates, these estimates may overcount the proportion of people who might potentially be served at lower levels of care, since the nursing home survey sample included an unknown number of facilities that might be more accurately characterized as RCFs. The survey did not disaggregate the certified intermediate care facilities providing only minimal levels of nursing care from facilities offering more care. Facilities offering minimal levels of care are likely to house residents with fewer ADL impairments than are facilities with higher levels of care.

Limitations in RCF supply may affect the number of persons who could be served in RCFs rather than nursing homes. RCF staffing levels and/or the RCF physical plants may not be capable of providing the level of care that might be needed by a nursing home relocation group. Most RCFs are small (that is, two-thirds have under nine beds) and many have no staff beyond the owner-operators and their families. Such limited staffing, it is argued, produces a resident-to-staff ratio that is two to three times that in nursing homes. Consideration of the other tasks — meal preparation, laundry, housework — that also must be provided with the same limited staffing raises a legitimate question about how much personal care can or should be provided.

Countering the argument that RCFs cannot substitute for nursing homes are the experiences of small facilities noted previously. Also, although most RCFs are small, the majority of RCF beds are in larger facilities (greater than 50 beds). Larger facilities have higher staff-to-resident ratios and more differentiated staff roles.

Although it may not be possible to estimate precisely the number of persons in nursing homes or in their own homes who might appropriately be served in RCFs, it is important to recognize that persons in need of assistance must be served at one level or another. Each state and community must consider this issue separately, because of the variation in RCF bed supply and because states vary in their willingness to admit to nursing homes only those with severe impairments. There is an inescapable reality: As greater restrictions are placed on admission to nursing homes, RCFs and community care services will experience greater demand to serve functionally impaired elderly people.

Residential Care Regulations and State Capacity

State and local government regulators have tried to differentiate the levels of care that can be provided in RCF versus nursing home settings. Resident needs for assistance in personal care and/or ambulation are conditions that highlight the ambiguous boundary between these levels of care. It is common for states to prohibit RCFs from administering medications and providing nursing care (or serving residents who receive regular nursing care elsewhere, for example, from a home health nurse). Both restrictions presumably limit access to RCF care, even when reimbursement is available under Medicaid waivers.

Another even more common restriction on RCFs is a requirement that residents be able to self-evacuate during a fire or other emergency. These standards affect either the design of facilities (requiring wheelchair accessibility, for example) or prohibitions against serving persons who are wheelchair-bound, or those who are confused. RCFs designed to meet such fire and life safety requirements look like nursing homes. This presumably affects the perceived residential nature of a facility and the age and impairment levels of its residents.

In evaluating the potential of RCFs to meet personal care and ambulation needs of residents, the complex and subtle influences of staffing, design, and services will require increased research attention. New data are needed to provide an understanding of the dynamic interrelationships involved, a comprehensive profile of the clientele served by various levels of care, and evaluation mechanisms for assuring quality of care and quality of life.

Little is known about the interrelationship of regulations and capabilities in the current care system. Most of the limited published work on this topic has focused on regulations and state administrative structure; fewer studies have examined how these elements affect the availability of care. This is an important gap in knowledge, because compliance with regulatory standards has operating cost implications for providers. These costs and standards can have direct effects on the supply of facilities, their size, and the level of care provided.[22]

Formal regulation involves a number of activities, including the licensing and/or certification of residential care facilities, the enforcement of explicit rules and regulations through both formal and informal sanctions, and the monitoring of facilities to ensure that operators adhere to the regulations. All states have some type of statutory authority and regulations addressing RCFs. Regulations are likely to cover such issues as staffing levels, administrator qualifications, the type of care allowed, and resident rights. (Fire and life safety codes, on the other hand, are often the province of local government.) States vary tremendously in the level of effort invested in licensing and regulation.[23] In addition, standards frequently vary within and between states. Some states use general licensing standards for all RCFs, whereas others have promulgated different standards by size and type of facility and by target population.

The regulatory process and administrative structure of state RCF programs nationwide form a continuum from total control of residential care facilities (in which facility supply and demand are determined by state policies) to a pure market model in which supply and demand are subject to competition and choice.[24] State programs targeted specifically for the mentally retarded adult tend to be the most formally and strictly regulated, with state and local agencies controlling recruitment and financing of providers as well as placement and oversight of residents. RCF programs for the mentally ill that are part of the state mental health system also appear to be heavily controlled by state policy.

Residential care facilities housing the elderly or a mixed adult population have been traditionally subject to minimal regulation and oversight. A nationwide survey of 118 state-administered board and care programs serving the aged or a mixed population identifies three common functions of a single state agency or combination of agencies: regulation of facilities; case management or placement of residents; and financial functions, including eligibility determination and reimbursement.[25]

The regulatory philosophy or approach adopted by a state arises from—and has implications for—state funding and administrative staffing levels. Some important barriers to effective oversight were identified by state administrators in a survey conducted by the Institute for Health and Aging, University of California.[26] These conditions included a lack of funding for licensing and inspection personnel; weak statutory enforcement authority; an encumbered legal process in revoking licenses and imposing penalties or sanctions; inadequate data bases regarding bed supply, client placements, and enforcement actions; fragmentation of responsibilities among the agencies responsible for the various populations served; and inadequate training among regulators and operators.

Innovative State Approaches

States have begun to recognize the various problems affecting the operation and quality of care in RCFs and the obstacles to regulation enforcement and financing. Many are exploring non-regulatory alternatives for expanding the supply of facilities and ensuring life safety and quality of care. These strategies make use of existing resources and attempt to provide low-cost, low-threat mechanisms to facilitate provider compliance. Previous reports have identified some state activities as "best practices."[27] Examples from these reports are summarized below, along with additional examples identified in a 1988 telephone survey of selected programs.[28] Few of the programs mentioned have been formally evaluated.

LICENSING

An apparent trend in enforcement is both to include more facilities and beds requiring licenses and to have regulations that allow varying stringency, depending on the size of the facility. An example of this approach is Wisconsin's Community-Based Residential Facilities Program, where if three or more persons are receiving personal care services in a facility, such as an apartment building, the facility must meet residential care licensing requirements.

EXTERNAL PARTICIPATION IN INSPECTION AND MONITORING

Provider organizations have begun to assume some responsibility for enforcing standards in several states. Methods include offering bimonthly training sessions for operators and monitoring the quality of care in member facilities. Some provider groups have begun to help states identify unlicensed facilities.

OPERATOR TRAINING AND CERTIFICATION

Most states mandate a minimum ongoing training requirement. However, a number of state agencies have gone further, with continuing education programs on topics such as financial management, home improvement, cardiopulmonary resuscitation, and nutrition. The curriculum being tested also includes information for operators on gaining access to community resources, establishing care management, and handling medications. This curriculum is implemented in various ways: self-training guides; a minimum number of hours of continuing education credit per year for operators; community college programs; and the use of trainers in each facility. Many states have begun to adopt procedures and to offer formal courses for operators to receive certification. The curriculum covers regulatory requirements, operational standards and procedures, and resident services, as well as ways to maximize resident dignity and well-being. However, these approaches may be more image than substance, in that training may not be very long or intensive.

REIMBURSEMENT

Typically, states rely on a flat rate prospective payment to RCF operators, who use it as they see fit. The rate may vary depending on type of client (mentally ill, developmentally disabled, alcoholic, or aged) or size of facility. Usually there is a higher rate for mentally ill and alcoholic clients, and a lower rate for clients in larger facilities. A few states are developing a supplemental prospective rate structure based on the level of care for individual residents. Facility operators would be expected to use existing community-based services to supply the services needed by residents at each level, if they cannot meet the service requirements with their own staff. Not all facilities would be licensed for all levels.

FINANCIAL INCENTIVES FOR DEVELOPMENT AND REHABILITATION

Financial incentives beyond RCF reimbursement rates is an important approach for increasing the supply of facilities while simultaneously ensuring quality of care and life safety among residents. These incentives have taken the form of low-interest loan and grant programs to assist operators in upgrading their physical plants. The loans are financed from bonds, housing authority reserves, or general fund revenues. Upgrading can include the installation of sprinklers and smoke alarm systems, elaborate remodeling, or new construction.

LOCAL ORDINANCES AND LAND USE

Local zoning regulations can affect the ability of an RCF to locate in a particular neighborhood. Several states have implemented zoning overrides that mandate the approval of small-scale residential facilities in residentially zoned areas.

SCREENING AND PLACEMENT

States have tried a number of approaches in this area, such as the development and use of facility directories.[29] More active approaches require persons who are publicly assisted to be assessed prior to placement in an RCF. In some communities, assessment is made through a central placement agency; in others, assessment is incorporated into nursing home preadmission screening programs. The assessment process is most common when RCF placement makes an individual eligible for state-financed assistance under a Medicaid waiver or other service funds (for example, a Social Services Block Grant, general revenues, or SSP).

MONITORING AND CASE MANAGEMENT

Developmentally disabled and mentally impaired RCF residents are typically in the caseloads of a community agency responsible for their treatment while in the facility. Aged residents, however, are not commonly in the caseloads of community agencies, but a few states have expanded the oversight of aged residents (and others) by assigning a case manager to them. Case managers periodically reassess resident needs and the appropriateness of care being received. Such programs reportedly have been effective in helping developmentally disabled and mentally impaired persons move to or remain in less restrictive settings. For the aged, case management is presumed to facilitate access to community services and to monitor the appropriateness of the level of care.

Financing Residential Care

The primary source of public financing for residential care programs is the federal Supplemental Security Income (SSI) program (Title XVI of the Social Security Act), which provides a guaranteed minimum income to persons who are aged, blind, or disabled.[30] States have the option of supplementing federal SSI payments with State Supplemental Payments (SSP). The SSI benefit levels are established nationally and provide uniform minimum payments in all states.

The maximum monthly benefit levels in 1987 were $340 for an individual and $510 for a couple.[31] The SSP income levels are more varied, with income levels depending on household size, housing type, and whether the person is aged, blind, or disabled. Some states tie the amount of SSP to specific types of licensed and sometimes unlicensed residential care facilities.[32]

Forty-three states provide some kind of supplementation for individuals with special needs. Thirty-six of these states provide SSP to persons who are in residential care or other supportive housing. Six states offer SSP to people living independently with personal care or nursing care.[33] Only eight states offer no SSP supplementation of any kind for domiciliary or in-home care benefits. In most states, total monthly payments (including both SSI and SSP) are between $450 to $600. In 1987, twenty-four states provided state supplemental payments of over $150 per month for an adult with nonmedical long-term-care needs in a residential care facility. At least sixteen states had monthly SSP levels of $200 or more for the aged and other eligible groups.

The income levels provided through the SSI/SSP programs operate as a direct income supplement to the low-income aged, blind, and disabled population. Recipients can use these funds to help pay the rent in RCFs. Government reliance on SSI/SSP benefit levels is, in effect, a "market" approach to influencing the supply, rent levels, and demand for RCF housing. This mechanism has been described as inadequate for encouraging the expansion of supply and the upgrading of facilities to meet life safety and quality of care standards.[34] One particularly important consideration is the difficulty experienced by low-income (publicly subsidized) individuals needing RCF housing in competing with unsubsidized, private-paying individuals seeking such housing. Access to RCF care is especially problematic when there is a high demand from private payers and a limited bed supply. Unless public subsidies are high enough to compete with private payers, low-income persons can be expected to have limited access. Approximately 320,000 SSP recipients live in some form of supportive housing.[35]

A few states have adopted procedures that directly affect the supply of and access to RCF housing. Such procedures are most commonly used to purchase RCF services for low-income clients not eligible for SSI, or for residents of states that do not offer optional supplementation payment. A few other states have found it possible to use Medicaid funds, because the intermediate care facility (ICF) classifications used in these states include some levels of residential care.

The use of Medicaid to fund RCFs is likely to be eliminated because of the Omnibus Budget Reconciliation Act (OBRA) of 1987. This act amended the Medicaid statutes to eliminate, by October 1, 1990, the distinction between skilled nursing facilities (SNFs) and intermediate care facilities (ICFs) (other than intermediate care facilities for the mentally retarded). OBRA revised and expanded the conditions of participation for SNFs and ICFs by combining these two levels of care into a single category of "nursing facility" under the Medicare and Medicaid programs. The ICFs that cannot meet the more stringent fire safety and life safety requirements of SNFs will need state waivers to operate as nursing facilities. It is likely that a number of ICF facilities with substandard physical plants will have to be downgraded to a lower category, because the necessary upgrading may be prohibitively expensive. Similarly, facilities not meeting the SNF nurse staffing requirements will not be eligible for Medicaid reimbursement without a waiver.

Conclusion

Although there is wide variation in size, staffing, levels of care, number of facilities, and terms used to describe residential care, there is ample evidence that RCFs are a substantial resource in the long-term-care delivery system. There is less consensus about who can and who should benefit from this level of care. A number of barriers have hindered consensus building: definitional ambiguities surrounding the concepts of residential care and quality of care; insufficient state and local resources for RCF programs; weak statutory authority and an encumbered legal process; fragmentation of responsibility; insufficient data on supply and residents; inadequate knowledge of the benefits and trade-offs associated with the long-term-care system; and the absence of a federal government role in tying RCF care into the long-term-care system.

Several states have attempted to overcome one or more of these barriers by expanding their statutory authority and by promulgating strict and explicit regulations. Others have begun to develop financial incentives for RCF operators and to expand and upgrade technical assistance and formal training for providers and for personnel responsible for licensure and inspection. These efforts, like traditional policy approaches, typically focus on RCFs as a discrete program. Few states explicitly tie RCFs to issues in the broader long-term-care system.

Actions to improve the knowledge base, the qualifications of staff, and access to appropriate levels of care are needed and long overdue. However, most basic are the needs to establish a clear boundary between RCFs and nursing homes and to set up equitable means of financing RCF services.

If RCFs are to fill critical gaps in the long-term-care continuum, federal and state policies must define levels of reimbursement as well as the types of clients who can be served at the different levels of care.

The federal government, except for mortgage insurance and tax incentives for investors, has exercised little direct influence on RCF use or quality. Its influence is reflected more in what it has not done than in positive action. For example, through Medicare and Medicaid, the federal government has the ability to cover a range of personal and other supportive care benefits; national policy, however, has severely limited such benefits except to those in nursing homes. If these benefits were based on need rather than place of residence, it is likely that many RCF residents would immediately be eligible for some covered services. Such flexible benefit eligibility would have added advantages; it would allow the public to select the manner in which they receive their care and reduce out-of-pocket costs for care in supportive housing settings.

In lieu of a direct service financing role, the federal and state governments have relied largely on an income strategy. This approach, exercised principally through SSI and SSP programs, provides supplemental income to poor persons needing assisted living. However, people have to be both income-qualified and willing to receive care in an eligible facility before they can benefit from this program.

In this context, state licensing regulations for nursing homes and residential care facilities ultimately determine who can and who cannot be served in RCFs. Within broad federal guidelines, state policy makes distinctions between residential care facilities and nursing homes, but there are numerous inconsistencies across states in the definition of facilities and levels of care.

At present, informed planning and policy-making regarding RCFs is impaired by the absence of consistent and timely knowledge about the RCF bed supply; poor understanding of the persons served by these facilities (where they come from, why they chose an RCF); and the effects of current regulations and financing mechanisms for all long-term-care services on RCF supply and demand.

The supply of RCF beds is directly affected by reimbursement rates for RCFs and nursing homes, by the costs of complying with licensure requirements, and by the costs of providing appropriate levels of care. In turn, the demand for RCF beds depends on the price and availability of beds and services at this and other levels of care. Thus, the supply of nursing home beds and other supportive care may affect the demand for RCF beds and vice versa. An understanding of the relationship between nursing home and RCF case mix (that is, resident need) across state jurisdictions would help to clarify the complex and dynamic interrelationships among the regulatory and market forces underlying supply and demand for beds at different levels of care.

As the attention of long-term-care planners turns to residential care, it seems reasonable and desirable to proceed with caution in imposing restrictions on these facilities and to avoid evaluating this care solely as a substitute for nursing homes. It is important to recognize the diversity of needs currently being met, to assess if and how the quality and appropriateness of residential care can be improved, and to determine if breakdowns in care are inherent in the RCF or if they stem from problems elsewhere in the long-term-care delivery system. Moreover, to be most effective, approaches to optimize supply and demand of RCFs need to be systemic, treating the RCF as an integral component of a multifaceted long-term-care system.

Notes

1. This estimate is based on the assumption that there are about as many unlicensed beds as licensed beds. There are about 500,000 licensed beds but no reliable data on the numbers of unlicensed beds.

2. One subcategory of (generally) unlicensed facilities is shared housing, both intergenerational and for the elderly. For a study on this subject, see Streib, G.F., W.E. Folts, and M.A. Hilker, *Old Homes — New Families: Shared Living for the Elderly*, New York: Columbia University Press, 1984.

3. Haske, M., and R. Cohen. *A Home Away from Home: Consumer Information on Board and Care Homes*. Washington, D.C.: American Association of Retired Persons, 1986.

4. Office of the Inspector General, U.S. Department of Health and Human Services. *Board and Care Homes: A Study of Federal and State Actions to Safeguard the Health and Safety of Board and Care Home Residents*. Washington D.C.: Office of the Inspector General, DHEW, 1982.

5. Lakin, K.C., R.H. Bruininks, B.K . Hill, and F.A. Hauber. *Sourcebook on Long Term Care for Developmentally Disabled People*. CRCS Report No. 17. Minneapolis, Minn.: University of Minnesota, 1982.

6. Janicki, M., T. Mayeda, and W. Epple. "Availability of group homes for persons with mental retardation in the United States." *Mental Retardation*, 21, 2:41–51, 1982.

7. Sherwood, C., and M.M. Seltzer. "Board and care literature review, evaluation of board and care homes." Task III Report. Boston: Boston University School of Social Work, 1981.

8. National Association of Residential Care Facilities (NARCF). Unpublished data. Richmond, Va.: NARCF, 1988.

9. Institute for Health and Aging (IHA). Data from 1983 Residential Care Facility Telephone Survey. San Francisco: IHA, University of California, 1984.

10. The following are examples of this research. On the mentally retarded/developmentally disabled: Baker, B.L., G.B. Seltzer, and M.M. Seltzer. *As Close as Possible: Community Residence for Retarded Adults*. Boston: Little Brown, 1977; Bruininks, R. H., F. A. Hauber, and M. J. Kudla. "National survey of community residential care facilities: A profile of facilities and residents in 1977." *American Journal of Mental Deficiency*, 84:470–478, 1980.

   The mentally ill: Melick, C.F., and C.O. Eysaman. "A study of former patients placed in private proprietary homes." *Hospital and Community Psychiatry*, 29, 9:587–89, 1978.

   The aged: Sherwood, S., V. Mor, and C. Gutkin. *Domiciliary Care Clients and the Facilities in Which They Reside*. Vols. 1–3. Boston: Hebrew Rehabilitation Center for the Aged, 1981; Dittmar, N., and J. Bell. *Board and Care for Elderly and Mentally*

Disabled Populations: Final Report. Vol. 2. Denver: Denver Research Institute, Social Systems Research and Evaluation Division, University of Denver, 1983.

Group home demonstration projects and state-specific studies, such as those in New Jersey: Gioglio, G., and R. Jacobsen. *Demographic and Service Characteristics of the Rooming Home, Boarding Home, and Residential Health Care Facility Population in New Jersey.* Trenton: Bureau of Research, Evaluation and Quality Assurance, Division of Youth and Family Services, New Jersey Department of Human Services, 1984a; *Ocean County Pilot Boarding Home Project: Progress Report.* Trenton: Ocean County Community Care Committee, New Jersey Department of Human Services, 1984b; *Sussex County Boarding Home Pilot Project: Progress Report.* Trenton: Sussex County Board of Social Services.

New York: Jacobsen, J., E. Silver, and A. Schwartz. "Service provision in New York's group homes." *Mental Retardation,* 22, 5:231–39, 1984.

Hawaii: Braun, K.L., and C.L. Rose. "The Hawaii Geriatric Foster Care Experiment: Impact evaluation and cost analysis." *The Gerontologist,* 26, 5:516–24, 1986.

Unlicensed facilities have been examined less frequently. The Comptroller General's Office (U.S. GAO, 1979) attempted to develop and test a methodology using SSI recipient records for identifying boarding homes. This approach was of limited value, and not all states were included. This approach was replicated to study a small sample of facilities in several states: Eckert, J. K., K. Namazi, and E. Kahana. "Unlicensed board and care homes: An extra-familial living arrangement for the elderly." *Journal of Cross-Cultural Gerontology,* 2:377–93, 1987.

11. Gioglio, G., and R. Jacobsen. *Demographic and Service Characteristics of the Rooming Home, Boarding Home, and Residential Health Care Facility Population in New Jersey.* Trenton: Bureau of Research, Evaluation and Quality Assurance, Division of Youth and Family Services, Department of Human Services, 1984.

12. Dittmar, N., and J. Bell. *Board and Care for Elderly and Mentally Disabled Populations: Final Report.* Vol. 2. Denver: Denver Research Institute, Social Systems Research and Evaluation Division, University of Denver, 1983.

13. Reichstein, K., and L. Bergofsky. "Domiciliary care facilities for adults: An analysis of state regulations." *Research on Aging,* 5, 1:25–43, 1983.

14. Dittmar and Bell, *Board and Care.*

15. Hill, B.K., and K.C. Lakin. "Classification of residential facilities for individuals with mental retardation." *Mental Retardation,* 24, 2:107–15, 1986.

16. Sherwood, S., V. Mor, and C. Gutkin. *Domiciliary Care Clients and the Facilities in Which They Reside.* Vols. 1–3. Boston: Hebrew Rehabilitation Center for the Aged, 1981.

17. Sherwood, S., and D. Morris. "The Pennsylvania Domiciliary-Care Experiment: Impact on quality of life." *American Journal of Public Health,* 73, 6:646–53, 1983.

18. Feder, J., W. Scanlon, J. Edwards, and J. Hoffman. *Board and Care: Problem or Solution?* Paper prepared for the Robert Wood Johnson Foundation and the American Association of Retired Persons. Washington, D.C.: Center for Health Policy Studies, 1988.

19. Sekscenski, E.S. *Discharges from Nursing Homes: Preliminary Data from the 1985 National Nursing Home Survey. Advance Data from Vital and Health Statistics.* DHHS Pub. No. (PHS) 87-1250. Hyattsville, Md.: U.S. Public Health Service, 1987.

20. Dittmar, N., G. Smith, J. Bell, C. Jones, and D. Manzanares. *Board and Care for Elderly and Mentally Disabled Populations: Final Report.* Vol. 1. Denver: Denver Research Institute, Social Systems Research and Evaluation Division, University of Denver, 1983.

21. Sekscenski, *Discharges from Nursing Homes.*

22. Benjamin, A.E., and R.J. Newcomer. "Board and care housing: An analysis of state differences." *Research on Aging,* 8, 3:388–406, 1986.

23. American Bar Association. *Board and Care Report: An Analysis of State Laws and Programs Serving Elderly Persons and Disabled Adults.* Report to the Department of Health and Human Services. Washington, D.C.: American Bar Association, 1983.

24. Stone, R., R.J. Newcomer, and M. Saunders. *Descriptive Analysis of Board and Care Policy in Fifty States.* Policy Paper No. 1. San Francisco: Institute for Health and Aging, University of California, 1983.

25. Reichstein, K., and L. Bergofsky. "Domiciliary care facilities for adults: An analysis of state regulations." *Research on Aging,* 5, 1:25–43, 1983.

26. Stone, et al. *Board and Care Policy.*

27. Feder, et al. *Board and Care: Problem or Solution?*

    Tiven, M., and B. Ryther. *State Initiatives in Elderly Housing.* Washington, D.C.: National Association of State Units on Aging and the Council of State Housing Agencies, 1986.

    Office of the Inspector General, *Board and Care Homes.*

    Harmon, C. "Board and care: An old problem, a new resource for long term care." Paper presented at the National Conference on Social Welfare and the U.S. Administration on Aging, Department of Health and Human Services. Washington, D.C.: Center for the Study of Social Policy, 1982.

    Stone, et al. *Board and Care Policy.*

28. Institute for Health and Aging (IHA). "State RCF Regulation and Financing Innovations Telephone Survey." Unpublished. San Francisco: IHA, University of California, 1988.

29. Tiven and Ryther, *State Initiatives.*

30. The U.S. Department of Housing and Urban Development (HUD) operates a number of programs to provide housing and related facilities for aged and/or disabled persons. Section 202 makes direct loans to private nonprofit sponsors to finance rental or cooperative housing. Section 238 provides mortgage insurance for private lending institutions to build or rehabilitate multifamily projects of eight or more units. The Congregate Housing Services Program (CHSP) makes grants to public housing authorities and Section 202 borrowers to provide meals and other supportive services for frail elderly persons to prevent or delay institutionalization. Section 8 provides rental assistance to low-income, elderly, and disabled persons to afford housing in the private market. Subsidies pay the difference between tenant contributions and rent charged for the unit (U.S. Department of Housing and Urban Development; Tiven and Ryther, *State Initiatives*).

31. U.S. Social Security Administration. *The Supplemental Security Income Program for Aged, Blind, and Disabled: Characteristics of State Assistance Programs for SSI Recipients, January 1987.* Washington, D.C.: U.S. Social Security Administration, 1987.

32. Meltzer, J. *Completing the Long-Term-Care Continuum: An Income Supplement Strategy.* Washington, D.C.: The Center for the Study of Social Policy, 1988.

33. U.S. Social Security Administration, *The Supplemental Security Income Program.*

34. Office of the Inspector General, *Board and Care Homes.*

35. Meltzer, J. *Long-Term-Care Continuum.*

CHAPTER SIX

CCRCs: An Option for Aging in Place

SYLVIA SHERWOOD,
HIRSCH S. RUCHLIN, AND
CLARENCE C. SHERWOOD

Social planners and policymakers have become increasingly concerned with devising effective strategies both to help maintain an independent life for the frail elderly and to contain, if not reduce, the costs of long-term care. Recognition of the increased housing options for elderly citizens has led to the proliferation of alternative living arrangements — from settings that cater to the fully independent elderly person to those that provide care to the very frail elderly.[1, 2] Continuing Care Retirement Communities (CCRCs), sometimes referred to as lifecare communities, represent one such alternative; they are planned communities that combine housing and a range of services including independent living, assisted living, and nursing home care.

Serving primarily middle- and upper-middle-class elderly, CCRCs developed as private sector ventures rather than as a result of governmental or philanthropic subsidy. They have depended financially on pooled risk through entry and monthly fees. The CCRC provides

This chapter draws on research supported in part by HCFA Grant #18-C-98672/1, "An evaluation of 'life-continuum of care' residential centers in the United States" and an NIA Teaching Nursing Home Award to the Hebrew Rehabilitation Center for the Aged, Boston.

an independent living unit (for example, an apartment) and specified services (meals, housekeeping, and so on) along with long-term-care insurance guaranteeing availability of nursing care at some time in the future, should it be needed. Most CCRCs have been sponsored by nonprofit organizations.

What Is a CCRC?

Special types of housing with health care arrangements for the elderly have been developing for a period of one hundred years or more. As noted by Winklevoss and Powell, many homes for the aged founded by religious and charitable organizations around the turn of the century in the United States took on the responsibility for medical care.[3] The development since the early 1900s of the concept of insurance against accident, sickness, and loss of income upon retirement also helped pave the way for the growth of CCRCs as an affordable option for the elderly. In the post–World War II era, CCRCs have experienced significant growth.

Considerable development during the 1950s and 1960s occurred in facilities sponsored and owned by religious organizations and operated on a not-for-profit basis.[4, 5] Types of sponsorship and ownership have broadened considerably, and greater interest has been exhibited by for-profit firms. Major hotel and nursing home chains, insurers, and banks are entering the field.[6, 7]

In some early CCRCs, the resident paid an initial fee and was guaranteed a place to live, services, and, if needed, nursing care for the rest of his or her life. Presumably due to actuarial miscalculations, inflation, and other factors, this arrangement did not prove financially feasible, and this type of CCRC has all but disappeared, although earlier contracts with residents in the community may still be honored. Virtually all CCRCs instituted an entry fee and monthly fees. This system has held great appeal for facility operators because it links revenue to the resident's longevity as well as to rates of inflation. In the landmark Wharton School survey, which reported on 207 responding CCRCs in existence as of December 1981, 94.2 percent indicated that a contract remains in effect for the resident's life.[8] This was the case despite the fact that, to be considered a CCRC in this survey, a community had only to offer a contract guaranteeing shelter and health care that lasted for more than one year. None of the responding facilities reported that they had ever asked a resident to leave because of inability to pay fees. Almost all of these CCRCs guaranteed residents of the independent units access to permanent nursing care, and many did not raise the monthly charges when the resident required permanent nursing care. Communities that charged for the full cost of health care services were not accepted in the Wharton survey definition as CCRCs.

The current definition of a CCRC, as promulgated by the American Association of Homes for the Aged (AAHA), recognizes not only communities in which health care services are at least partially prepaid by the resident as part of the entrance and monthly fees, but also those in which a full-cost fee-for-service arrangement for nursing care is included.[9, 10] Although with this model facility owners minimize or even eliminate their risk for care beyond the levels implicit in the fees, we know of no instance in which residents have been asked to leave a CCRC because of inability to pay the fees. Furthermore, according to the 1988 AAHA directory of CCRCs, the nursing facilities of about half of the listed CCRCs are Medicaid-certified and therefore, at least theoretically, use Medicaid to finance care after the individual's assets become exhausted. Those that do not rely on Medicaid may accumulate contributed funds to subsidize residents in the health center when necessary. More information is needed on how CCRCs handle these problems.

A further refinement in financing CCRC care is the introduction of entry fee refund policies. Most CCRCs have offered at least partial refunds if the resident left the community within a specified period of time, but now many CCRCs offer refunds whenever the resident leaves. However, to accommodate such a policy, fees are likely to be higher.

It appears that more than 650 CCRCs are currently in operation and house about 200,000 elderly residents.[11, 12] A 1987 report identified 683 CCRCs.[13] However, there is reason to believe that this figure understates the number in actual operation. For example, the survey in the 1987 report identifies 34 communities in the state of California. But another recent study of state regulations reports 63 such facilities in the state.[14] Similar or greater discrepancies were found for other states that regulate CCRCs.

The financial relationships between residents and management in continuing care retirement communities have been evolving. In the early years of CCRC development, the resident paid a large entrance fee in cash and the organization assumed the entire financial responsibility for providing housing, nursing care, and other services. The resident's only risk was the financial viability of the CCRC — and for a few early CCRCs this turned out to be a substantial risk indeed.[15] In present-day CCRCs, through monthly fees, fee-for-service arrangements, and the power of the CCRC to raise these fees, the financial burden of increased costs is passed on to residents.

Despite the fact that CCRCs have been part of our social landscape for many years, the term "CCRC" implies no standard set of financial and service arrangements. Facilities vary in the services provided, the length of a contract, and the payment arrangements. However, they all share a basic set of characteristics. The American Association of Homes for the Aging (AAHA) defines the essential characteristics of a CCRC as follows:

> *Long-term contracts.* A continuing care retirement community is distinguished from all other housing options for senior citizens (such as rental units, assisted living facilities, or nursing homes) by its offer of a long-term contract that provides residence, services, and nursing care: a continuum of care.
>
> *Commitment to a community.* The continuing care contract is intended to remain in effect for more than one year, usually for the rest of one's lifetime, and represents the long-term commitment of the continuing care providers to the community resident.
>
> *Residential and nursing care in one community.* The continuing care contract provides housing, services, and health care, usually in one location, coordinated or directly managed by a single administrator responsible to the community's board of directors.
>
> *Guaranteed nursing care.* The continuing care contract is secured by an entrance fee plus monthly fees that prepay some or all services and care, a form of insurance for one's later years. At a minimum, the contract guarantees access to health care services; at a maximum, it covers the full cost of nursing care.[16]

This definition accommodates widely divergent CCRCs. For example, housing and health care are fairly broad labels that can encompass many services. The AAHA 1984 CCRC Director enumerates various services (for example, meals, apartment cleaning, and linens) and amenities (bank, beauty salon, cable television, and so on), that can be provided by CCRCs for residents.[17]

CCRC Contracts

There are different types of contracts between the facility and the resident. Two basic types have been designated by AAHA as all-inclusive plans and fee-for-service plans. An all-inclusive plan provides an independent living unit, residential services, amenities normally associated with retirement communities, and health-related services and long-term nursing care in return for a specific price, paid as a lump-sum entrance fee and monthly payments. Under such a contract, after moving to the nursing unit the resident continues either to pay the same fee previously paid for the independent unit or to pay the monthly fee of the smallest apartment unit. With such a contract the CCRC insures the resident against catastrophic nursing care costs.

A fee-for-service plan provides an independent living unit, residential services, and amenities, and guarantees access to nursing care. However, residents pay a per diem rate for any and all health and nursing care they require, except for minimal health services such as twenty-four-hour emergency care and possibly a few days of infirmary care that may be included in the basic monthly fee.

Between these two polar contracts, various arrangements are possible that provide the resident with some but not all care covered by the monthly fee. AAHA characterizes such contracts as modified service plans.

Currently, at least, CCRC contracts of all three types are quite unique in one particular way. Despite entry fees, which in many cases are substantial, residents do not own the residential unit and cannot sell it.

The CCRC concept, as initially developed, consisted of a unique combination of features: (1) a multilevel community (independent housing and nursing home arrangements within the same location) in which residents do not own their units and cannot sell them; (2) a contract between resident and management giving the elderly person access to appropriate living arrangements (whether in an apartment or in a nursing home facility); and (3) the provision of long-term-care insurance to the resident through pooled risk (through an entry and monthly fees). Until recently, options that did not embrace the community and shared risk concepts were not included in the CCRC domain. For example, a common view regards CCRCs as a form of long-term-care insurance with a primary goal of preventing impoverishment.[18, 19] Thus, in the Wharton School survey, communities operating totally on a fee-for-service basis for nursing care were not considered in the CCRC domain even if other aspects were in place.[20] Based on developments in the field, however, AAHA has expanded its definition to include fee-for-service facilities.

CCRCs vary in other ways as well. For purposes of description and comparative analysis it is important to develop meaningful classifications of key ways (for example, size, age, and fees) in which CCRCs differ. Lomanno, for example, classifies facilities by proportion of nursing home beds, suggesting that CCRCs with fewer than two apartments per nursing care bed be regarded as "oriented toward nursing care."[21]

To understand better how CCRCs function as a mechanism for aging in place, particularly as compared to other options, it is important to limit the kinds of facilities to be considered in the CCRC domain. In addition to providing housing and the form and spirit of a community, a CCRC should supply independent living units and nursing beds adequate for providing multiple levels of care to its residents. Thus, facilities that do not have a large enough number of either independent living units or nursing care beds should not be classified as CCRCs. In lieu of formal guidelines in this area, we illustrate two types of situation that we believe disqualify an enterprise from being considered a CCRC. First, a 100-bed nursing home that owns a few apartments, say 10, and offers a service contract to the residents of those apartments that includes meals and other housing-related services should not be considered a CCRC, because of its concentration on nursing home care. Second, a facility with 150 housing units that owns or contracts for 10 nursing home beds and provides a service contract for residential housing and nursing care to its housing unit residents also should not be considered a CCRC. We would also exclude facilities established on a rental basis with no entry fee required, since a central feature of the CCRC — shared risk among the residents — is absent.

Recently, a new service delivery program, Life Care at Home, has been initiated that seeks to provide much of the same care as a CCRC but does not provide housing.[22] This may be a less expensive approach to providing care, as it excludes the cost of housing construction and maintenance. However, the development of the Life Care at Home option is now in a demonstration phase; how it will fare in the long run is not known. Although the program is an interesting and potentially important development in long-term insurance, it does not provide new (that is, new to the individual) residential housing. It also lacks the community feature integral to the CCRC concept. We therefore believe that Life Care at Home should also be excluded from the CCRC domain.

Some CCRCs admit persons directly from the community into their nursing care facilities. We believe that persons included on this basis differ in many respects from those who enter from their CCRC independent living units. Persons in the latter group reflect the established concept of CCRCs—that residents receive a continuum of care *within the same community* as their needs change. Those who move directly into the CCRC nursing care facility from the outside community are primarily selecting a desired, presumably high-quality, nursing home facility. It does not represent selection of a community continuum of care arrangement, even though persons choosing to move to such a facility from the outside community may pay the required CCRC fees. In our view, lack of participation in the continuum of care arrangement would disqualify such persons from inclusion in the CCRC population. These distinctions are also important in describing the characteristics of CCRC populations.

CCRC Residents

Very little hard data are available on characteristics of CCRC residents, their reasons for entering CCRCs, or their satisfaction with this type of living arrangement. Information published to date consists mainly of: (1) demographic characteristics of residents from various mail surveys sent to CCRC operators/sponsors, particularly the Wharton School study[23] and the 1986 survey of CCRCs[24] by AAHA and the firm of Ernst & Whinney; (2) case histories of one or a few selected CCRCs and their residents;[25] and (3) a Brandeis University Bigel Institute survey of 988 persons on the waiting lists of two suburban Northeast CCRCs offering all-inclusive contracts.[26] In addition, a survey of random samples of over 2,000 CCRC apartment dwelling residents is currently being completed by the Department of Social Gerontological Research at the Hebrew Rehabilitation Center for the Aged (HRCA) in Boston as part of a larger study of 19 selected CCRCs in Florida, Pennsylvania, Arizona, and California.[27] This HRCA sample, for analytic purposes, distinguishes residents by length of time in the CCRC community.

CHARACTERISTICS OF CCRC RESIDENTS

Both short and longer-standing CCRC residents tend to be drawn from the older segments of the elderly population.[28] As compared with 38 percent of persons sixty-five and over nationally,[29] nearly 90 percent of CCRC residents are seventy-five years of age or older. The average age of CCRC residents, regardless of region, tends to be eighty or older. As might be expected for this age group, the majority of CCRC residents (usually over 70 percent) are female, and only a minority are married, although in the HRCA sample more than fifty percent who were in the CCRC community for less than a year were married.

Data on number of children and residential propinquity of residents and offspring are sparse. In the HRCA sample, 34 percent of those who were in the CCRC community for less than one year, and 42 percent of those living in the community for a year or longer, had no children. Moreover, 66 percent of recent entrants and almost 74 percent of those living in the CCRC community for a year or more had no children living nearby.

Although the majority of residents are women in the over-seventy-five age group, data from the HRCA sample indicate that most CCRC residents had been in the workforce during most of their adult life; only about five percent of the longer-tenured residents and six percent of the more recent entrants reported "housewife" as their occupation. The majority were white-collar workers: 56 percent of the longer-time residents and 47 percent of the recent entrants had been professionals during their working years, 13 percent of the longer-time and 17 percent of the recent residents had been proprietors or managers, and about 22 percent of both groups had been sales or clerical workers.

CCRCs tend to serve well-educated white middle- to upper-middle-class elders.[30] Few nonwhites have been found among CCRC populations, regardless of region in the United States. In the AAHA/E&W survey, the largest proportion of nonwhite CCRC residents (4 percent) were found in the Great Lakes region. In the HRCA sample, as many as 52 percent of recent CCRC residents and 44 percent of residents who had been in the CCRC community for a year or longer had an annual income of over $30,000. Forty-seven percent of more recent residents and 53 percent of longer-standing residents had graduated from college.

These data on CCRC residents are interesting in light of current demographic trends. For the first time in the United States, the median educational level in 1980 of those sixty to sixty-four was above a high school education (12.1 years of school), a level roughly similar to younger adults and considerably higher than that of persons seventy-five and older, who had a median educational level of 8.4 years.[31] This cohort of emerging elderly also had higher income levels than their counterparts in prior eras. Income and educational level have implications not only for lifestyle and ability to afford living arrangements such as CCRCs, but also for health status: Higher income and higher educational groups generally enjoy better health.[32] These trends suggest that, even aside from sheer increased numbers of persons surviving to the advanced age groups, an expanding market for CCRCs may be expected.

To a large extent, the description of the emerging elderly corresponds to empirical findings and anecdotal descriptions in the literature of typical CCRC residents. This resemblance is apparent despite the fact that the typical CCRC resident, even at entrance, is part of the old-old (seventy-five and older) of today. Besides possessing educational and economic advantages, this group represents a relatively healthy segment of the older age group, which may not be surprising, since CCRCs have health status entrance requirements for persons applying for an independent living unit.

These conclusions are supported by (1) age-stratified comparisons of characteristics in the HRCA samples of recent and longer-tenured CCRC residents seventy-five and older across the nineteen sites; and (2) a random sample of over 1,200 Massachusetts community elderly seventy-five and older (for whom data were gathered in 1984 to 1985 as part of another HRCA longitudinal study).[33] As can be seen from Table 6-1, demographic characteristics

Table 6-1. Residents in CCRCs for Less than One Year, Longer-Term Residents, and the Massachusetts Community Sample: Characteristics by Age and Sample (Percent)

	75–79 years			80–84 years			85 + years		
	CCRC Less Than 1 Year	CCRC 1 Year or More	Mass. Community	CCRC Less Than 1 Year	CCRC 1 Year or More	Mass. Community	CCRC Less Than 1 Year	CCRC 1 Year or More	Mass. Community
	(N = 165)	(N = 285)	(N = 653)	(N = 183)	(N = 465)	(N = 360)	(N = 100)	(N = 573)	(N = 236)
DEMOGRAPHICS									
Children nearby	30.5	21.4	61.2	33.9	25.2	69.1	42.0	29.6	70.3
Live alone	38.2	55.1	8.4	53.0	65.4	8.8	61.0	75.0	6.3
EDUCATION									
Less than high school	10.3	7.4	48.7	10.4	9.3	56.4	22.0	12.7	64.6
High school	20.0	15.4	29.7	15.4	13.8	24.0	15.0	18.1	21.7
Some college	24.2	25.3	9.1	28.0	20.7	10.2	17.0	22.8	4.7
College grad	45.5	51.9	12.5	46.2	56.3	9.4	46.0	46.3	9.0
ANNUAL INCOME†									
Less than $20,000	19.7	24.7	95.4	15.7	25.8	95.7	26.2	30.7	96.6
$20,001–$30,000	29.3	30.9	3.1	28.1	30.4	3.1	28.6	25.8	2.4
$30,001–$50,000	26.2	23.6	1.1	32.0	24.6	.7	29.7	28.0	.9
Over $50,000	24.8	20.8	.5	24.2	19.2	.4	15.5	15.5	.1

Table 6-1. Residents in CCRCs for Less than One Year, Longer-Term Residents, and the Massachusetts Community Sample: Characteristics by Age and Sample (Percent) (cont.)

	75–79 years			80–84 years			85+ years		
	CCRC Less Than 1 Year	CCRC 1 Year or More	Mass. Community	CCRC Less Than 1 Year	CCRC 1 Year or More	Mass. Community	CCRC Less Than 1 Year	CCRC 1 Year or More	Mass. Community
	(N = 165)	(N = 285)	(N = 653)	(N = 183)	(N = 465)	(N = 360)	(N = 100)	(N = 573)	(N = 236)
FUNCTIONAL STATUS									
ADL Index‡									
One or more ADL problems	16.4	13.0	18.3	9.3	15.3	18.7	24.0	22.8	35.4
IADL Index:§									
One or more IADL problems	43.0	47.0	52.5	54.4	63.4	71.4	63.0	72.3	81.6
Mobility-ability to:									
Climb stairs	95.3	92.1	84.2	96.8	89.7	79.1	90.6	82.6	65.9
Walk ½ mile	90.0	88.2	62.8	91.0	83.2	45.2	77.3	69.2	29.2
Walk 20 feet	97.0	97.5	89.1	97.8	96.3	83.3	97.0	92.0	75.3
MSQ:‖									
No. of incorrect responses	98.8	99.3	83.9	95.6	97.2	76.5	93.0	90.6	68.0
1 or more incorrect	1.2	.8	16.1	4.3	2.8	23.5	7.0	9.4	32.0
2 or more incorrect	1.2	.4	0.0	2.1	1.0	1.6	2.0	4.0	2.5

Table 6-1. Residents in CCRCs for Less than One Year, Longer-Term Residents, and the Massachusetts Community Sample: Characteristics by Age and Sample (Percent) (cont.)

	75–79 years			80–84 years			85+ years		
	CCRC Less Than 1 Year	CCRC 1 Year or More	Mass. Community	CCRC Less Than 1 Year	CCRC 1 Year or More	Mass. Community	CCRC Less Than 1 Year	CCRC 1 Year or More	Mass. Community
	(N = 165)	(N = 285)	(N = 653)	(N = 183)	(N = 465)	(N = 360)	(N = 100)	(N = 573)	(N = 236)
ACTIVITIES									
Venture out of house	98.2	97.2	85.1	98.4	95.1	76.5	96.0	91.8	63.2
Time spent visiting/ phoning friends:									
Little	30.3	18.6	30.6	31.3	22.4	33.6	41.0	24.1	44.7
Some	38.8	38.6	33.1	46.7	38.3	38.5	33.0	41.3	35.2
Considerable	30.9	42.8	36.3	22.0	39.4	28.0	26.0	34.5	20.1
Time spent visiting/ phoning family:									
Little	38.7	41.1	22.2	34.3	41.3	20.5	36.0	43.4	22.5
Some	32.7	28.8	22.4	35.4	29.7	27.7	36.0	29.6	29.6
Considerable	28.5	30.2	55.4	30.4	29.0	57.8	28.0	27.0	47.9
INDEPENDENCE									
Makes own decisions	84.8	83.3	79.2*	76.4	77.5	69.1	68.0	65.4	48.5

Table 6-1. Residents in CCRCs for Less than One Year, Longer-Term Residents, and the Massachusetts Community Sample: Characteristics by Age and Sample (Percent) (*cont.*)

	75–79 years			80–84 years			85 + years		
	CCRC Less Than 1 Year	CCRC 1 Year or More	Mass. Community	CCRC Less Than 1 Year	CCRC 1 Year or More	Mass. Community	CCRC Less Than 1 Year	CCRC 1 Year or More	Mass. Community
	(N = 165)	(N = 285)	(N = 653)	(N = 183)	(N = 465)	(N = 360)	(N = 100)	(N = 573)	(N = 236)
SUPPORT-RELATED CONCERNS									
Feels has enough to live with no trouble	93.3	85.2	50.2	89.5	86.1	47.4	89.8	88.4	41.8
If needed: Confident that family and friends could provide financial help	50.9	43.9	57.8	49.7	46.6	61.8	63.3	55.5	56.8*
Very confident of getting more help with everyday needs from family and friends#	62.8	59.2	64.0	65.6	56.2	58.3	72.0	56.5	59.8
Concerned about becoming a burden#	15.7	15.1	31.4	21.5	16.0	37.5	14.6	15.5	37.5

Sources: HRCA Study of CCRCs and HRCA study of elderly residents in the community.

Note: All comparisons are statistically significant except where noted with an asterisk (*).

†N's were somewhat smaller because of greater number of refusals.

‡ADL (Activities of Daily Living) include dressing, bladder control, personal care, and medications. Score ranges from 0 to 8.

§IADL (Instrumental Activities of Daily Living) include housework, meals, chores, and shopping. Score ranges from 0 to 8.

‖MSQ (Mental Status Quotient) questions asked: What year is it? What month is it? Where are we now? Score ranges from 0 to 3.

#These questions were not asked of proxies; N's were therefore somewhat smaller.

related to lifestyle are very different for CCRC residents when compared with their age counterparts in the general population (at least as represented by the Massachusetts elderly). For each of the age groups, CCRC residents were significantly less likely than Massachusetts elderly to have children nearby; they were much more likely to live alone; they had achieved much higher levels of education; and they were better off economically. CCRC residents had also better functional status[34] and were more likely than their Massachusetts counterparts to venture out of the house and to spend time with friends; but they spent less time with their families. Although, for the cohorts under eighty-five, Massachusetts elders tended to be more confident than CCRC residents that financial aid from family or friends would be available if needed, CCRC residents across the board were less concerned about their financial status or about becoming a burden to family or friends, and were more likely to make their own decisions.

A key characteristic of residents in the overall CCRC sample is their rejection of dependence on others. The majority (68 percent of recent entrants and 61 percent of residents in the community for a year or longer) felt that, in general, it was not right to expect family to help them; even larger percentages (almost 86 percent of the more recent and over 84 percent of longer-stay residents) felt that, for themselves, it was unacceptable to depend on family. The personal values of dependence on self and retention of locus of control were undoubtedly prime factors in motivating them to move into a CCRC. About 91 percent of the shorter-term and 90 percent of the longer-term residents responded that they "felt in control of important things and events most of the time"; the overwhelming majority — 85 percent of the shorter-term and 84 percent of the longer-term residents — indicated that when making plans, most of the time they are certain that they can make them work.

Studies indicate a positive relationship between ability to manipulate key aspects of the environment and physical and mental health outcomes[35] and, conversely, that loss of control of the environment is related to unfavorable outcomes.[36] Thus, based on functional, economic, and educational status, as well as apparent ability to affect important aspects of their environment, the life chances of CCRC residents tend to be better than those of their counterparts in the general population, even apart from any benefits that may be contributed by the CCRC environment.

REASONS FOR ENTERING CCRCs

The very high proportion of CCRC elderly of all ages who make their own decisions, coupled with the resistance of this population to dependence on family, strongly indicate that the decision to enter the CCRC was their own. Data from the HRCA sample of CCRC residents indicate that the advantage assumed by proponents of CCRCs—that these facilities are a type of health and social insurance affording protection and security—is among the important reasons that CCRC residents enter into this living arrangement. Of the eight areas queried, access to current and future services was cited most frequently in both the more recent (ninety percent) and the longer-tenured resident (82 percent) groups,[37] followed by the protection accorded in the contract (84 percent and 78 percent, respectively, in the two groups).

About 70 percent of each group considered living within one's means also to be important. Avoiding pressure or demands on family and friends appeared more important for new entrants (74 percent) than for those in the CCRC for a year or more (61 percent). The remaining items queried were desirable apartment or location; living with close friends or family; compensating for lack of helper; and desire to be with people like oneself. Interestingly, for both groups, "desire to be with people like oneself" was considered important by the fewest (46 percent and 48 percent, respectively, in the newer and longer-tenured groups).

The respondents of the Brandeis Bigel Institute survey of 988 persons on CCRC waiting lists represented a younger age group (69 percent under seventy-five). Nevertheless, of fifteen reported reasons for choosing CCRCs, access to the following services was among those cited most frequently: services to maintain independence (94 percent); nursing home services (73 percent); and medical services (72 percent). Over half of the respondents cited five additional reasons as very important: fear about being a burden on other family members (74 percent); financial protection against costs of long-term care (68 percent); having staff nearby (66 percent); assurance that spouse is cared for (61 percent); and proximity to spouse if he or she ever needs nursing home care (61 percent).[38]

SATISFACTION AND CONCERNS

Over half of the sample (55 percent) in the Brandeis study expressed no serious concerns about moving into a CCRC. Of ten concerns reported, only five were considered serious by more than 10 percent of the respondents: ability to keep up with fee increases (21 percent); size of entrance fee (19 percent); size of monthly charge (15 percent); moving from the family home (15 percent); living near too many old people (11 percent).

Although case histories exist that indicate points of satisfaction and dissatisfaction,[39] survey data on concerns and satisfaction with CCRC living are sparse. In the HRCA sample, a large proportion of residents — 85 percent of those who had entered within the year and 82 percent of those in the CCRC community for a year or more — expressed distinctly positive feelings. Only 1 percent of the more recent residents and 3 percent of the longer-term residents expressed distinctly negative feelings. As many as 65 percent of the more recent residents and 57 percent of the longer-term residents described the level of assistance with activities of daily living (that is, the combination of formal and informal services in the community) as "just about perfect." Most persons were satisfied with activities; that is, 94 percent of the more recent entrants and 94 percent of those who had entered the CCRC a year or more ago. Moreover, 76 percent of the more recent and 66 percent of the residents of longer standing felt that they had the opportunity to influence management decisions.

Although only a minority of the residents expressed concerns about CCRC fees, significant differences were found between residents who had entered the CCRC within the year and those who had entered at a prior date. A higher proportion of the more recent entrants (20 percent) than the longer-term residents (13 percent) considered the entry fee too high. Conversely, a higher proportion of longer-tenured residents (28 percent) than newer entrants (20 percent) considered the monthly fee too high. This situation is undoubtedly a function of expectations and circumstances at the time of entrance and thereafter.

Organizational Characteristics of CCRCs

It is difficult to portray accurately the operating characteristics of the CCRC industry. The industry is changing. Published surveys often do not clearly state the criteria used to define a CCRC and are based on less than robust response rates. Despite these caveats, such studies provide the only available data bases on the CCRC industry. The most recent and comprehensive survey of CCRCs was conducted by AAHA and Ernst & Whinney (AAHA/E&W) and presents a profile of the industry as of 1986.[40] These organizations compiled a list of 1,090 facilities believed to be CCRCs and sent each a detailed questionnaire. Of this universe, 417 facilities indicated that they did not meet the definition of a CCRC used by the survey. Responses were received from about 400 of the remaining 673 facilities.

Responding CCRCs were located in all regions of the country: 24 percent in the Southeast; 19 percent in the Northeast; 19 percent in the Central region; 20 percent in the Great Lakes region; and 17 percent in the West. With one apparent exception, the definition of a CCRC in this survey coincides with our concept of a CCRC. It appears that some facilities without independent living units and some without nursing care beds were included in the survey; in the data cited, as many as 11 percent of the responding CCRCs had no independent living units, and about 12 percent either reported that they had no nursing home beds or made no response.

PREVALENCE OF VARIOUS CONTRACT TYPES

One-third of 394 responding AAHA/E&W survey CCRCs provided all-inclusive contracts, 28 percent offered fee-for-service contracts, and 31 percent offered modified contracts (8 percent could not be classified). All-inclusive contracts were the modal agreement type offered by CCRCs in the Northeast and the Southeast. Fee-for-service contracts appeared to predominate among CCRCs in the Great Lakes region. Modified contracts were the most prevalent agreement form in the Central states. The survey found that all three types of contracts were in use, however, in all five regions of the country. (Although not dealt with in the AAHA/E&W survey, it is not uncommon for a CCRC to have many different types of contracts, whether they are offered concurrently or accrue from changes in types of contracts offered over the years.)

AGE, FACILITY SIZE, AND CONFIGURATION

Twenty-four percent of the CCRCs responding to the AAHA/ E&W survey began operations before 1963; 25 percent opened between 1963 and 1974; 40 percent opened between 1974 and 1985; and 11 percent began operations in the 1985 to 1987 period. Fifty-one percent of CCRCs with all-inclusive contracts were built between 1974 and 1987. CCRCs built prior to 1970 are more likely to offer fee-for-service contracts.

Older facilities are likely to be serving their second and possibly third generation of residents, since it takes about twenty years for a complete generation of residents to pass through the continuum of care. It is likely that these facilities offered all-inclusive or modified plan contracts when they first commenced operations, as the fee-for-service plan seems to be a relatively new development. It is possible that the experience of older facilities, particularly if they were contractually limited in their ability to raise fees, motivated them to switch to a fee-for-service contract, which places them at less financial risk. However, the number of changes from all-inclusive and modified plan contracts to fee-for-service contracts is not known.

Among the CCRCs who responded to the AAHA/E&W survey, those offering all-inclusive contracts were the largest, despite the fact that fee-for-service CCRCs tended to have more nursing beds. Forty-two percent of all-inclusive and 15 percent each of modified and fee-for-service CCRCs were very large—that is, with 321 or more combined independent living units (ILUs) and nursing care beds. As many as 57 percent of the responding all-inclusive CCRCs have 201 or more ILUs as compared with only 28 percent of the modified and 17 percent of the fee-for-service CCRCs.

Fifty-seven percent of the responding CCRCs had over 120 ILUs; over a third had 201 or more ILUs. These CCRCs offer residents a choice among a variety of independent living quarters—from studios to apartments with more than two bedrooms. One-bedroom ILUs appear to be the most common.

About half of all CCRCs have personal care/assisted living units—specially designed rooms, usually with private baths but without kitchens, for residents who require some supervision and assistance with dressing, bathing, and taking medications. About 30 percent of CCRCs in the survey provided personal care and assistance to residents who remained in their apartments, or ILUs (including some of the CCRCs with special assisted living units).

The majority of AAHA/E&W survey CCRCs have sixty or more nursing care beds; 60 percent have skilled nursing care beds and 40 percent have intermediate care beds. Although some CCRCs may have both types of beds in their nursing care units, the survey classifies CCRCs according to one of these two categories without indicating the mix of beds.

MEALS AND SELECTED OTHER SERVICES

Most of the reporting CCRCs in the AAHA/E&W survey provide meal service, but meals are not always included in the monthly fees. In fee-for-service facilities, over half include at least one meal per day as part of the monthly fee. As many as one-quarter or more provide all three meals as part of the contract—35 percent, 35 percent, and 25 percent in the all-inclusive, modified, and fee-for-service CCRCs, respectively.

Approximately 75 percent of these CCRCs include social service in their monthly fees. Recreational therapy is covered by 79 percent of the all-inclusive contracts, 56 percent of the modified, and 52 percent of the fee-for-service contracts. Although about two-thirds of all-inclusive CCRCs include costs connected with treatment of Alzheimer's disease, only one-third of the modified CCRCs include this coverage. Fifty percent or more of CCRCs of all types make available for an additional fee the following health-related services: podiatrist, physical therapy, speech therapy, physician care, and prescription drugs.

FEES

Median entry fees in 1986 reported by AAHA/E&W survey CCRCs, by type of independent living unit, were: studio, $29,625; one-bedroom, $45,300; two-bedroom, $65,000; and larger units, $82,950. Over the 1985–86 period, entrance fees were raised an average of 6.6 percent (based on data provided by only 117 respondents). Prorated refunds are provided by two-thirds of the CCRCs upon termination of the contract by the resident or, under certain circumstances, upon the resident's death. Median monthly fees were: studio, $628; one-bedroom, $715; two-bedroom, $808; and larger units, $852. Fees varied also by type of contract offered; CCRCs with all-inclusive contracts had higher fees, and CCRCs with all services paid for individually had substantially lower fees.

Our analysis of a random sample of CCRCs that had submitted complete information to both the 1984 and the 1988 AAHA Directories indicates that CCRC fees increased during the period 1983–86 at a faster rate than did the Consumer Price Index (CPI) or its housing component.[41] Table 6-2 lists fee changes over this period. The increases in the CPI and two of its relevant components for the same time period are: CPI, 8.8 percent; housing component, 9.7

Table 6-2. CCRC Fee Changes, 1985 to 1986

	1983	1986	% Increase
CCRCS WITH ALL-INCLUSIVE PLANS			
Entrance fee	$38,995	$43,667	12.0
Monthly fee	662	760	14.8
Nursing care fee	651	743	14.1
CCRCS WITH MODIFIED OR FEE-FOR-SERVICE PLANS			
Entrance fee	$23,603	$27,592	16.9
Monthly fee	583	663	13.7
Nursing care fee	1,338	1,729	29.2

percent; and medical care component, 21.4 percent. As can be seen, the CCRC increases are considerably higher than the indexes, except for nursing care in CCRCs with the all-inclusive plan.

Research is needed to identify factors, other than inflation, that may be contributing to these increases in fees. For example, it might be expected that monthly fees in CCRCs with all-inclusive plans would increase over time even without inflation, since as residents get older a higher proportion are likely to need nursing care. Either the nursing care unit will be more fully occupied and fewer patients will be accepted from outside the CCRC, or the nursing care component of the CCRC will have to be expanded, and the increased cost burdens are likely to appear in increased monthly fees.

UTILIZATION PATTERNS

CCRCs responding to the AAHA/E&W survey generally reported relatively high occupancy rates. Over two-thirds of CCRCs under all three contract types reported occupancy rates of 95 percent or higher, but 6 percent reported occupancy rates below 75 percent. (About 2 percent reported occupancy levels below 50 percent.) Facility age (the number of years a CCRC had been in operation) was not found to be related to level of occupancy.

Of the responding CCRCs, 24 percent indicated immediate availability for their one-bedroom units; 35 percent reported a one-year waiting period; and 6 percent reported a waiting interval of six or more years. The waiting list for a two-bedroom unit was generally longer than for a one-bedroom unit. Respondents reported average occupancy levels of about 83 percent for their nursing care beds. This rate was fairly uniform across all three contract types. Among those CCRCs with assisted living/personal care, the occupancy rate for such units was 97 percent. (The average number of such units in CCRCs with this service was forty-eight.) The annual attrition or turnover rate in independent units was about 13 percent: Deaths accounted for 4 percent, permanent transfer to nursing or personal care, for 7 percent, and resident move-out, for 2 percent.

CCRC residents occupied a little more than half of all nursing care beds: 45 percent of beds were filled by permanent transfers and 13 percent by temporary transfers. Outside patients (non-CCRC contract holders) used 42 percent of beds and accounted for 38 percent of nursing home utilization in CCRCs with all-inclusive contracts and for 65 percent of such use in those with fee-for-service contracts. In CCRCs with a modified contract, this group represented 41 percent of total facility utilization. Average length of stay within the nursing care unit was about 27 days for temporary transfers and 425 days for permanent transfers. On the basis of the data in the AAHA/E&W report, type of contract has no relationship to either of these two statistics.

Economic Characteristics of the CCRC Industry

Information on economic and financial characteristics of CCRCs is just beginning to emerge in the literature. An ongoing survey in this area, conducted annually since 1981 by the accounting firm of Laventhol & Horwath, is based on small samples of CCRCs; for example, for 1982, N = 81[42] and for 1984, N = 102.[43] The reports do not identify the method of sample selection. More in-depth knowledge of CCRCs' economic and financial characteristics are provided by the AAHA/E&W survey and three additional studies.[44]

OPERATING COSTS BY COST CENTER

The Laventhol & Horwath reports provide some fragmentary information on the cost of operating a CCRC. Median 1984 costs illustrate the type of information presented in these reports: Raw food cost per meal = $1.38; utilities expense per square foot = $1.23; cost of food management service per meal = $0.18; dietary payroll per meal = $1.52; housekeeping payroll per square foot = $0.66; maintenance payroll per square foot = $0.45; total number of residents and patients per employee = 2.6; annual medical cost per apartment resident = $319; and total reserves per resident = $7,194.[45]

The 1982 report provides additional data on the distribution of medical costs per apartment resident by type of cost. The types and their percent of the total are: prescriptions, 13 percent; medical supplies, 5 percent; costs not paid by Medicare, 32 percent; Medicare deductibles, 7 percent; and other, 43 percent.[46]

Data for 1986 in the AAHA/E&W study cover some of the 1982 and 1984 cost categories appearing in a 1986 Laventhol & Horwath report[47] and indicate, at least for those categories, that costs did not rise much over this period of time. Average utility cost per square foot, for 171 CCRCs in the AAHA/E&W survey providing this data, was $1.29. Average raw food cost per meal was $1.40 (N = 138). Among the respondents in this AAHA/E&W survey, salary costs were 56 percent of total expenses.

As part of the nineteen-site CCRC study we are conducting, average unadjusted daily operating costs per resident[48] from July 1985 to June 1986 were $39.56.[49] Daily costs ranged from a low of $18.32 in one CCRC to a high of $59.75 in another. By type of living arrangement, the average cost per resident day in the residential sector of the CCRC was $32.93, and the average cost per bed day in the health center was $74.70. Three of the nineteen sample CCRCs reported health center per diem costs above $100 (the highest two being $116 and $177). Only two CCRCs reported per diem nursing care center costs below $50.

This analysis of operating costs was based on self-reported data for ten distinct cost centers. These cost centers and their percent of the total daily average cost of CCRC living of $39.56 were: administration, 10.5 percent; housekeeping, 5.5 percent; plant operating and maintenance, 13.8 percent; dietary, 16.8 percent; medical and nursing services, 20.9 percent; social and community activities, 1.9 percent; interest, 17.2 percent; depreciation, 8.1 percent; amortization, 4.2 percent; and taxes, 1.1 percent.

COST OF CCRCs VERSUS OTHER
LONG-TERM-CARE OPTIONS

It is difficult to compare the cost of CCRC living with other long-term-care options because no other comparable option exists. However, one can compare each of the two CCRC components — independent living units and nursing care — to other such services in the economy at large. The annual cost of living in the residential units is $12,019 ($32.93 x 365). This figure includes rent, utilities, some transportation, some food, housekeeping, emergency response systems, grounds and apartment appliance maintenance, and some recreation costs that would be incurred by individuals in community residences. A good data set for comparable living arrangements in the community (for example, service-rich condominiums) is not available. A second-best source is the higher-level budget for a retired couple published in 1981 by the U.S. Department of Labor, Bureau of Labor Statistics.[50, 51] The 1985–86 cost for a couple for food and housing is projected to be $10,149. Assuming that the cost for a single person is 75 percent of that for a couple, the annual housing and food cost for a single person in the community under a high budget would be $7,612 in the 1985–86 period. Even if the statistic for a couple is used as the base for comparison, CCRC living appears to be more expensive than the Department of Labor's estimate for people with a "high" budget.

The annual cost of nursing home care in the United States in 1985–86 is believed to be about $25,000.[52] Translated to a daily cost, this equals $68.50. The average cost per CCRC bed day reported earlier ($74.70) exceeds this estimate. However, Medicaid reimbursement rates frequently determine nursing home costs. Private pay charges, which form a better comparison base, can run as high as $100 a day. From this vantage point, the costs of CCRC nursing care are probably comparable to community-wide self-pay levels.

METHODS OF FINANCING CCRC CONSTRUCTION

Respondents to the AAHA/E&W survey who planned or had capital expansion programs underway indicated the following expected sources of finance (the number of CCRCs reporting each source is in parentheses): conventional financing (seventy-eight); charitable contributions (seventy); tax-exempt financing (forty-two); equity (twenty-seven); taxable bonds (eleven); and joint ventures (seven). Financing mechanisms are not mutually exclusive, and many CCRCs use more than one type. This pattern closely resembles that found in the Wharton study for the 1981 period.[53]

THE FINANCIAL VIABILITY OF CCRCs

Using 1981, 1983, and 1985 annual financial report data for a sample of 109 CCRCs drawn from a universe of 232 CCRCs in operation since 1981 and listed in AAHA's 1984 CCRC Directory, Ruchlin noted that one-third or more of the respondents reported operating losses (negative net income) in each of the three study years.[54] Similarly, a third of the sample or more reported a negative fund balance (defined as total liabilities in excess of total assets) in each of the three periods. Over 16 percent of all CCRCs studied reported both operating losses and a negative fund balance in each period.

Additional indicators of possible financial trouble also were found. Total asset turnover, which indicates the amount of revenue generated by a facility's assets, was quite low. On average, a dollar of assets generated only $0.35 in revenue. Furthermore, facility liquidity, as measured by the current ratio (calculated by dividing current assets by current liabilities), was below the commonly accepted critical value of two. A facility with relatively low liquidity is expected to have trouble meeting its short-term financial obligations. Evidence from the economy at large and the acute care hospital sector indicates that such financial indicators seem to be extremely good diagnostic measures in the prediction of bankruptcy.[55]

CCRCs classified as offering all-inclusive contracts had a poorer financial profile than those with fee-for-service or modified contracts — 82 percent of CCRCs in the latter group (N = 49) had a positive fund balance profile, but only 42 percent in the former group did (N = 60).[56] This pattern emerged despite the fact that CCRCs with all-inclusive contracts had higher entry and monthly fees for independent living units than CCRCs with modified or fee-for-service contracts.

Various reasons can be offered to explain this situation: underestimates of the amount of care that will be needed, underestimates of resident longevity, poor actuarial analyses, and the limited risk pool inherent in a population of 200 to 300 people. A reluctance to earn "profits" has also been noted among many not-for-profit providers in the CCRC industry.[57] Another hypothesis is that the all-inclusive plan CCRCs still have residents who entered under an entry-fee-only plan or whose contracts curtail increases in monthly fees sufficient to cover increases in costs. Whatever the reasons, these data illustrate the difficulty of assuming financial risk *and* remaining financially viable in an era of escalating health care costs and increased resident longevity.

Potential Problem Areas

Very little information exists on the pitfalls of CCRC living, and what is known about such problems is mainly anecdotal. The actual occurrence of major problems may be rare; nevertheless, a number of areas may be of potential concern to residents. Financial solvency of the CCRC is one obvious problem area.

Contract termination is another area of concern. Equity problems have arisen when contracts have been terminated due to death or to other reasons.[58] Continuing care contracts often allow for the termination of the contract, without cause, by either the resident or the community during a specified and usually short period after occupancy begins. Some allow the resident to terminate the contract at any time, providing notice has been given, and permit the community to terminate the contract at any time, but only for cause. What constitutes "cause" and how the decision is made may not be clear. Refunding of some or all of an entrance fee can also be an issue in the termination process, and legal suits have arisen when refunding arrangements have not been clearly specified. Questions have arisen as to whether death, when it occurs during the probationary period, constitutes termination as specified in the contract. The courts, however, have established a legal precedent in this area by rejecting suits brought by heirs.[59] Currently there is insufficient data on how often these termination issues constitute real problems for CCRC residents.

Giving up the independent unit and transferring to the nursing care center may not be experienced as a problem by the vast majority of persons so transferred, but it is an area of potential concern to residents. Contracts may specify that the resident must give up a residential unit after some specified number of days in the nursing care facility, or after the CCRC's physician or administration has determined that the move is permanent. However, the decision-making process for transferring a resident to the nursing care facility may be ambiguous. Little is known about the extent to which residents understand the necessity for transfer or about the pressures they face to acquiesce to a permanent transfer. More research is needed concerning the decision-making process and the way in which circumstances other than the actual health condition of the resident enter into such decisions. For example, the availability of space in the two components of the CCRC and the net gain or loss to the facility may influence transfer decisions.

The adequacy of nursing care also is a potential problem. As reflected in the guidelines developed by the recently formed accrediting commission for CCRCs, the philosophy of care and its implementation, the professional competence of health care staff, nursing staff hours per patient, and the number of beds are all matters of importance.[60] In the start-up phases of the CCRC, unless patients are accepted directly from the community, a large nursing facility is neither financially feasible nor administratively sensible. During later stages of their development, some CCRCs have added health care units. Unless the organization's long-range planning has taken this potential problem into account, competition for nursing beds may arise. As a result residents may remain in their residential units when they should be receiving nursing care, or the organization may be forced to place some of its residents in outside nursing homes. In the latter circumstance, the advantage of being able to select a nursing facility prior to need has been seriously impaired. Arrangements with outside nursing homes may change at any time, perhaps without notice. In addition, the CCRC management may be less able to observe the conditions in an off-site facility than they may in an on-site facility. And the quality of the off-site nursing care facility may deteriorate over time. Even when recognizing this situation, the CCRC may be unable to change it if CCRC clients account for only a small proportion of the nursing care facility's population. Furthermore, in the more traditional CCRC, in which the nursing unit is part of the total community, the residents themselves have an opportunity to detect developing problems in nursing home care, should they occur. To the extent that residents have some management input, they are also in a position to take action.

Ideally, an ongoing projection-of-needs system should be in force, with sufficient lead time for appropriate planning and implementation. How well needs are projected affects the ability of management to honor its "guarantee" of nursing care for residents. This is another area of CCRC operations that merits research.

Regulation of CCRCs

Calls for government regulation of CCRCs arise from the distinctive financial and contractual characteristics of the industry. Moreover, proprietary operators are entering the continuing care field in increasing numbers. Advocates of regulation believe, based on lessons learned from the nursing home industry, that the marketplace is an inadequate mechanism for protecting residents' interests.[61]

The federal government at present has no role in regulating CCRCs, with one minor exception. To the extent that CCRCs seek Medicare and/or Medicaid certification for their nursing home beds, they may be required to meet federal standards for care. But such standards are not directed specifically at CCRCs. The one exception to this overall pattern is the tax treatment of refundable entrance fees paid to CCRCs by residents. Prior to 1984, part of the nonrefundable entry fees were tax-deductible since they were considered as prepayment for lifetime medical care. No ruling had been made about refundable fees, as this mechanism was quite new. In 1984, the Internal Revenue Service declared that refundable fees were to be considered as "no interest loans" under Section 7872 of the Tax Code and thus subject to taxation. Public Law 99-121, enacted in 1985, modified this ruling by exempting the first $90,000 of any "loan" given to a qualified CCRC.[62]

STATE GOVERNMENT

A survey of states concerning the regulation of CCRCs revealed that, by 1986, twenty states had passed some type of legislation regulating CCRCs, six states had bills in progress or were considering legislation, and two more had the subject under study.[63] In examining CCRC state regulations, AAHA found that most require: (1) application by sponsors for a permit or certificate of authority before fees can be accepted or contracts signed with prospective residents; (2) disclosure of financial and development information regarding new facilities; (3) placement in escrow accounts of all deposits and entry fees paid by prospective residents to new facilities; and (4) a designated period of time after signing or occupancy within which a resident has the right to rescind a contract.[64]

At the same time, state statutes vary widely in purpose, coverage, registry or certification requirements, disclosure provisions, mandatory contract contents, provisions concerning escrow of entry fees, reserve fund requirements, and agencies designated to implement the regulations.[65] Furthermore, not all states seek to regulate the same entity. Although definitions in some states encompass the overall concept of continuing care activities, definitions in the majority of states are more limited, focusing only on specific aspects of CCRCs. In regulations of the seventeen states in the Netting and Wilson study, of thirty-three contract items covering issues of financing, services, preadmission, postadmission, and general considerations, only one state's regulations addressed twenty-five of the items; the remaining states regulate less than half, with nine addressing ten or fewer of these contract items.[66] Furthermore, some states have encountered substantial problems in implementing CCRC regulations due to lack of authority and limited appropriations. Fewer than half of the responding state officials indicated that their state's regulations had a definite impact. In these cases the regulations offered greater uniformity of resident protection or improved the conditions of homes that might have been in financial trouble.

VOLUNTARY SELF-REGULATION

Accreditation by professional organizations and special commissions has contributed significantly to the health field, by establishing and maintaining standards to ensure appropriate operating procedures, maintain quality of care, and protect the interests of patients. As the CCRC industry has matured, the need for oversight has been increasingly recognized. In 1986, AAHA agreed to sponsor an independent national accrediting commission for CCRCs, the Continuing Care Accreditation Commission (CCAC). This commission designs standards to assure consumers that accredited communities meet acceptable criteria for governance and administration, disclosure, resident life, financial operations, and provision of quality health care.[67] The accreditation program is voluntary. By July 1988, forty-six CCRCs in fifteen states had already been accredited and over fifty were under review.[68] The CCAC accreditation program also can be used by states as either a component of or substitute for state regulations.[69]

The American Academy of Actuaries also is interested in developing standards and in conducting a comprehensive study that will enable both licensing agencies and prospective residents to estimate the extent to which prices are likely to rise over the next decade. Currently, the CCAC is working with the American Academy of Actuaries to develop further standards and methods to assess CCRCs.[70] However, unless all states demand accreditation, some form of protection may still be needed for residents of those CCRCs that have not applied for or that have been denied accreditation.

Future Outlook

There is little question that the CCRC industry is growing. The dramatic increase in the size of the elderly population is an important factor in this growth, as is their increasing affluence. Current predictions indicate that not only the number of people over the age of sixty-five will double by the year 2025 but that, equally significant, the income of this group will increase at a faster rate than that of younger cohorts. It has been estimated that less than 1 percent of the elderly currently reside in CCRCs and less than 5 percent of the elderly may live in such settings in the future.[71] If this estimate is accurate, there may eventually be as many as a million people living in CCRCs. Assuming an average of 300 residents per CCRC, over 3,000 CCRCs will be needed to fill this predicted demand.

The for-profit sector has evinced increasing interest in the CCRC industry. With the aggressive marketing techniques these groups are employing, CCRCs will become more widely known, thereby creating additional demand.

Some major changes are also taking place in refund policies. In the past, the pattern generally has been to allow very limited refunds, providing for a kind of probationary period after which no refunds are possible. Some CCRCs now offer very large refunds that are not dependent on length of residency.[72] If this practice becomes widespread, more prospective residents may be attracted to CCRCs. However, since large refunds may be accompanied by higher entrance and monthly fees, these policies will make such CCRCs affordable for fewer and fewer of the elderly. Research is needed to obtain information on the relationships among refund policies, entry fees, monthly fees, and costs, distinguishing between refunds due to death and those due to expulsion or voluntary withdrawal.

A further development that could increase the market for CCRCs is the potential growth of long-term-care insurance. Through this risk-pooling method, some of the financial uncertainty about future costs for care can be minimized. If CCRC residents are indeed healthier and use less nursing care than elders in the community, as proponents of CCRC care allege, then CCRCs may be able to get more favorable rates for such insurance. Furthermore, small CCRCs may use this mechanism to attain a better risk-sharing experience than they can achieve with their own limited population. The purchase of such insurance may have a calming effect on the apparent trend of CCRCs to shift the risk for care to the individual resident. AAHA is currently trying to develop such an insurance product.

Recently, Johnson & Higgins has developed an insurance program for CCRCs. In the CCRCs that participate in this program, residents in the independent living units are required to contract with the company for long-term-care insurance. For example, in eight of ten CCRCs sponsored by American Baptist Homes of the West in this program, a resident under eighty-five pays $98 per month; persons eighty-five and older pay $166 per month. When such residents need nursing care, the insurance company will pay $1,000 per month toward such care, even if the resident stays in the nursing unit for the rest of his or her life. In the seven CCRCs operated by Ohio Presbyterian Retirement Services, the individual pays $125 per person per month and $200 per couple, regardless of age. When nursing care is needed, the company will pay $1,500 per month toward that care for life.

The premiums in these examples are high. However, if insurance programs such as these prevent or reduce what would otherwise be even higher fees, they may increase the number of people who can afford CCRC care.

Policy Considerations and Recommendations

As the CCRC industry continues to grow and evolve, two major issues merit attention: the need for additional regulatory initiatives and the inadequate knowledge base in this small but potentially important industry.

NEW REGULATORY INITIATIVES

Even for the more affluent elderly, joining a CCRC often entails transferring a large bulk of their assets to the CCRC. Once this transfer has been completed, the resident has limited power to influence the operating decisions of the CCRC. Although a resident who is dissatisfied is free to leave the CCRC, returning to the community with a fraction of one's assets, or even no assets, is a very unappealing option. We therefore believe that some additional protection to CCRC residents may be in order.

States should assume the major regulating role, but there may be at least two important roles for the federal government. The first is to create an insurance system to protect the individual's investment in CCRCs. There are two models for this. One is the insurance on bank savings accounts that insures them for up to $100,000. A second model is the Pension Benefit Guarantee Corporation, which insures defined benefit pension plans. The proposed insurance program should be voluntary, and the cost of such insurance should be part of the CCRC's operating costs. It is likely that this cost will be passed on to residents through higher charges. We believe that the costs of this program will be modest if it is adopted by most CCRCs. The federal government may wish to consider subsidizing this insurance since ex-CCRC residents with no or few assets may be prime candidates for the Medicaid spend-down process.[73] If such insurance becomes available, CCRCs should be required to inform current and prospective residents about whether the facility carries this type of insurance.

The second potential federal role is informational and educational. It should be directed at informing the elderly of what to look for in joining a CCRC, the need to understand what the contract does and does not provide, and what the individual may forfeit if discharged from a facility. A possible vehicle for disseminating such information is the Medicare program.

AAHA has expressed a clear preference for regulation of CCRCs by states rather than the federal government and has provided examples and recommendations for eleven general areas: (1) definitions; (2) registration procedures; (3) the resident contract; (4) disclosure; (5) refund provisions and termination rights; (6) escrow of entry fees; (7) reserve funds; (8) the regulatory agency; (9) enforcement; (10) advertising; and (11) the establishment of residents' associations.[74] For most of these areas AAHA has suggested specific regulatory language with examples drawn from the regulations of a number of states, especially those of Arizona, California, Florida, and Pennsylvania. The guidelines are comprehensive and any state adopting all of the recommended provisions would undoubtedly have a model set of regulations.

Finally, although the extent of problems pertaining to transfer is not known, we believe that the state could be helpful when problems do arise by designating a special ombudsman who can serve as an advocate for the resident in transfer decisions. Hearings should take place within a reasonable period of time (for example, thirty days) and while the hearing is pending the CCRC should be prohibited from renting or selling the resident's independent living unit. The services of the ombudsman should also be available in cases where CCRCs wish to evict a resident.

NEED FOR ADDITIONAL RESEARCH

Despite the substantial amount of information about CCRCs summarized in this chapter, there is still much to be learned. We have indicated throughout a number of areas that need research. It is probably fair to say that even the number of CCRCs, however defined, is not known. AAHA has made a valiant effort in this regard, but participation in its surveys is voluntary and therefore its listings are by no means complete. Responses generally are from only about two-thirds of those solicited, and the solicitation list was probably incomplete. Additionally, because the industry is growing so rapidly, such lists are quickly out of date. Surveys conducted by others have even greater limitations.

We believe that the time is ripe for greater efforts to identify, establish, and maintain a systematic basic minimum data set on this industry, on more than a purely voluntary basis. Working out just how this might be done constitutes a major undertaking. Obtaining a consensus as to what a CCRC is, developing a procedure for requiring registration, and the schism that separates not-for-profit and for-profit providers in the nursing home industry may hamper any private sector initiative in this area. We recognize the current economic constraints confronting the federal government; nonetheless, we suggest that this activity be seriously considered as a new program worthy of federal support.

Finally, the CCRC industry is growing in size and changing. For example, for-profit providers are entering the field, and their numbers are likely to increase in the future. Will this result in changes in the contractual commitment to the resident? Will what was initially an industry that provided life care and assumed much if not all of the financial risk for such care become an industry with a time-limited commitment, providing care on a fee-for-service basis as long as the resident can afford to pay for such care? We believe that there is reason to be concerned about the possibility of such changes. To the extent that CCRCs are shifting in these directions, the "heart" of the industry that appealed to social planners may be endangered.

Equally troubling is the charge structure that may become inherent in the modern CCRC. Entry fees that approach and exceed $100,000 and monthly fees well in excess of $1,000 place CCRCs out of reach for many middle-class people.[75] Obviously, everyone needs adequate housing and health services—the economically advantaged and the disadvantaged—and CCRCs represent a valuable way to address these needs for those with sufficient assets and income. But facilities with high entrance and monthly fees will not address the needs of the bulk of the elderly population. Research is needed to identify the trends, if any, that are taking place and incentives and mechanisms for maintaining CCRCs as an option for aging in place for persons of more modest assets and income. It is unclear what can be done about this. We encourage all parties interested in the needs of people with middle and lower incomes to consider ways of broadening the potential market for CCRCs.

Notes

1. Sherwood, S., C.E. Gutkin, T.G. Lewis, and C.C. Sherwood. "Housing alternatives for an aging society. A legislative agenda for an aging society: 1988 and beyond." Paper presented at the Congressional Forum convened by the House Select Committee on Aging, the House Subcommittee on Health and Long Term Care, and the Senate Special Committee on Aging, November 16, 1987.

2. Weeden, J.P., R.J. Newcomer, and T. O. Byerts. "Housing and shelter for frail and nonfrail elders: Current options and future directions." In R.J. Newcomer, M.P. Lawton, and T.O. Byerts (Eds.), *Housing an Aging Society.* New York: Van Nostrand Reinhold Company, 1986.

3. Winklevoss, H.E., and A.V. Powell and Associates. *Continuing Care Retirement Communities: An Empirical, Financial, and Legal Analysis.* Homewood, Ill.: Richard D. Irwin, 1984.

4. Ibid.

5. Some CCRCs that have the name of a religious denomination in their corporate name have no legal ties with a church or the denomination.

6. Netting, F.E., and C.C. Wilson. "Current legislation concerning life care and continuing care contracts." *The Gerontologist,* 27, 5:645–51, 1987.

7. "Marriott Corporation moves into life-care communities." *Geriatric and Residential Care News,* 13, 3:1301, 1988.

8. Winklevoss, et al., *Analysis.*

9. American Association of Homes for the Aging. *National Continuing Care Directory.* Washington, D.C.: American Association of Retired Persons, 1988.

10. Raper, A.T. (Ed.). American Association of Homes for the Aging *National Continuing Care Directory.* Glenview, Ill.: Scott, Foresman and Company, 1984.

11. Winklevoss, et al., *Analysis.*

12. Estes, C.E., and P.R. Lee. "Social, political, and economic background of long-term care policy. In C. Harrington, R.J. Newcomer, C.E. Estes, et al. (Eds.), *Long Term Care of the Elderly: Public Policy Issues.* Beverly Hills, Calif.: Sage Publications, 1985.

13. American Association of Homes for the Aging and Ernst & Whinney. *Continuing Care Retirement Communities: An Industry in Action.* Washington, D.C.: American Association of Homes for the Aging, 1987.

14. Netting and Wilson, "Current legislation."

15. U.S. Senate, Special Committee on Aging. *Life Care Communities: Promises and Problems.* Washington, D.C.: U.S. Government Printing Office, 1983.

16. American Association of Homes for the Aging. *National Continuing Care Directory.* Washington, D.C.: American Association of Retired Persons, 1988, p. 3.

17. See Raper, *NCCD.*

18. Branch, L.G. "Continuing care retirement communities: Self-insuring for long-term care." *The Gerontologist,* 27, 1:4–8, 1987.

19. Combined Jewish Philanthropies of Greater Boston. *Solving the Puzzle: A Consumer's Guide to Long-Term Care Insurance.* Boston: Combined Jewish Philanthropies, 1987.

20. Winklevoss, et al. *Analysis.*

21. Lomanno, M.V. "The lifecare industry—1983." In *Lifecare Industry 1983*. Philadelphia: Laventhol & Horwath, 1983, pp. 13–34.

22. Tell, E.J., M.A. Cohen, and S.S. Wallack. "Life care at home: A new model for financing and delivering long-term care." *Inquiry*, 24, 4:245–52, 1987.

23. Winklevoss, et al. *Analysis*.

24. American Association of Homes for the Aging and Ernst & Whinney. *Industry*.

25. Morrison, I.A., R. Bennett, S. Frisch, and B.J. Gurland (Eds.). *Continuing Care Retirement Communities*. New York: Haworth, Press, 1986.

    Stephens, M.A.P., J.M. Kinney, and A.E. McNeer. "Accommodative housing: Social integration of residents with physical limitations." *The Gerontologist*, 26, 2:176–79, 1986.

    Elliott, F.E., and S.H. Elliott. "Evolving management structure: A case study of a life care village at Pine Run, Doylestown, Bucks County, Pennsylvania." *Journal of Housing for the Elderly*, 3, 1/2:73–98, 1985.

    Barbaro, E.L., and L.E. Noyes. "A wellness program for a life care community." *The Gerontologist*, 24, 6:568–71, 1984.

    Hunt, M.E., A.G. Feldt, R.W. Marans, L.A. Pastalan, and K.L. Vakalo. "Continuing care retirement communities: Friendship Village, Schaumberg, Illinois." *Journal of Housing for the Elderly*, 1, 3/4:205–47, 1983.

    Pynoos, J., V. Regnier, and T.K. O'Brien. "Continuum of Care Retirement Community Project final report." Institute for Policy and Program Development, Andrus Gerontology Center, University of Southern California, Los Angeles, 1983.

    Peterson, W.A., C.E. Longino, and L.W. Phelps. "A study of security, health and social support systems, and adjustment of residents in selected congregate living and retirement settings." Center on Aging Studies, Institute for Community Studies, University of Missouri-Kansas City, 1979.

    Hartwigsen, G. "The appeal of the life care facility to the older widow." *Journal of Housing*, 2, 4:63–75, 1984–85.

    Thompson, B., M. Swisher. "An assessment, using the Multiphasic Environmental Assessment Procedure (MEAP) of a rural life care residential center for the elderly." *Journal of Housing*, 1, 2:41–56, 1983.

26. Tell, E.J., M.C. Cohen, M.J. Larson, and H.J. Ballen. "Assessing the elderly's preferences for lifecare retirement options." *The Gerontologist*, 27, 4:503–509, 1987.

27. Sherwood, S., C.C. Sherwood, and S.A. Morris. "Baseline information on residents in 20 sites cooperating in the study of continuing care retirement communities across the nation." Boston: Department of Social Gerontological Research, Hebrew Rehabilitation Center for the Aged, 1987.

    Sherwood, S., S.A. Morris, H. Ruchlin, and C.C. Sherwood. "Factors associated with quality of life of CCRC residents." Paper presented at the 40th Annual

Scientific Meeting of the Gerontological Society of America, Washington, D.C., November 18–22, 1987.

Morris, S.A., J.N. Morris, and S. Sherwood. "Quality of life and living environment: CCRCs versus other community residences." Paper presented at the 40th Annual Scientific Meeting of The Gerontological Society of America, Washington, D.C., November 18–22, 1987.

Morris, S.A., S. Sherwood, and C.C. Sherwood. "Characteristics of residents of continuing care retirement communities." Paper presented at the 39th Annual Scientific Meeting of the Gerontological Society of America, Chicago, Illinois, November 19–23, 1986.

28. Winklevoss, et al. *Analysis;* American Association of Homes for the Aging and Ernst & Whinney, *Industry*; Sherwood, S., et al., "Baseline information"; Morris, et al., "Quality of life."

29. U.S. Department of Health and Human Services. "Health statistics on older persons, 1986: Analytical and epidemiological studies." Series 3, No. 5. In *Vital and Health Statistics,* DHHS Publication No. (PHS) 87-1409. Washington, D.C.: DHHS, 1987.

30. American Association of Homes for the Aging and Ernst & Whinney, *Industry.*

Peterson, et al., "Adjustment of residents."

Sherwood, S., et al., "Baseline information."

Marans, R.W., M.E. Hunt, and K.L. Vakalo. "Retirement communities." In I. Altman, M.P. Lawton, and J.F. Wohlwill (Eds.), *Elderly People and the Environment.* New York: Plenum Press, 1984.

31. Serow, W.J., and D.V. Sly. "The demography of current and future aging cohorts." Paper presented at the Symposium on the Social and Built Environment sponsored by the National Research Council/Institute of Medicine Committee on the Aging Society, Washington, D.C., 1985.

32. Ibid.

33. This work was undertaken under the NIA Teaching Nursing Home grant to HRCA.

34. To avoid unanticipated costs, some CCRCs require a medical exam or physician's report for persons applying for admission, and some CCRCs specify pre-existing conditions for which the CCRC will not be financially responsible.

35. Slivinske, L.R., and V.L. Fitch. "The effect of control enhancing interventions on the well-being of elderly individuals living in retirement communities." *The Gerontologist,* 27:176–81, 1987.

36. Barbaro and Noyes, "Wellness program."

Slivinske and Fitch, "Control."

Birren, J.E., and V.J. Renner. "Concepts and issues of mental health and aging." In J.E. Birren and R.B. Sloane (Eds.), *Handbook of Mental Health and Aging.* Englewood Cliffs, N.J.: Prentice-Hall, 1980.

37. That access to services was ranked first by both groups is in line with the findings on elderly persons in other community settings. The availability of medical services in particular seems to be of concern to elderly persons, whether they currently need them or not. See, for example, Lawton, M.P., "Supportive services in the context of the housing environment. *The Gerontologist,* 9, 1:15–19, 1969.

38. Tell, et al., "Assessing preferences."

39. Elliott and Elliott, "Management structure"; and Peterson, et al., "Adjustment of residents."

40. American Association of Homes for the Aging and Ernst & Whinney, *Industry.*

41. Since many CCRCs submitted information to either one or the other of the directories, but not both, this is a very "particular" collection of facilities; the data, therefore, probably contain biases in unknown directions.

42. Laventhol & Horwath. *Lifecare Industry 1983.* Philadelphia: Laventhol & Horwath, 1983.

43. Laventhol & Horwath. *Lifecare Retirement Center Industry 1985.* Philadelphia: Laventhol & Horwath, 1985.

44. Ruchlin, H.S. "Analysis of CCRC operating costs." Boston: Department of Social Gerontological Research, Hebrew Rehabilitation Center for the Aged, 1988 (mimeographed).

    Ruchlin, H.S. "Are CCRCs facing a promising future or potential problems?" *Healthcare Financial Management,* 41, 10:54–60, 1987.

    Ruchlin, H.S. "Continuing care retirement communities: An analysis of financial viability and health care coverage." *The Gerontologist,* 28, 2:156–62, 1988.

45. Laventhol & Horwath, *Lifecare 1985.*

46. Laventhol & Horwath, *Lifecare 1983.*

47. Laventhol & Horwath. *Lifecare Industry 1986.* Philadelphia: Laventhol & Horwath, 1986.

48. As part of our ongoing research, an attempt will be made to adjust for the imputed cost of resident volunteer labor in areas where an outside person would be hired to perform a task if volunteer labor were not available, and for low occupancy rates that are considered a one-time, short-term phenomenon and lead to unrealistically high per diem rates.

49. Ruchlin, "Analysis of CCRC operating costs."

50. This data series was discontinued in 1980. For the purpose of this study, the data reported are projected to 1985–86 levels, based on changes in the food and housing components of the Consumer Price Index.

51. U.S. Department of Labor, Bureau of Labor Statistics. *Three Budgets for a Retired Couple.* Autumn 1980, USDL81-384. Washington, D.C.: U.S. Department of Labor, 1981.

52. U.S. Senate, Special Committee on Aging. *Developments in Aging: 1987.* Washington, D.C.: U.S. Government Printing Office, 1988.

53. Winklevoss, et al., *Analysis.*

54. Ruchlin, "Promising future?"

55. Cleverly, W. O. "Financial ratio analysis." In W. O. Cleverly (Ed.), *Handbook of Health Care Accounting and Finance, Vol. 1.* Rockville, MD: Aspen Systems Corporation, 1982.

56. Ruchlin, "Analysis of CCRC operating costs."

57. Winklevoss, H.E. "Continuing care retirement communities: Issues in financial management and actuarial prediction." In I.A. Morrison, R. Bennett, S. Frisch, and B.J. Gurland (Eds.), *Continuing Care Retirement Communities: Political, Social and Financial Issues.* New York: Haworth, 1986.

58. Cohen, D. "Continuing-care communities for the elderly: Potential pitfalls and proposed regulation." *University of Pennsylvania Law Review,* 128, 4:883–936, 1980.

59. Ibid.

60. Continuing Care Accreditation Commission. *Continuing Care Accreditation Commission Self-Study Manual.* Washington, D.C.: American Association of Homes for the Aging, March 1987.

61. Cohen, "Pitfalls."

62. American Association of Homes for the Aging and Ernst & Whinney, *Industry.*

63. Netting, F.E., and C.C. Wilson. "Current legislation concerning life care and continuing care contracts." *The Gerontologist,* 27, 5:645–51, 1987. Netting and Wilson have reported more recently that twenty-seven states are now regulating CCRCs (information presented at the 1987 Annual Meeting of the Gerontological Society of America).

64. American Association of Homes for the Aging. *Current Status of State Regulation of Continuing Care Retirement Communities.* Washington, D.C.: American Association of Homes for the Aging, May 1987.

65. Netting and Wilson, "Current legislation."

American Association of Homes for the Aging, *State Regulation.*

American Association of Homes for the Aging. *Guidelines for Regulation of Continuing Care Retirement Communities.* Washington, D.C.: American Association of Homes for the Aging, May 1987.

66. Netting and Wilson, "Current legislation."

67. Continuing Care Accreditation Commission. *Continuing Care Accreditation Commission Handbook*. Washington, D.C.: American Association of Homes for the Aging, March 1987.

68. Personal communication from Ann Gillespie, CCAC Director.

69. Continuing Care Accreditation Commission, *Handbook*.

70. "Continuing care retirement communities can benefit from accreditation and a comprehensive actuarial study." In *AARP Housing Report*. Washington, D.C.: AARP, 1988, p. 3.

71. Tell, et al., "Assessing preferences."

72. Branch, "Self-insuring."

73. Since the number of such residents is unknown, this issue merits research.

74. American Association of Homes for the Aging, "Guidelines for regulation of CCRCs."

75. Cohen, "Pitfalls."

PART THREE

The Policy Setting

CHAPTER SEVEN

Public Policy and Aging in Place: Identifying the Problems and Potential Solutions

JON PYNOOS

"Aging in place" is an idea whose time has come. Although not yet embodied in major legislation, the phrase has achieved broader recognition since its initial coinage in the early 1980s and has surfaced in recent discussions on policies designed to meet the housing needs of aging Americans.[1] However, the term has yet to be identified as a major aspect of long-term-care policy.

Aging in place has several connotations beyond the rather simple phenomenon of older persons remaining in their current housing. The concept encompasses individual aging, implying changing needs over time. These changes are generally accompanied by increasing frailty (often due to declining health and income), increased age and disability levels, changes in marital status and informal supports, or a combination of such factors, and by subsequent risk for relocation.

Aging in place also connotes the aging of the residential setting itself, its unsuitability or physical deterioration, and this extends to a person's neighborhood or community. Thus, aging in place is a dynamic concept that implies aging of both inhabitant and

---

[1]The author is indebted to Phoebe Liebig for her conceptual and editorial contributions to this chapter.

167

residential setting, which requires periodic reassessments of the adaptive fit of each to the other.

Aging in place also refers to an emerging social policy aimed at helping older persons to remain in their current housing as long as possible. This requires identifying ways in which a given residence and its surroundings promote or inhibit this goal, and in which needed assistance can be integrated with current housing. "Current" can mean the place where older persons have lived all or most of their adult lives or the residence to which they have made a subsequent move. Residences of older Americans are predominantly single- and multiple-family homes and apartments, as well as age-segregated housing projects. Approximately 93 percent live in independent housing of this sort (see Chapter 1). Moving across the residential continuum toward greater dependence, residences include congregate housing, residential care facilities, continuing care retirement communities, and nursing homes.

Aging in place is a strongly held preference of older persons. A recent survey found, for example, that 70 percent of older persons age sixty-five and above, especially women over eighty, agreed with the statement "What I'd really like to do is stay in my own home and never move."[2] Such strong attachment to place is associated with the benefits of familiarity, access to neighborhood services, proximity of friends, psychological attachments to the home, and, especially for homeowners, financial security. It is also motivated by fears that a decline in income or health or changes in marital status may force premature moves to less desirable and/or more institutional settings. Thus, aging in place also implies that individuals want to be able to make residential changes volitionally rather than be forced to move because there are no good alternatives.

There is no coherent public policy for promoting "aging in place." The two key components, housing and long-term-care policies, have developed without a shared history or perspective. Housing policy has traditionally focused on improvement of overall structural quality and on affordability, rather than on suitability over time. Little attention has been paid to the role housing can play in promoting "aging in place" through the addition of social and health-related services, or to its central relationship to long-term-care policy. Long-term-care policy, on the other hand, has almost exclusively focused on financing of nursing home care, despite the recognized need for a continuum of care. Although private and public insurance reimbursements are gradually including more home-based care, even the relatively small amount of federal assistance allocated to in-home services has not been closely coordinated with housing. According to a recent study, the result is "a patchwork of services with large gaps between fully independent living and the near total dependence that often characterizes nursing home care."[3] A better understanding of the role of housing in the organization and financing of long-term-care services is essential if aging in place is to move from a social concern to an effective policy.

To assess the potential of policy that can promote aging in place, this chapter describes the extent of the problem, outlines goals in this area, analyzes current barriers, and evaluates several strategies for reform.

The Nature of the Problem

Aging in place is emerging as an identifiable social problem for several reasons. First, mounting evidence suggests that housing units, which fit the needs of persons when they initially moved into them at younger ages, are not designed to meet the physical, social, and service needs of their occupants as they age and become more frail.[4,5] As a result, some older persons move to more supportive environments in spite of their preference to remain in their current homes. Others do stay in unsafe and unsupportive environments.

Second, studies suggest that many older persons in nursing homes could be cared for in noninstitutional settings, including their own residences, if home care services and other supports were more available.[6] Gradual shifts in reimbursement for more days of home health care, as opposed to more costly acute care, also add to this perception.

Third, forces such as tight housing markets, rising rents and repair costs, and increased property taxes can affect the ability of older persons to stay in and maintain their homes.

Goals for Aging in Place Policy

The goals of an aging in place policy have not yet been well articulated and may consist of underlying principles that appear to be contradictory. The first level of goals relates to desired outcomes for *individuals* that are aimed at encouraging older persons to age in place. Six desirable goals can be identified:

1. House individuals in the least restrictive setting.
2. House individuals in settings that accommodate or adapt to their capabilities, promote independence, and ensure safety.
3. House individuals in settings that accommodate or adapt to their changing needs as they become more frail.
4. Provide services that enable individuals to remain in their current settings by linking services to group settings and providing uncoupled services in other places.
5. Provide environments that prevent medical or social problems that could result from premature moves.
6. Provide a range of housing and service options that meet changing needs as individuals age and move from independence to dependence (and sometimes back again).

Such outcome goals justify services and programs promoting aging in place.

A second order of goals relates to the desired outcomes of the broader *system.* Such goals might include the following:

1. Increase supportive features in new and existing housing.
2. Restore public funding for housing programs and increase funding for in-home services that relieve family caregiving burdens.
3. Effectively coordinate housing and services.
4. Ensure that programs, policies, and activities do not unnecessarily displace persons.
5. Ensure equity of access to housing benefits and services for renters and owners.
6. Target public benefits to those most in need.
7. Provide programs that are cost-effective.
8. Increase affordability of housing.
9. Delay deterioration of and increase the suitability of existing housing stock.

Policy and Systems Barriers to Aging in Place

Political, financial, and organizational barriers currently block progress toward the goals of aging in place policy. Several particularly troublesome problems emerge in seeking new directions or making current programs more responsive to the problem of aging in place.

POLITICAL AND FINANCIAL BARRIERS

Political and financial barriers arise from the nature of the policy-making process and resulting policy domains, principles concerning the appropriate role of government, the federal deficit, and the lack of focused advocacy.

Multiple policies and policy domains. An overriding political barrier to a cohesive aging in place policy is the policy-making process itself. Public policies affecting health care, housing, social services, welfare, and income support are dealt with by different congressional committees that are zealous in maintaining their independence and authority. Moreover, each policy domain is administered by a separate bureaucracy, each with its own specific mandate and subculture. Because aging in place is not a high enough priority on the agenda of any one federal legislative committee or agency, there is no overarching, coordinating policy that encourages its development. The House and Senate aging committees play important roles by serving as forums for exploring the impact of current policies and programs affecting older Americans. They do not, however, have legislative control over program development and financing.

This same pattern of fragmented and disjointed policy-making is evident at the state and local government levels. Several legislative committees and several departments deal with housing, health and long-term care, social services, and welfare programs. State Units on Aging (SUAs) and local Area Agencies on Aging (AAAs) usually lack the political clout to bridge these gaps among policy domains.

Consequently, there is a confusing set of uncoordinated policies and programs at all levels of government, with differing priorities, differing eligibility requirements, and separate service delivery systems. Thus, the programs needed to foster aging in place successfully emanate from governmental subsystems that differ considerably in their conceived roles and responsibilities with regard to older persons. For example, at the most elemental level an older person is defined by the health system as a patient, by the public housing system as a tenant, by the personal care system as a client, and by the social security system as a recipient.[7] These semantic differences reflect deep differences in agency role concepts.

Furthermore, the policies of various agencies often appear to be in conflict. Some legislation and programs encourage aging in place, but others provide incentives for moving to different settings. Similarly, many important programs are left dangling among different agencies or languishing for lack of support and direction.

Program inflexibility. Where a combination of services and programs is necessary to solve problems, solutions may be easier to achieve if there is flexibility within programs. Many programs, however, are the product of legislation with very specific, categorical purposes. Flexibility often is further reduced by regulations. Although the advantages of defining specific agency activities and providing for greater accountability may result, less flexible and innovative approaches to problem solving and a mindset that resists even small changes in mission or program activities can be engendered. For example, in some public housing and Section 202 projects, the Congregate Housing Services Program recently added services to assist frail elderly residents to continue to age in place. This was done on a demonstration basis. But some upper-level HUD officials did not adjust easily to this change in mission, raising many objections about the desirability of the program.

Other program rigidities arise from specific orientations. For example, the largest entitlement programs such as Medicare and Medicaid do not provide reimbursement for many nonacute services or environmental modifications. In California, both programs reimburse hospital bed rentals only if a physician certifies that the patient is confined to bed *and* requires the positioning of his or her body in a way not feasible in an ordinary bed, or if attachments are required which could not be used on an ordinary bed. But Medicare does not cover grab bars in bathrooms, which are considered a nonmedical self-help device, and Medicaid covers only grab bars that are *not* fixed to the walls. Both deny reimbursement for telephone arms or elevator devices which, even though they may promote independence, are considered nonmedical convenience items.

Program inflexibility can also stem from management-related problems. Reductions in staff or new programs without additional staff can prevent programs from carrying out tasks easily and efficiently. Similarly, budgetary constraints often result in limited opportunities for staff training.

Role of government. Other political barriers derive from rethinking the appropriate role of government in general and the federal government in particular. Epitomized by the Reagan administration's laissez-faire principles and the "taxpayer's revolt," nearly a decade of retreat from proactive government of the New Deal and the Great Society eras has occurred. This swing in political philosophy has centered on a freer rein on market forces, the privatization of government-provided services, a devolution of national programs to the state and local governments, and reduced federal outlays for nondefense programs. Welfare policies have been subjected to intense scrutiny at all levels of government.

Federal government withdrawal and the increased reliance on market forces has severely reduced the availability and affordability of housing and services for the poor and near poor. These policies have also put greater pressure on the voluntary, nonprofit sector to fill gaps, and have thrust subnational governments into new or unfamiliar program areas. Although many innovative programs have been created, these organizations have been attempting to fill increasing needs for resources without benefit of federal funds or the broad tax capacity of the national government. The impact on vulnerable subgroups of the population has been severe, especially on the frail elderly.

The federal deficit. The increase in the federal budget deficit has accompanied this period of renewed emphasis on less government involvement. The deficit has been used as a rationale for cutting programs and for inhibiting the initiation of new ones. A flurry of demonstration programs, judged primarily on their ability to reduce costs, has been the alternative to creating permanent new programs. The deficit has also curtailed the expansion of existing programs unless "revenue neutrality" can be achieved.

Thus, the large federal deficit has reduced the political will to create solutions to emerging problems such as aging in place; sometimes it appears to preclude any serious exploration of important new programs. The mention of costs often tables serious discussion or calls to action; costs constitute a mote in our vision of the future.

Fragmented advocacy. The lack of focused advocacy is a major political barrier to placing aging in place high on the public policy agenda. Because of multiple policy domains and territoriality, no single legislative committee or agency is likely to exercise leadership or promote interagency cooperation, particularly if faced with staff reductions. Also contributing to the advocacy problem is the relative newness of the aging in place idea, and our only recently acquired ability to frame concepts and pose appropriate research questions. Unfortunately, the ability to address these questions is hampered by the lack of integrated housing and long-term-care data and the reduction in federal data collection.[8]

A final factor in effective advocacy is the extent to which (1) the public and policymakers understand and are aware of an issue; (2) the issue is seen as related to other concerns receiving more attention; and (3) a broad constituency exists. "Aging in place," unlike the "homeless," is not yet a household phrase. Important aging advocacy groups, such as AARP, have not yet given this issue a top priority compared with issues of income and health, although the linkage has been made between housing and long-term care.[9]

This lack of high priority is understandable because housing itself has not been high on the agenda of aging interest groups. In contrast to the major business-related interest groups such as the National Association of Home Builders, which has dozens of lobbyists, no major organization involved in aging has had more than two staff persons assigned to housing as a specialty. This clearly is a handicap in an arena where there are dozens of complex programs and in which the private profit-making sector is extremely active.[10]

Elderly housing interests generally have been represented by a small but active nucleus of three types of groups: multimission national organizations, nonprofit sponsors of elderly housing, and coalitions. Up until the mid-to-late 1970s, elderly housing interest groups focused primarily on Section 202 housing, but in response to the changing federal agenda they began to broaden their housing perspective. Nevertheless, Section 202 continues to consume much of their energies because it continually faces elimination or reduction in its size and features.

The lower priority assigned to housing can also be explained by the fact that different subgroups of older persons experience different types of housing problems. For example, approximately 75 percent of older persons are homeowners, the overwhelming majority of whom have paid off their mortgages and reaped the benefits of deducting interest payments from income tax—by far the largest housing subsidy program. Owners report general satisfaction with their housing. Their problems are related to maintenance and property taxes. Renters, on the other hand, tend to pay a higher percentage of their income for housing and live in housing stock that is in worse repair. In response to such problems, the government has created a large number of relatively small programs, such as public housing, Section 8, and Section 202, that have benefited only about 3 percent of the elderly.

Long-term care, on the other hand, is a source of widespread concern because the costs of nursing home care can easily push a family into poverty. With the large growth of persons over age seventy-five, it has become a national agenda item for major aging and nonaging organizations. However, long-term-care advocacy programs, such as Long-Term-Care '88, have not identified housing and aging in place as a major component.

ORGANIZATIONAL BARRIERS

Political and financial barriers give rise to organizational barriers, which include service system fragmentation, poor coordination, gaps in needed services and supportive housing, and biases leading to inappropriate or conflicting results.

The service system is fragmented. Frail older persons often require multiple supports to age in place, such as home modifications, in-home services, and financial assistance. Although some progress has been made over the last decade in improving coordination, the system of supports still suffers from high fragmentation in financing and delivery.[11] A multitude of agencies and programs at the federal, state, and local levels provide services that help older persons age in place, but without centralized responsibility at any one level. Policies and programs in at least nine areas directly impact aging in place:

housing; long-term care; income assistance; taxation; health care; social services; community facilities; transportation; energy assistance; and land use. At the federal level alone, eight major departments including Housing and Urban Development, Health and Human Services, Energy and Agriculture, as well as the Veterans Administration, administer nearly one hundred major programs that can affect aging in place (see Table 7-1).

Some departments fund similar services whereas others are distinct. Each program tends to have its legislatively mandated eligibility requirements, benefit coverage, regulations for provider participation, administrative structure, and service delivery mechanisms.[12] Moreover, programs operate fairly independently at each level of government. The differences among Section 8, Title XX, Title III, Medicaid, and SSI programs are especially important because they represent the problems of fitting together the necessary housing, social services, and health and income supports of an effective aging in place system for the very poor elderly.

Programmatic fragmentation has resulted in a service delivery system whose wide variety of disconnected housing types, services, providers, and sponsors is linked only by informal ties. Consequently, older persons with multiple needs may find some services unavailable or they may be eligible for one program (for example, weatherization) but not for another (such as home care). Even if needed services are available, without a coordinator or case manager some older persons may be unable to put together a package of supports that addresses their problems, and thus may find it easier to move from their own homes into housing environments that offer physical supports and social services.

Housing and services are poorly coordinated. Coordination is particularly troublesome when housing and services need to be linked because of the different orientations of funding agencies. For example, HUD housing programs for new construction have focused their limited resources on the physical environment, providing only limited space and few resources for services and activities not viewed as within its jurisdiction. As Lawton points out, federal policy has actually discouraged the production of service-rich environments.[13]

In the face of new problems, such as meeting the needs of an increasingly frail older population, HUD has been extremely reluctant to take on new responsibilities, such as providing social services.

Table 7-1. Inventory of Federal Programs Related to Aging in Place

Program Number	Program Name	Summary of Authorization	Description	Type of Assistance	Type of Service	Type of Applicant	FY86	FY87	FY88
10.410	Very Low and Low Income Housing Loans	Title V of the Housing Act of 1949	Below Market rate loans to obtain, construct or repair housing.	Direct Loans	FIN	Individual	1,155,418	1,339,800	0
10.411	Rural Housing Site Loans	Housing Act of 1949	Two year loans to buy land and make improvements on sites to be sold to low income households.	Direct Loans	FIN	Nonprofit	0	600	0
10.415	Rural Rental Housing Loans	Housing Act of 1949	Financing for the purchase, construction, repair or improvements for rental cooperative housing and related facilities for independent living	Guaranteed/ Insured Loans	FIN	Individual Local State U.S. Ter.	652,348 nonprofit,	669,900	0
10.417	Very Low Income Housing Repair Loan and Grants	Title V of the Housing Act of 1949	Home repair loans to repair existing homes including weatherization.	Program Grants Direct Loans	FIN	Individual	13,891 6,992	13,891 11,335	0 0
10.550	Food Distribution	Older Americans Act of 1965	Provides food for qualifying households and organizations.	Sale, Equipment	NON-FIN	State U.S. Ter. Federal Tribal	2,325,613	2,311,658	2,302,774
10.551	Food Stamps	Food Stamp Act of 1977	Coupons to buy food or seeds and plants to produce food for personal consumption.	Direct Payments for Specified Use	FIN	State U.S. Ter.	10,626,339	10,675,641	10,023,560
10.567	Needy Family Program	Agricultural Act of 1949, Food Stamp Act of 1977	Distributes donated food to needy persons living in or near the Indian reservations.	Program Grants Sale, Equipment	COMB	State Federal Tribal	53,995	56,432	52,891
10.850	Rural Electrification Loans and Loan Guarantees (REA)	Titles I and III of the Rural Electrification Act of 1936 Guarantees (REA)	35 year loans to ensure that people in rural areas have access to electric services.	Guaranteed/ Insured Loans	FIN	Individual Local Nonprofit	1,819,445	808,874	1,024,000
10.851	Rural Telephone Loans and Loan Guarantees (REA)	Titles II and III of the Rural Electrification act of 1936 as amended	35 year loans to ensure that people in rural areas have access to telephone service comparable in reliability and quality to the rest of the nation.	Guaranteed/ Insured Loans	FIN	Individual Nonprofit	183,340	134,718	106,000

Sources: U.S. Office of Management and Budget, *Catalogue of Federal Domestic Assistance*, Washington, D.C.: U.S. Government Printing Office, 1987; Dumouchel, R.J., *Government Assistance Almanac*, 1988, Regency Gateway, Inc., Washington, D.C.: Foggy Bottom Publications; Newcomer, R.J., M.P. Lawton, and T.O. Egerts, *Housing an Aged Society: Issues, Alternatives and Policy*, New York: Van Nostrand Reinhold, 1986.

Table 7-1. Inventory of Federal Programs Related to Aging in Place (*continued*)

Program Number	Program Name	Summary of Authorization	Description	Type of Assistance	Type of Service	Type of Applicant	FY86	FY87	FY88
10.852	Rural Telephone Bank Loan (Rural Telephone Bank)	Title IV of Rural Electrification Act of 1936	35 year loans to extend and improve telephone service in rural areas.	Direct Loans	FIN	Individual Local Nonprofit State U.S. Ter. Federal Tribal	127,897	148,511	93,000
13.633	Special Programs for the Aging—Title III, Part B-Grants for Supportive Services and Senior Centers	Older Americans Act of 1965, Title IV	Assistance to State and area agencies in in supporting programs for the elderly.	Formula Grants	FIN	State U.S. Ter.	253,605	270,000	0
13.635	Special Programs for the Aging—Title III, Part C—Nutrition Services	Older Americans Act of 1965 as amended	Provides meals, nutrition education and other nutritional services for the elderly.	Formula Grants	FIN	State U.S. Ter.	386,502	422,000	0
13.655	Special Programs for the Aging—Title VI—Grants to Indian Tribes	Older Americans Act of 1965	Provides services to older Indians comparable to services provided under Title III.	Program Grants	FIN	Local Federal Tribal	7,178	7,500	0 Tribal
13.667	Social Services Grant	Social Security Act, Title XX	Grants to states such that the states may be able to provide service best suited for their needs.	Formula Grants	FIN	State U.S. Ter.	2,583,900	2,700,000	2,700,000
13.668	Special Programs for the Aging—Title IV—Training, Research and Discretionary Projects and Programs	Older Americans Act of 1965	Improves the quality of life for the elderly through research training, educational programs and demonstration.	Program Grants	FIN	Nonprofit	23,921	12,500	0
13.714	Medical Assistance Program	Title XIX, Social Security Act	Financial assistance to states for payments of medical assistance on behalf of recipients of cash assistance.	Formula Grants	FIN	Local State	24,826,246	26,700,000	26,864,000

Table 7-1 (continued).

Program Number	Program Name	Summary of Authorization	Description	Type of Assistance	Type of Service	Type of Applicant	FY86	FY87	FY88
13.766	Health Financing Research, Demonstration and Evaluations	Social Security Act, Title XI	Improves the administration of the medicare and medicaid programs through research, experiment, demonstration and pilot projects.	Program Grants	FIN	Nonprofit	30,055	28,000	36,000
13.773	Medicare—Hospital Insurance	Social Security Amendments of 1965 Title XVIII	Medical insurance for hospitals and related facilities for covered services to persons age 65 and over and to certains disabled persons.	Direct Payments for Specified Use	FIN	Individual	49,685,171	48,273,280	49,067,432
13.774	Medicare—Supplementary Medical Insurance	Social Security Amendments of 1965 Title XVIII	Supplements benefits obtainable under 13.773.	Direct Payments for Specified Use	FIN	Individual	25,166,156	28,936,600	33,035,600
13.777	State Survey and Certification of Health Care Providers and Suppliers	Title XVIII, Social Security Act	Financial assistance in monitoring of Compliance by health care providers and suppliers with regulatory health and safety standards and conditions of participation in Medicare and Medicaid programs.	Formula Grants Project Grants	FIN	State	82,209	101,045	114,238
13.789	Low Income Home Energy Assistance	Low Income Home Energy Assistance Act of 1981, Title XXVI	Payments to or for low income households for their energy bills (heating, cooling). May also receive weatherization assistance.	Formula Grants	FIN	State U.S. Ter. Federal Tribal	2,007,560	1,822,265	1,237,000
13.792	Community Services Block Grant	Omnibus Budget Reconciliation Act 1981	Grants to fund community based anti-poverty programs and projects such as elderly services and health care.	Formula Grants	FIN	State U.S. Ter. Federal Tribal	320,595	335,000	282,100
13.793	Community Services Block Grant—Discretionary Awards	Omnibus Budget Reconciliation Act of 1981 Budget	Alleviates the causes of poverty on distressed communities.	Direct Payments for Specified Use	FIN	Nonprofit	31,167 State	30,736	27,900
13.795	Community Services Block Grant Discretionary Awards—Community Food and Nutrition	Omnibus Budget Reconciliation Act of 1981	Coordinates the existing private and public food assistance resources to better serve the low income population.	Formula Grants Direct Payments for Specified Use	FIN	Local State U.S. Ter.	0	2,500	0

Table 7-1. Inventory of Federal Programs Related to Aging in Place (continued)

Program Number	Program Name	Summary of Authorization	Description	Type of Assistance	Type of Service	Type of Applicant	FY86	FY87	FY88
13.802	Social Security—Disability Insurance	Social Security Act of 1935	Replaces part of earnings lost due to physical or mental impairment which prevents a person from working (Spouses 62 and over may be beneficiary).	Direct Payments with Unspecified Use	FIN	Individual	19,638,881	19,912,804	20,720,000
13.803	Social Security Retirement Insurance	Social Security Act of 1935	A replacement of part of the earning lost due to retirement.	Direct Payments with Unspecified Use	FIN	Individual	134,766,599	141,577,514	148,642,000
13.804	Social Security—Special Benefits for Persons Aged 72 and over	Tax Adjustment Act of 1966	Monthly cash benefits for persons 72 years and older who had little or no opportunity to earn Social Security Protection during their working years.	Direct Payments with Unspecified Use	FIN	Individual	49,000	39,000	31,000
13.805	Social Security—Survivors Insurance	Social Security Act of 1935	A replacement of part of the earnings lost to dependents due to worker's death	Direct Payments with Unspecified Use	FIN	Individual	40,349,000	42,259,000	44,617,000
13.807	Supplementary Security Income	Social Security Act of 1935 Title XVI	Supplemental income to persons aged 65 or over, blind or disabled individuals with incomes below specified levels	Direct Payments with Unspecified Use	FIN	Individual	9,395,156	9,790,000	11,210,000
13.812	Social Security—Research and Demonstration	Social Security Act of 1935, Title II and Title XVI	Cost sharing for various research and demonstration projects to improve management, administration, and effectiveness of SSA programs.	Project Grants	FIN	Individual Nonprofit State	2,516	10,800	10:100
13.866	Aging Research	Public Health Service Act	Funding for biomedical and behavioral research and research training concerning the aging process, diseases, special problems and needs of the elderly.	Project Grants	FIN	Individual Local Nonprofit State	113,641	124,820	124,134
13.888	Home Health	The Orphan Drug Act, Preventive Health Amendments of 1984	Supports home health services and the training of paraprofessionals.	Project Grants	FIN	Individual	1,432	0	0

Table 7-1 (continued).

Program Number	Program Name	Summary of Authorization	Description	Type of Assistance	Type of Service	Type of Applicant	FY86	FY87	FY88
14.103*	Interest Reduction Payments—Rental and Cooperative Housing for Lower Income Families.	National Housing Act	Mortgages for projects housing the low and moderate income households and and provides subsidies to reduce interest costs.	Direct Payments for Specified Use	FIN	Individual Nonprofit	633,390	619,987	619,119
14.108	Rehabilitation Mortgage Insurance	National Housing Act	30 year mortgages for one to four unit residential buildings to cover the cost of rehabilitation.	Guaranteed/ Insured Loans	FIN	Individual	10,783	17,985	14,535
14.116	Mortgage Insurance Group Practice Facilities	National Housing Act	25 year mortgage loans to help develop group practice facilities.	Guaranteed/ Insured Loans	FIN	Nonprofit	0	0	0
14.122	Mortgage Insurance— Homes in Urban Renewal Areas	Housing Act of 1954	Helps families with a 30 year mortgage to purchase or rehabilitate homes in urban renewal areas.	Guaranteed/ Insured Loans	FIN	Individual	6,437	9473	7,656
14.123	Mortgage Insurance— Housing in Declining Areas	National Housing Act	A long term mortgage to assist in the purchase or rehabilitation of housing in older, declining areas.	Guaranteed/ Insured Loans	FIN	Individual	141,134	78,208	134,276
14.124	Mortgage Insurance— Investor Sponsored Cooperative Housing	National Housing Act, Housing Act of 1956	40 year mortgage for new or rehabilitated multifamily housing to be sold to nonprofit housing cooperatives.	Guaranteed/ Insured Loans	FIN	Individual Nonprofit	0	0	0
14.126	Mortgage Insurance— Management Type Cooperative Projects	National Housing Act	40 year mortgage to develop housing projects to be operated as management type cooperatives.	Guaranteed/ Insured Loans	FIN	Nonprofit	0	1,005	813
14.127	Mortgage Insurance— Manufactured Home Parks	National Housing Act as amended	40 year mortgage for mobile home park development.	Guaranteed/ Insured Loans	FIN	Individual	0	0	0
14.134	Mortgage Insurance— Rental Housing	National Housing Act as amended	40 year mortgage insurance to profit motivated sponsors for rental housing for middle income families.	Guaranteed/ Insured Loans	FIN	Individual Nonprofit	1,386	9,696	8,491
14.135	Mortgage Insurance— Rural Housing for Moderate Income	National Housing Act as amended	40 year mortgages to profit motivated sponsors for rental housing for middle income households.	Guaranteed/ Insured Loans Families	FIN	Individual Nonprofit	0	0	0

Table 7-1. Inventory of Federal Programs Related to Aging in Place (*continued*)

Program Number	Program Name	Summary of Authorization	Description	Type of Assistance	Type of Service	Type of Applicant	FY86	FY87	FY88
14.137	Mortgage Insurance—Rental Cooperative Housing for Moderate Income Families, Market Interest Rate	National housing Act as amended	40 year mortgages for rental or cooperative housing for middle income households.	Guaranteed/Insured Loans	FIN	Individual Nonprofit	1,026,143	484,804	353,786
14.138	Mortgage Insurance—Rental Housing for the Elderly	National Housing Act as amended	40 year mortgages for nonprofit and public sponsors for new or rehabilitated rental housing for the elderly or handicapped.	Guaranteed/Insured Loans	FIN	Individual Nonprofit	15,722	16,160	14,151
14.139	Mortgage Insurance—Rental Housing in Urban Renewable Areas	National Housing Act as amended	40 year mortgages for new or rehabilitated housing in urban renewal, code enforcement and other public program areas.	Guaranteed/Insured Loans	FIN	Individual Nonprofit	185,513	64,640	56,606
14.149*	Rent Supplements—Rental Housing for Lower Income Families	Housing and Urban Development Act of 1965	Rent Supplements for lower income tenants of certain HUD insured housings.	Direct Payments for Specified Use	FIN	Individual Nonprofit	46,577	43,128	43,769
14.151	Supplemental Loan Insurance—Multifamily Rental Housing	National Housing Act as amended	To expand or improve existing multi-family housing, group practice facility, hospital or nursing home insured by HUD or held by HUD.	Guaranteed/Insured Loans	FIN	Individual Nonprofit	2,171	16,160	14,151
14.155	Mortgage Insurance—Purchase or Refinancing of Existing Multifamily Housing Projects	National Housing Act as amended by the Housing and Community Development Act of 1974	10- to 35- year mortgages to purchase or refinance existing multifamily housing.	Guaranteed/Insured Loans	FIN	Individual Local Nonprofit State U.S. Ter. Federal Tribes	37,508	0	0
14.156	Lower Income Housing Assistance Program	Housing Act of 1937 as amended by the Housing and Community Development Act of 1974	Rent supplements paid to property owners to cover the difference between the low income renters' adjusted rent and the market rent for a dwelling.	Direct Payments for Specified Use	FIN	Individual Local Nonprofit State	7,430,234	7,841,560	8,238,255

Table 7-1 (continued).

Program Number	Program Name	Summary of Authorization	Description	Type of Assistance	Type of Service	Type of Applicant	FY86	FY87	FY88
14.157	Housing for the Elderly or Handicapped	Housing Act of 1959 as amended by the Housing and Community Development Act of 1974	40-year loan for the construction or rehabilitation of rental or cooperative housing and related facilities for the elderly or handicapped.	Direct Loans	FIN	Individual Nonprofit	555,741	592,661	35,864
14.163	Mortgage Insurance—Cooperative Financing	National Housing Act	30 year mortgages to purchase the Cooperative Certificate and Occupancy Certificate in cooperative housing projects which gives the purchaser the right to occupy the unit.	Guaranteed/ Insured Loans	FIN	Individual	0	0	0
14.164	Operating Assistance for Troubled Multi-family Housing Projects	Housing and Community Development Act of 1978	Assistance to restore or maintain the physical and financial soundness of subsidized multifamily rental projects.	Program Grants Direct Payments for Specified Use	FIN	Individual Nonprofit	11,405	86,491	86,491
14.169	Housing Counseling Assistance Program	National Housing Act as amended	Counseling for homeowners, home-buyers, and tenants under HUD programs to assure successful homeownership and tenancy.	Program Grants	FIN	Individual Local Nonprofit State	3,312	3,500	0
14.170	Congregate Housing Services Program	Congregate Housing Services Act of 1978	Support of a service delivery arrangement in certain housing projects designed to prevent premature institutionalization of the elderly.	Program Grants	FIN	Local Nonprofit	2,821	5,942	0
14.171	Manufactured Home Construction and Safety Standards	National Manufactured Housing Construction and Safety Standards Act	Consumer protection through the enforcement of standards regarding the safety, quality and durability of manufactured housing.	Dissemination of Technical Information	NON-FIN	Individual Local Nonprofit State U.S. Ter. Federal Tribes	5,374	6,628	6,979
14.174	Housing Development Grants	Housing Act of 1937	Supports the construction or the rehabilitation of rental housing in areas that are short of rental units.	Program Grants	FIN	Local	82,648	99,550	0

Table 7-1. Inventory of Federal Programs Related to Aging in Place (*continued*)

Program Number	Program Name	Summary of Authorization	Description	Type of Assistance	Type of Service	Type of Applicant	FY86	FY87	FY88
14.176	Section 221(d) Coinsurance for the Construction or Rehabilitation of Multifamily Housing Projects	National Housing Act	40 year mortgages for new construction or rehabilitation of multifamily housing projects for middle income families.	Guaranteed/ Insured Loans	FIN	Individual Nonprofit	230,568	808,006	778,330
14.177	Housing Voucher Program	Housing Act of 1937	Rent subsidies paid to very low income families.	Direct Payment for Specified Use	FIN	Local Nonprofit State	0	0	0
14.220	Section 312 Rehabilitation Loans	Housing Act of 1964 as amended	Loans for persons with incomes of 80% of the area median or below for the rehabilitation of residential, non-residential or mixed use properties.	Direct Loans	FIN	Individual	40,411	85,000	0
14.230	Rental Housing Rehabilitation	National Housing Act of 1937 as amended	Grants for private owners to rehabilitate housing for occupancy by lower income tenants.	Formula Grants	FIN	Local State	90,532	220,193	85,000
14.400	Equal Opportunity in Housing	Civil Rights Act of 1968 as amended by the Housing and Community Development Act of 1974	Conducts investigations and provides information to enforce fair housing laws.	Information, Counseling	NON-FIN	Individual	0	0	0
14.401	Fair Housing Assistance Program State and Local	Civil Rights Act of 1968 as amended by the Housing and Community Development Act of 1974	Grants to support agencies to whom HUD must refer Title III complaints to develop an effective work force to ensure complaints are properly and efficiently handled	Program Grants	FIN	Local State	4,700	4,448	4,000
14.402	Non-Discrimination in Federally- Assisted Programs (On the Basis of Age)	The Age Discrimination Act of 1975	Enforcement of the Age Discrimination Act of 1975 as it relates to housing.	Information, Counseling	NON-FIN	Individual Local Nonprofit State U.S. Ter. Federal Tribal	0	0	0

Table 7-1 (continued).

Program Number	Program Name	Summary of Authorization	Description	Type of Assistance	Type of Service	Type of Applicant	FY86	FY87	FY88
14.406	Non-Discrimination in the Community Development Block Grant Program (On Basis of Race, Color, National Origin, Sex, Handicap or Age)	Title I of the Housing and Community Development Act of 1974 as amended	Prohibits discrimination on the basis of race, color, national origin, sex, handicap or age.	Information, Counseling	NON-FIN	Individual Local Nonprofit State U.S. Ter. Federal Tribal	0	0	0
14.507	Mortgage Insurance-Experimental Homes	National Housing Act as amended	Mortgages to help finance the development of homes which incorporates new or untried construction concepts designed to reduce housing costs, raise living standards and improve neighborhood design.	Guaranteed/ Insured Loans	FIN	Individual Local Nonprofit State U.S. Ter. Federal Tribal	0	0	0
14.509	Mortgage Insurance-Experimental Rental Housing	National Housing Act as amended	Mortgages to help finance the development of multifamily housing which incorporates new or untried construction concepts designed to reduce housing costs, raise living standards and improve neighborhood design.	Guaranteed/ Insured Loans	FIN	Individual Local Nonprofit State U.S. Ter. Federal Tribal	0	0	0
14.550	Solar Energy and Energy Conservation Bank	Energy Security Act	Financial assistance for the purchase and installation of conservation and solar means.	Program Grants	FIN	State	9,654	2,200	0
16.103	Fair Housing and Equal Credit Opportunity	Civil Rights Act of 1968 Title VIII	The enforcement of the provisions of the Civil Rights Act regarding equal housing opportunities.	Provision of Specialized Services	NON-FIN	Individual Local Nonprofit State U.S. Ter. Federal Tribal	1,861	1,973	2,063
20.509	Public Transportation for Nonurbanized Areas	Urban Mass Transportation Act of 1964	Improves, initiates, or continues public transportation services to nonurbanized areas.	Formula Grants	FIN	Individual Local Nonprofit State	101,223	75,011	64,900

Table 7-1. Inventory of Federal Programs Related to Aging in Place (*continued*)

Program Number	Program Name	Summary of Authorization	Description	Type of Assistance	Type of Service	Type of Applicant	FY86	FY87	FY88
20.511	Human Resource Program	Urban Mass Transportation Act of 1964	Assistance for public transportation activities particularly for minorities and women's needs.	Program Grants Dissemination of Technical Information	COMB	Individual Local Nonprofit State U.S. Ter. Federal Tribal	2,385	2,000	1,100
20.512	Urban Mass Transportation Technical Assistance	Urban Mass Transportation Act of 1964	Improves mass transportation services by sharing the cost for training, demonstrations, systems development and service innovations.	Program Grants Dissemination of Technical Information Training	COMB	Nonprofit	17,098	17,590	14,200
21.006	Tax Counseling for the elderly	Revenue Act of 1978	A network of trained volunteers to provide free tax information and assistance to elderly taxpayers.	Direct Payments for Specified Use	FIN	Local State	2,200	2,400	2,500
64.007	Blind Veterans Rehabilitation Center	38 U.S.C 610	Personal and social adjustment programs and medical or health related services for blind veterans at certain VA hospitals maintaining blind rehabilitation centers.	Provision of Specialized Services	NON-FIN	Individual	8,783	9,309	9,794
64.008	Veterans Domiciliary Care	Public Laws 89-358 and 94-581 38 U.S.C 601 and 610	Provides medical care and physical, social and psychological and dental services for veterans. Rehabilitates them of his/her return to the community after hospitalization.	Provision of Specialized Services	NON-FIN	Individual	99,270	110,270	118,812
64.009	Veterans Hospitalization	38 U.S.C. Chapter 17	Provides inpatient, medical, surgical and neuropsychiatric care and related medical and dental services.	Provision of Specialized Services	NON-FIN	Individual	5,303,057	5,481,002	5,601,964
64.011	Veterans Outpatient Care	38 U.S.C. Chapter 17	Outpatient medical and dental services, medicines and medical supplies. Includes home based care, prosthetic appliances and transportation.	Provision of Specialized Services	NON-FIN	Individual	452,397	504,108	573,205

Table 7-1 (continued).

Program Number	Program Name	Summary of Authorization	Description	Type of Assistance	Type of Service	Type of Applicant	FY86	FY87	FY88
64.012	Veterans Prescription Service	38 U.S.C. 612 Public Laws 91-500, 93-82 and 94-581	Provides prescription drugs and prosthetic medical supplies for veterans	Sale, Equipment	NON-FIN	Individual	381,336	404,727	426,115
64.013	Veterans Prosthetic Appliances	38 U.S.C. Section 362, 601, 610, 612, 613, 614, 617, 619, 1504, 1901, 1902, 1903 and 5023	Provides prosthetic appliances, equipment and services to disabled veterans so that they may live as productive citizens.	Formula Grants	FIN	State	51,307	55,366	60,200
64.018	Sharing Specialized Medical Resources	Public Laws 89-785, 91-496, 93-82 and 96-151, 38 U.S.C. 5051-5053	Exchange or mutual use of specialized medical techniques and resources for the care and treatment of veterans.	Provision of Specialized Services	NON-FIN	Local Nonprofit State	17,796	18,775	19,807
64.019	Veterans Rehabilitation Alcohol and Drug Dependence	38 U.S.C. Chapter 17	Medical, social and vocational rehabilitation to alcohol and drug dependent Veterans.	Provision of Specialized Services	NON-FIN	Individual	260,352	276,096	290,496
64.022	Veterans Hospital Based Home Care	Public Laws 93-82, 94-581 38 U.S.C. 612	Medical, nursing, social and rehabilitation.	Formula Grants	FIN	State	2,816	2,850	2,992
64.100	Automobiles and Adaptive Equipment for Certain Disabled Veterans and Members of the Armed Forces	38 U.S.C. Chapter 39	Financial assistance to veterans to purchase an automobile or other conveyance and for adaptive equipment deemed necessary to insure the individual will be able to operate the vehicle.	Direct Payments for Specialized Use	FIN	Individual	15,785	15,695	15,398
64.102	Compensation for Service Connected Deaths for Veterans Dependents	38 U.S.C. 321, 341	Compensation for surviving dependents of veterans.	Direct Payments with Unspecified Use	FIN	Individual	27,118	23,300	20,100
64.103	Life Insurance for Veterans	War Risk Insurance Act as amended	Life insurance protection for veterans of WWI, WWII, Korean conflict and service disabled veterans separated from active duty on or after April 25, 1951. Also mortgage protection life insurance for veterans receiving specially adapted housing	Direct Loans	FIN	Individual	1,806,801 115,069	1,926,060 127,117	2,002,520 124,915

Table 7-1. Inventory of Federal Programs Related to Aging in Place (*continued*)

Program Number	Program Name	Summary of Authorization	Description	Type of Assistance	Type of Service	Type of Applicant	FY86	FY87	FY88
64.104	Pension for Non-Service Connected	38 U.S.C. 511, 512, 521	Pensions for wartime veterans with total and permanent non-service connected disabilities.	Direct Payments with Unspecified Use	FIN	Individual	2,502,162	2,479,129	2,470,923
64.105	Pension to Veterans Surviving Spouses and Children	38 U.S.C. 541, 542	Assistance to surviving spouses and children of deceased war-time veterans whose deaths were not service related.	Direct Payments with Unspecified Use	FIN	Individual	1,347,904	1,347,971	1,369,077
64.106	Specially Adapted Housing for Disabled Veterans	Public Laws 80–702, 96–385 and 97–66 38 U.S.C. 801–806	Assistance to severely disabled veterans in obtaining suitable housing units with special fixtures and facilities made necessary by the nature of the veterans' disabilities.	Direct Payments for Specified Use	FIN	Individual	14,498	13,910	13,170
64.109	Veterans Compensation for Service Connected Disability	38 U.S.C. 310, 311	Compensation to veterans who are disabled due to military service.	Direct Payments with Unspecified Use	FIN	Individual	8,406,343	8,434,333	8,289,180
64.110	Veterans Dependency and Indemnity Compensation for Service Connected Death	38 U.S.C. 410–415	Compensation to surviving spouses, children and parents for the death of any veteran who died on or after Jan 1, 1957 because of a service connected disability.	Direct Payments with Unspecified Use	FIN	Individual	1,993,563	2,039,097	2,042,720
64.115	Veterans Information and Assistance	38 U.S.C. 212, 230, 231, 240–243	Information and assistance to veterans about benefits to which they are entitled	Advisory Services and Counseling	NON-FIN	Individual	67,822	67,138	68,089
64.118	Veterans Housing Direct Loans for Disabled Veterans	38 U.S.C. 1811	Loans for severely disabled veterans to purchase, construct or improve homes with specially adapted features and facilities.	Direct Loans	FIN	Individual	119	190	190
64.119	Veterans, Housing Manufactured Home Loans	38 U.S.C. 1819	15 to 25 year loans for veterans and service persons and certain unmarried surviving spouses of veterans for the purchase of a manufactured home.	Guaranteed/Insured Loans	FIN	Individual	133,059	315,731	331,513

This hesitancy, evidenced by HUD's opposition to the Congregate Housing Services Program (CHSP), is partly understandable in light of HUD budget cuts totaling approximately 70 percent during the Reagan administration. In addition, some administrators and policy-makers have argued that CHSP provides disincentives because HUD pays for the program, but any Medicaid-related savings accrue to HHS. Consequently, as older persons have aged in government-sponsored housing such as Section 202 or public housing, the responsibility for providing additional services or environmental modifications has been unclear, leading to poor coordination and gaps in services. As a result, some programs and services support older persons in aging in place, and others encourage their movement to more institutional settings when their abilities decline.

Supportive housing environments and services are lacking. Most housing is designed for young persons, with little regard for incorporating features that facilitate aging in place. Consequently, the housing stock does not provide adequate support for an increasingly frail population. Only about two percent of older persons, most of whom reside in government-sponsored housing, have features such as space for services, handrails, and wheelchair accessibility. Instead, the overwhelming proportion of older persons live in housing that itself is older and may present problems for them and care providers, such as inaccessible and unsafe bathrooms and kitchen facilities.[14] Currently, no comprehensive programs are available for modifying facilities or homes, and not enough persons are trained to identify deficits in the physical environment.[15]

Because many supports needed for aging in place are not reimbursed by entitlement programs, there are serious gaps and considerable variation in program availability. Some needed services such as respite care remain generally unavailable in almost all communities, and others may be available in one area but not in an adjoining jurisdiction. The variability in available services extends even to similar housing facilities for the elderly, such as public housing, some of which may be service-rich and others, service-poor, depending on the practices of management and community agencies.[16]

Market forces and government policy often result in displacement. During the 1950s and 1960s, urban renewal dislocated poor persons, many of whom were elderly, from residences and neighborhoods in which they had resided for many years. Although these projects have greatly diminished, private market trends such as "gentrification" continue to dislocate the elderly and push up rents in many cities.

Older tenants in federally subsidized housing face similar problems. Landlords of many low- and moderate-income housing developments financed through programs such as Section 221(d)(3) (Below Market Interest Rate) and Section 236 (Rent Subsidy) are legally allowed to pay off the balance of their federally subsidized mortgage loans after twenty years, permitting them to convert their properties into condominiums or market rate rentals. According to a recent study, older households occupy 12.4 percent of Section 221(d)(3) units, 24 percent of Section 236 units, and 48 percent of Section 515 Farmers Home Administration units.[17] A General Accounting Office study has estimated that of the 361,000 units at risk of prepayment by 1995, nearly 115,000 units or almost a third are occupied by older households.

An equally troubling potential problem is the expiration of more than a million federal rental subsidy contracts in programs such as Section 8. Currently there are two million privately owned, federally subsidized units and almost a million additional units whose occupants receive federal rent subsidies. Contracts will run out on more than 700,000 units by 1995 and 1.4 million units by the year 2000, a large proportion of which are occupied by the elderly.

Long-term-care expenditures focus on nursing home care. Although older persons have a strong preference for aging in place, there are strong reimbursement incentives to institutionalize older persons. Of the $11.5 billion spent by government on long-term-care services in 1980, over 80 percent or $9 billion was paid by Medicaid for nursing home and other institutional services for the elderly. Only about one-quarter of frail older persons with similar incapacities residing in the community received in-home services, suggesting a large, unmet need for assistance.

Strategies for Reform

The current system does not support aging in place because of enormous gaps, organizational roadblocks, and incentives to house persons in more restrictive settings than they need. In fact, it could be argued that there is no coherent aging in place policy because there is no coherent housing *or* long-term-care policy on which to build.

A number of proposals, however, have begun to surface. Some call for incremental changes to existing policy by improving and targeting specific programs, merging existing programs, or marginally expanding specific programs. Others propose substantial expansion of existing programs, totally new programs, or new administrative approaches. Some strategies emphasize meeting the individual and system level goals enumerated earlier, whereas others focus more on overcoming policy and systems barriers.

PROGRAM STRATEGIES

Several program strategies have the potential to help achieve aging in place goals.

A supportive housing modernization program. Approximately 25 percent of older persons are renters, the majority of whom live in multiunit apartment complexes. As of 1980, the elderly occupied approximately one million units in HUD-subsidized apartment complexes.[18] This concentration of older persons offers opportunities to organize efficient service arrangements that enable the frail to age in place. Most buildings occupied by the elderly, however, were not designed for frail older persons.

A supportive housing modernization program could address this problem by providing direct grants to nonprofit sponsors and loans to private developers. The funds would be used for building renovations to accommodate meal, recreational, and social service programs. They could also be used to convert parts of residential facilities into assisted living units, so that older persons who need more supervision and personal care services than their own units can provide may remain in the complex by moving into an assisted living unit.

Congregate housing services. Approximately 300,000 older persons live in federally subsidized congregate housing, apartment complexes, or group accommodations that provide varying amounts and types of supportive and social services, but not nursing care.[19] Efforts to introduce additional services into federally subsidized congregate housing for the elderly have been resisted by HUD. After more than ten years of advocacy, the Congregate Housing Services Program (CHSP) finally came into existence in 1978 as a demonstration program. It was designed to prevent premature admission to nursing homes of almost 3,000 elderly and handicapped residents in sixty-three federally subsidized sites by providing meals and other nonmedical in-home services. Evaluation of CHSP resulted in inconclusive findings. HUD contended that the CHSP yielded only limited success and said that the evaluation did not address the questions of cost-effectiveness and the prevention of premature institutionalization. Program proponents, on the other hand, cited numerous instances of participants who entered the program directly from nursing homes—where they had been supported by Medicaid—with substantial cost savings. Despite HUD opposition, congregate housing advocates were successful in convincing Congress to authorize approximately $10 million as part of the 1987 Housing Act to continue the program beyond the demonstration period.

The CHSP approach raises issues about how to pay for and organize services. One proposal would increase the rent to provide an in-home services insurance pool, a variation of the "life care at home" concept. The federal rent subsidy could be increased to cover the costs for those unable to afford the premiums. Such a proposal, however, has several drawbacks because services are tied to the setting rather than to the older person, and older persons might lose their benefits if they have to move elsewhere. There is also an equity question: Targeting benefits only to residents in federally subsidized housing does not help other older people living in different settings who may be equally in need.

Home modification programs. A variety of home repair programs have been supported by all levels of government over the last twenty years.[20] Many federal programs have had neighborhood preservation as their major goal. Because the elderly have been thought to undermaintain their property, older homeowners have often been a target group of such programs. A number of states and localities also currently offer low-cost loans that can be used for repair and maintenance costs. Many of these programs permit homeowners to defer payment of principal and interest for a specified term or until the house is sold.

Homeowners can use equity in the home to obtain a loan or convert the equity into a benefit that will allow them to do remodeling. Interest on home equity loans can be deducted on income tax returns. In addition, even though not widespread, local programs exist that will make loans to homeowners to upgrade their properties.

One proposal to stimulate remodeling of existing homes would create a National Housing Investment Corporation, capitalized with an appropriation of approximately $2.1 billion for each of seven successive years, which could lend the elderly up to $15,000 for home rehabilitation and remodeling.[21] Thereafter, the program would be self-financing as loans would be repaid with interest when older persons vacated their homes. It is estimated that approximately 140,000 elderly homeowners could be served annually by such a program.

An effective home modification program, however, must also address the needs of low-income homeowners with little equity and renters who do not have equity on which to draw. Renters often have landlords who are reluctant to make changes outside the unit or to allow physical changes within units because they prefer to have frail older persons move out. This overall situation could be improved by expansion of Medicare and Medicaid funding for home modifications accompanied by legislation and/or regulations guaranteeing tenants the right to make modifications at least within their own units. Stronger accessibility codes and enforcement of such regulations could also prove beneficial to frail older persons living in rental buildings.

The expansion of publicly financed benefits for home modification would also need to address consumer protection. Currently, home modifications are made by older persons themselves or by relatives, friends, medical supply companies, handymen, and repair programs set up by city agencies and nonprofit corporations. The expansion of benefits could bring in a variety of other home improvement contractors into the field, raising important consumer protection issues.

Home equity conversions. Housing is usually not mentioned in discussions of long-term-care policy that concern financing and organization of services. The one exception is reverse annuity mortgages, which primarily generate funds to purchase long-term-care insurance or otherwise pay for long-term-care services.

The concept of home equity conversion has been promoted for approximately twenty years. Home equity conversion would allow an older person to stay in his or her own home and draw down its cash value through a monthly stipend. The loan is then repaid, with interest, when the home is vacated. Theoretically, the older person is guaranteed lifetime tenancy. Proponents argue that almost half the elderly at risk of needing health and personal care service living in single-family dwellings and using home equity conversions would be able to finance the long-term-care they need over their lifetimes. One estimate suggests that over one-third of the elderly near poor could receive at least $2,000 annually based on the equity in their homes for the rest of their lives.[22]

Home equity conversion has not yet had the impact that proponents had hoped. First, many older persons have been reluctant to participate because of their desire to pass on their property to heirs and fears that they might lose their homes or eventually be forced to move.

Second, banks have not been enthusiastic because of the capital that could be tied up in such a program and concerns about return on investment.

Third, although a number of states such as Connecticut, Arkansas, California, and New York have experimented with home equity conversion, there are not enough data yet to know how many elderly will participate and for what purposes the generated income would be used. Preliminary findings from current projects suggest that many older persons have used the money for home repairs and modifications.

Fourth, even if federal insurance for reverse annuities were tied to the use of funds generated for long-term care or home modifications—a stipulation that is not in the current demonstration authorized by the 1987 Housing Act—it would not address the needs of renters for similar support.

Fifth, most older persons with low incomes typically have low housing wealth. Given the complexities of the program, the issues of equity, and the limited demand for the instruments, it does not seem likely in the short run that reverse annuity mortgages will have a large impact on the ability of older persons to age in place.

Life span housing. Life span or universal housing refers to the inclusion of features in new housing that meet the needs of users throughout their life span or adapt to their needs if they become more frail or disabled.[23] Life span housing should be easy to use and maintain; compensate for changes associated with aging such as poor vision or arthritis; be safe and forgiving if one had an accident such as a fall; provide easy accessibility to cabinets, surfaces, and equipment; allow for maximum control over features such as temperature and lighting; and promote communication with the outside world in case of emergencies.

Life span housing incorporates special features in houses when they are initially built, such as wheelchair-accessible entryways, kitchens and bathrooms; single lever faucets; nonslip flooring in kitchens and bathrooms; and grab bars by tubs and toilets. Although many such features are found in specially designed elderly housing, they are not generally provided in single-family homes where the great majority of older persons live.

Policies encouraging life span housing design face a number of barriers. Because housing is primarily a private market enterprise, such features would have to appeal enough to consumers to be marketed by developers. A recent survey found substantial interest for specific features.[24] Nearly two-thirds indicated that they would be willing to pay for items such as single-lever faucets, custom-made pantries, grab bars, and nonslip concrete sidewalks. On the other hand, market interest was marginal for nonslip kitchen flooring, covered porches, and front-door package shelves. Nevertheless, about 64 percent of the respondents indicated that they would be willing to pay the $1,400 for the entire design package if they were buying a new house.

To have significant impact on the housing stock, such features would have to be purchased not just by older persons, who represent a very small percentage of the new housing market. They would also need to appeal to younger households, who form the majority of new home buyers and who show some interest in "baby proofing" houses to increase safety. If features such as nonslip flooring are perceived as improving the safety and functioning of all age groups, they may find a broader market and more widespread political support. Otherwise, they may not seem as desirable for younger persons, whose concern with housing affordability tends to emphasize short-term savings rather than long-term investment to help them age in place twenty to thirty years down the road. As with earlier housing quality changes, life span housing may require a large educational campaign, tax incentives, or changes in building codes. Even so, a long period of time will be required for such changes to have an impact because of the relatively small percentage of the housing stock represented by new construction each year.

Long-term care and housing block grants. Problems with categorical federal programs have led to proposals for consolidating federal long-term care and housing expenditures into block grants that would provide states with a fixed amount of funds to organize and develop services and housing. From the federal perspective, a capped long-term-care block grant has the advantage of predictable expenditures. From the state perspective, these block grants could enhance flexibility and allow states to decide how best to organize and deliver services and how to appropriate funds among different housing options (for example, housing for younger persons, congregate housing, home modifications, and vouchers). Block grants in both housing and long-term care could provide the opportunity to coordinate them efficiently, bypassing problems created by categorical programs.

There is some evidence that, without federal restrictions, states have been more innovative than the federal government, entering territory in which there has been little past federal involvement. Until the early 1980s, state-level public policies in elderly housing were largely derived from federal policy.[25] With the relatively sudden elimination of federal funds for new construction,[26] a number of states recognized housing needs as a special area of concern.[27] Consequently, housing programs have received not only a larger share of state general revenues but also new sources of funds from tax-free bonds, real estate taxes, fees on new development, and the use of excess housing-finance agency (and other agency) reserves and community loan funds.[28]

State policy initiatives have aimed at expanding new construction, converting or rehabilitating housing, creating new housing types such as shared or echo housing and accessory apartments, and providing rental assistance.[29,30] These initiatives have been shaped by various factors: the extent to which the federal government's withdrawal has been viewed as temporary; the lobbying efforts of developers who had been beneficiaries of federal new construction programs; and advocacy by aging interest groups.

The disadvantages of the block grant approach relate to the amount of funds available to states, pressures to continue funding existing programs, and issues of equity.[31] States are especially concerned that a long-term-care block grant will eliminate the entitlement nature of Medicaid and fix expenditures at an unrealistically low level.[32] These concerns stem from the perception that federal expenditures for housing — reduced 70 percent since 1980 — are very much less than what is needed. Also, it is unclear how a block grant would affect the mix of programs. In the absence of new funds, institutional and provider pressures could result in a relatively stable mix of program expenditures. In the area of housing, although states and localities have funded programs such as home modifications, accessory apartments, and house-sharing, the overwhelming majority of their housing funds are still spent on new construction. And although state housing activity has increased options for older persons, the issue of affordability has not been substantially addressed.

Social/health maintenance (S/HMO) organizations. The S/HMO attempts to expand the HMO acute model of case management and prepaid fees to encompass long-term care.[33] The model includes four essential features. First, one organization is responsible for organizing acute and chronic care. Second, the S/HMO is intended to enroll a cross-section of the community. Third, the S/HMO operates on a prepaid fee basis with fees paid by individuals and third parties such as Medicare and Medicaid. Fourth, because it is "at risk" for service costs, the S/HMO has an incentive as gatekeeper to find the least costly, most efficient use of its limited resources, especially in chronic care.

One potential advantage of an S/HMO for aging in place is that older persons do not need to move to obtain in-home long-term-care services. However, the S/HMO's ability to assist older persons to age in place is dependent on the type and amount of community-based services it offers. The federal government is sponsoring a demonstration project involving four geographic sites to test and evaluate the S/HMO concept. Owing to the risk factor, the relatively low per capita fees provided by the federal government, and the newness of the concept, the four experimental sites are offering only a limited long-term-care package with few benefits for home modifications. Moreover, the long-range potential of S/HMOs is still untested as the demonstrations have been slow to get off the ground.

Housing vouchers. The federal government has been moving away from what it considers a relatively expensive housing production program to a less costly direct cash housing assistance payments program that subsidizes eligible individuals. These voucher programs have the advantage of potentially allowing persons greater freedom of choice, especially to stay in their own residences, and could be applied to homeowners as well as renters. However, voucher programs require a participant to live in a unit that meets certain housing standards. Thus, elderly persons who generally reside in older housing units may not qualify unless they move, or use the voucher, if it is large enough, as an incentive to upgrade their unit.

The experience with vouchers suggests that many eligible elderly do not participate in the program, move as often, or upgrade their units as much as younger persons. Instead, the voucher is used primarily to reduce their rent burden. However, vouchers appear to generate approximately 60 percent higher levels of repair by older homeowners than were undertaken previously, leading one analyst to suggest that this approach is at least roughly comparable to the provision of in-kind maintenance services.[34]

There are approximately 5 million homeowners and almost 3 million older renters who would be eligible for vouchers. But actual program participation is estimated to be 1.6 million older owners and 700,000 older renters, compared with the approximately 1.5 million renters of all ages now receiving assistance. Using a figure of about $2,200 per household, Struyk estimates a total program cost of $5.1 billion.[35]

An entitlement program based on vouchers has a number of potential advantages. First, if adequately funded, it would reduce the inequities between those who now receive assistance and those who are eligible but do not receive help due to lack of funds. Second, because of its flexible use, a housing voucher program might be easier to coordinate with long-term care than other existing housing programs. Third, if units can be brought up to standard, a housing voucher that does not tie the subsidy to a particular setting allows older persons to age in place.

An expanded home care program. For many years advocates of home care and congregate housing services have argued that such programs would not only improve the quality of life for older persons but also more than pay for themselves in terms of reduced hospital and nursing home usage. The various administrations and Congress, reluctant to fund costly new programs, responded by launching several demonstrations in the 1970s and early 1980s to test the cost-effectiveness of additional funds for case management, day care, in-home supports, and congregate housing services.

Evaluations of these demonstrations have been somewhat inconclusive. Analysts have pointed out that such demonstrations suffer from inadequate targeting, the lack of potential power of the interventions, and the limited span and scope of authority over resources. The inability of such demonstrations to create significant savings has led many proponents to stress quality of life issues, including reduction of caregiver stress, rather than purely economic justifications.

The continuing concern over the institutional focus of Medicare and Medicaid and the unmet need for community-based services have led to the introduction of several bills in Congress to reform long-term care. One such bill was H.R. 3426 (the Pepper/Roybal bill), which was defeated in the spring of 1988. This bill would have expanded the Medicare program to cover long-term-care services such as nursing home care, homemaker/home health aide services, medical social services, rehabilitation therapies, medical supplies, patient and caregiver education, and training and counseling. The program would have been financed by eliminating the $45,000 cap on income exposed to the 1.45 percent Medicare payroll tax.

Although H.R. 3426 represented a significant expansion of Medicare-reimbursed home care, it had an implicit medical orientation. For example, by basing eligibility on the need for assistance with the activities of daily living rather than including instrumental activities of daily living (for example, the ability to cook and clean), it left out services such as doing laundry and other chores and home-delivering meals that can help promote independent functioning. Given that some home adaptations for wheelchair-bound persons can be costly, even if medical supplies include modifications, the bill's Medicare cap would probably have necessitated a separate provision to ensure their availability. In contrast to many other proposals, however, the Pepper/Roybal bill was universal in its coverage, thereby reducing the stigma of a means-tested program such as Medicaid. It also dealt with the problem of affordability that private long-term-care insurance presents for low-income elders.

CRITERIA FOR EVALUATING PROGRAM STRATEGIES

Several criteria can be used to evaluate alternative program strategies for enhancing aging in place. Aging in place policy should include programs that develop new types of housing with supportive features and programs that increase supportive features in existing housing. Aging in place policy needs to provide more funds for in-home services and to stimulate major expansion of such services in areas where they are scarce and initiate them in areas where they do not now exist. It must improve the coordination of housing and services. Aging in place policy should provide states and localities with some flexibility and incentives for creating innovative programs. It also needs to address complex issues of equity in relation to the circumstances of tenants and owners and assist those deemed to be in need. To provide maximum benefits and choice, financing of services should be uncoupled from housing settings. Program financing mechanisms need to draw on a variety of public and private sources, and attention should focus on the political feasibility as well as the time horizon of different strategies. In short, an aging in place policy needs to fulfill many of the system goals proposed earlier.

THE NEED FOR A MULTIFACETED APPROACH

A comparative analysis of aging in place program strategies suggests that no one approach is likely to address all objectives (see Table 7-2). Aging in place policy, therefore, will most likely continue to face the legislative and bureaucratic problems that have plagued program development in the past: multiple congressional committees and implementation by a variety of administrative agencies. Some of the proposed strategies, however, may produce benefits that should at least lessen these problems. For example, if an expanded home care bill included a wider range of supports than those in the

Table 7-2. Comparative Analysis of Aging in Place Program Strategies

Program	Develops new types of housing with supplementary features	Increases supportive features in existing housing	Improves coordination among programs	Provides states & localities with flexibility & incentives	Benefits low-income persons	Coverage Renters	Coverage Owners	% of population in need likely to be served	Financing mechanism	Time horizon	Type of change
Supportive housing modernization	Low	High	Medium	Medium	High	High	Low	Low	Local, state, federal	Medium	Incremental
Congregate housing services	Low	Medium	Medium	Medium	High	High	Low		Local, state, federal	Short	Incremental
Home modification programs	Low	High	Medium	High	Medium	Medium	High	Medium	Individual's local, state, federal loans	Short	Incremental
Home equity conversion	Low	Unknown	Low	Medium	Low/Medium	Low	High	Medium	Individual's	Medium	Incremental
Life span housing	High	Low	Low	Medium	Low	Low	High	Low	Individual's	Long	Incremental
Social service, long-term care, and housing block grants	Low	Medium	High	High	Medium	Medium	Medium	Medium	Local, state, federal	Medium	Incremental
S/HMOs	Low	Low	High		Medium	High	High	Low/Medium	Individual's	Medium	Incremental
Housing vouchers	Low	Medium	Low	Low	High	High	Low	Medium	Federal	Short	Incremental
Expanded home care	Low	Medium	Medium	Low	High	High	High	High	Federal Medicare	Medium	Major

"High" means performs well in terms of this criterion; "low" means performs poorly.

Pepper/Roybal bill, it could reduce the necessity of a separate CHSP. Many of the smaller-scale programs such as CHSP, however, have had continual uphill fights because of their limited target groups. Thus, it may be appropriate to push for more major universal change.

POLICY STRATEGIES AND ACTIONS

Several systematic barriers inhibiting the development of a more cohesive aging in place policy must be addressed. These include policy territoriality, governmental roles, the deficit's preemption vis-à-vis new program approaches, and lack of effective advocacy.

Reducing policy territoriality. Although it is not possible, and perhaps not even desirable, to overhaul the policy-making process totally, several actions might improve policy coordination and reduce multiple policy domains. The saving grace of the early 1990s is the opportunity afforded by a change in administration and the introduction of major housing and long-term-care legislation at approximately the same time. This coincidence could allow for greater coordination in the drafting of legislation and its implementation. For example, those promoting a new housing bill are seriously considering inclusion of a statutory HUD assistant secretary for supportive housing to make the provision of services a visible HUD concern. The bill's sponsors thought that raising the responsibility to the assistant secretary level also would facilitate coordination with HHS. The proposal is supported by AARP and other organizations.[36]

Joint hearings on aging in place policy by the House and Senate aging committees could clarify the importance of the issue and also promote enhanced coordination. The hearings could explore the often contradictory impacts of current and proposed housing and long-term-care policies and programs on the abilities of older Americans to age in place. In addition, they could serve as a springboard for the discussion of aging in place policy at the fifth White House Conference on Aging, to take place in the early 1990s. Commission on Aging in Place, appointed by the president in 1989, might serve a similar function.

At the federal and state levels interagency task forces should be created, composed of departments with jurisdiction over programs affecting aging in place. These task forces would examine policies in light of their ability to promote or inhibit aging in place and would explore opportunities for the establishment of joint programs. Experience shows that task force deliberations can lead to greater flexibility within—and collaboration among—programs. State task forces have played important and successful roles in promoting policy coordination in areas such as Alzheimer's disease and geriatric education. At the federal level such a task force could act as a sounding board for the proposed assistant secretary for supportive housing and other high-level administrators. It could identify ways in which the national government can encourage state and local government efforts to promote aging in place.

Reassessing government roles. Citizens look to one or more levels of government to provide programs and services. Because of cutbacks in federal housing policy and programs in the 1980s, states have tried to fill these gaps for the elderly, often encouraging or requiring local government collaboration, accompanied by different or better ways to use limited resources to promote aging in place. Their experiences can serve as the basis for a new national housing policy that supports aging in place, as can the deliberations of groups such as the Housing Task Force of the National Conference of State Legislatures and the Council of State Housing Agencies. To capitalize on these diverse experiences, the federal government must reaffirm its role as a leader in creating solutions to the country's housing problems[37] and developing new federal/state and federal/local partnerships that help older persons stay in their homes.[38]

Through renewed leadership, support, and assistance, the federal government can foster initiatives by state and local governments to work with private sector and nonprofit partners to enable older persons to age in place. Identification of aging in place as a major policy endeavor through congressional hearings and the creation of commissions or task forces would signal federal commitment and willingness to exercise leadership. In its role as a catalyst, the federal government should leverage state and local government efforts, through mechanisms such as matching funds for states with housing assistance corporation laws and for local initiatives (for example, housing trust funds) that rehabilitate or convert properties to provide rental housing, shared housing, or supportive group homes for frail elderly.

The federal government can also demonstrate its commitment to aging in place by the creation of initiatives designed to be self-funding over the long term. These could include mortgage insurance for home equity conversions[39] or deferred loans for property rehabilitation or home modification through the National Housing Investment Corporation (NHIC) proposed by Schwartz et al.[40] Increased federal regulation of reverse annuity mortgages could be developed to ensure lifetime tenancy, return of unborrowed equity, and full disclosure.

Countering the deficit dilemma. Federal deficit pressures also are a barrier to the creation of a meaningful aging in place policy and can be overcome by developing mechanisms that move toward self-funding by those able to afford it, and by leveraging state and local initiatives, as discussed earlier. This overall strategy may prove the key to a successful aging in place policy. The federal government can promote aging in place, without adding substantial federal fiscal burdens, by overcoming the problems associated with home equity conversions; creating new approaches such as federal deferred loans for home rehabilitation, a National Elderly Housing Trust Fund to administer revolving accounts to finance elderly housing programs,[41] and a dedicated federal bond program; and promoting policies and programs that encourage the greatest amount of nonfederal assistance. These strategies can also enhance responsibility and support for aging in place as a public policy.

Broadening advocacy. A final barrier to be overcome is unfocused and limited advocacy. Countering strategies include introducing of the aging in place concept into deliberations on housing and long-term-care policies and broadening efforts to combine with other groups, young as well as old, to command more universal support. These efforts should also link, where appropriate, organizations representing frail elderly and younger, disabled persons.[42]

The idea that supportive housing is the missing link in long-term care and forms the basis of aging in place policy[43] must become part of our national thinking. Major aging consumer organizations (such as AARP, NCOA, and NCSC), working in concert with foundations such as Villers and other organizations with an important stake in aging in place (The American Association of Homes for the Aging (AAHA), the National Association of State Units on Aging (NASUA), the National Association of Area Agencies on Aging (NAAAA), the Gerontological Society of America, and the

American Society on Aging), can encourage this idea by identifying its impact in diverse areas. These include its relevance for the development of state and local long-term-care plans, pre- and post-retirement planning, and the training of case managers and discharge planners. The Leadership Council of Aging Organizations should develop a joint plan of focused advocacy, including a policy statement about aging in place.

In addition, these organizations should seek to develop aging in place as a more universal issue for consumers and producers and to generate broader political support to affect a major change in policy.[44] For such a strategy to succeed, housing—especially supportive and decent housing—must become part of the long-term-care policy and a high priority for other age groups. The recent report of the National Housing Task Force, existing housing and long-term-care coalitions, and reports and surveys stressing intergenerational solidarity (e.g., the Gerontological Society's *The Ties That Bind*)[45] can provide the foundations for such efforts.

A number of demographic and political factors are now converging that enable us to address aging in place in a deliberate and concerted fashion. The foundation has been laid, for today and tomorrow's older Americans, to make aging in place a reality—indeed, to make it an idea whose time is now.

Notes

1. American Association of Homes for the Aging. *Partnership in Creating Communities That Care: Meeting the Housing Needs of Aging Americans: Recommendations for the Reform of Federal Housing Policy.* Washington, D.C.: AAHA, 1987.

2. American Association of Retired Persons. *Understanding Senior Housing: An AARP Survey of Consumer's Preferences, Concerns and Needs.* Washington, D.C.: AARP, 1987.

3. Subcommittee on Housing and Consumer Interests, Select Committee on Aging, U.S. House of Representatives. *Dignity, Independence, and Cost-Effectiveness: The Success of the Congregate Housing Services Program.* Washington, D.C.: U.S. Government Printing Office, 1988.

4. Lawton, M.P. "The changing service needs of older tenants in planned housing." *The Gerontologist,* 25:258–64, 1985.

5. Pynoos, J., E. Cohen, L.J. Davis, and S. Bernhardt. "Home modifications: Improvements that extend independence." In V. Regnier and J. Pynoos, *Housing*

the Aged: Design Directives and Policy Considerations. New York: Elsevier Science Publishing Company, 1987.

6. Subcommittee on Housing and Consumer Interests, *Dignity.*

7. Callahan, J., and S. Wallack. "Major reforms in long-term care." In Callahan and Wallack (Eds.), *Reforming the Long-Term Care System.* Lexington, Mass.: Lexington Books, 1981, pp. 3–10.

8. See Chapters 1, 11. Also, National Housing Task Force. *A Decent Place to Live — The Report of the National Housing Task Force.* Washington, D.C.: NHTF, 1988.

9. American Association of Retired Persons. *Proposals of the AARP on National Housing Policy.* Washington, D.C.: AARP, 1987a.

10. Pynoos, J. "Setting the elderly housing agenda." *Policy Studies Journal,* 13:173–84, 1984.

11. Morris, R., and P. Youket. "The long-term-care issues: Identifying the problems and potential solutions." In J. Callahan and S. Wallack (Eds.), *Reforming the Long-Term Care System.* Lexington, Mass.: Lexington Books, 1981, pp. 11–28.

12. Ibid.

13. Lawton, "Changing needs."

14. Newman, S. "Housing and long-term care: The suitability of the elderly's housing to the provision of in-home services." *The Gerontologist,* 25, 1:35–40, 1985.

15. Pynoos, et al. "Home modifications."

16. Holshouser, W., and F. Waltman. *Aging in Place: The Demographics and Service Needs of the Elderly in Urban Public Housing.* Boston: Citizens Housing and Planning Association, 1988.

17. Gaberlavage, G. *Prepayment and the Potential for Displacement of Older Tenants.* Washington, D.C.: American Association of Retired Persons, 1987.

18. Zais, J., R.J. Struyk, and T. Thibodeau. *Housing Assistance for Older Americans.* Washington, D.C.: The Urban Institute Press, 1982.

19. See Chapter 1.

20. Struyk, R., and B. Soldo. *Improving the Elderly's Housing: A Key to Preserving the Nation's Housing Stock and Neighborhoods.* Cambridge, Mass.: Ballinger Publishing Company, 1980.

21. Schwartz, D., R. Ferlauto, and D. Hoffman. *A New Housing Policy for America: Recapturing the American Dream.* Philadelphia: Temple University Press, 1988.

22. Jacobs, B., and W. Weissert. "Home equity financing of long-term care for the elderly." In P. Feinstein, M. Gornick, and J. Greenberg (Eds.), *Long-Term Care*

Financing and Delivery Systems: Exploring Some Alternatives. Washington, D.C.: U.S. Government Printing Office, 1984, pp. 82–84

23. Ruschko, B. "Universal design: for today and tomorrow." In *Park Edition: A Quarterly Monograph for Gerontology Professionals.* Portland, Ore.: Park Place Living Center and Regency Park Living Center, 1988.

24. Heald, G., and J. Rayburn. *Market Interests in Various Age Specific Design Improvements in New Home Construction.* Tallahassee, Fl.: Communication Research Center, Florida State University, 1987.

25. Schwartz, D. "Housing and America's elderly: A state-level policy perspective." *Policy Studies Journal,* 13:157–71, 1984.

26. Pynoos, "Housing agenda."

27. Stegman, M., and J. Holden. *Nonfederal Housing Programs.* Washington, D.C.: The Urban Land Institute, 1987.

28. Schwartz, et al. *New Policy.*

29. Tiven, M., and B. Ryther. *State Initiatives in Elderly Housing.* Washington, D.C.: Council of State Housing Agencies and National Association of State Units on Aging, 1986.

30. Lammers, W., and J. Pynoos. "State roles in aging policy: Lessons from the 1980s." *Generations,* 12, 3:35–38, 1988.

31. Hudson, R. "Restructuring federal/state relations in long-term care: The block grant alternative." In Callahan and Wallack (Eds.), *Long-Term Care System,* pp. 31–60.

32. Rivlin, A., and J. Weiner. *Caring for the Disabled Elderly: Who Will Pay?* Washington, D.C.: The Brookings Institution, 1988.

33. Greenberg, J.N., and W.N. Leutz. "The social health maintenance organization and its role in reforming the long-term care system." In P. Feinstein, M. Gornick, and J. Greenberg (Eds.), *Long-Term Care Financing and Delivery Systems: Exploring Some Alternatives: Conference Proceedings,* Health Care Financing Administration Conference, Washington, D.C., January 24, 1984.

34. Struyk, R.J. "Housing-related needs of elderly Americans and possible federal responses." Testimony presented at hearings of the U.S. Senate Select Committee on Aging, Boston, April 23, 1984.

35. Struyk, R.J. "Future housing assistance policy for the elderly." *The Gerontologist,* 25:41–6, 1985.

36. AARP, *Proposals.*

37. NHTF, *A Decent Place to Live.*

38. Schwartz, et al., *New Policy.*

39. AARP, *Proposals.*

40. Schwartz, et al., *New Policy.*

41. AAHA, "Partnership."

42. Torres-Gil, F., and J. Pynoos, "Long-term care policy and interest group struggles." *The Gerontologist,* 26, 5:488–95, 1986.

43. Pynoos, "Housing agenda."

44. Ibid.

45. Kingson, E.R., B.A. Hirshorn, and J.M. Cornman. *The Ties That Bind.* Cabin John, Md.: Seven Locks Press, 1986.

CHAPTER EIGHT

Financing Long-Term Care in Residential Environments

MARK R. MEINERS

Housing is a key component of long-term care, but it is often overlooked. In part this is a problem of perceived priorities. When we focus on issues of the elderly, health care looms large in the discussion. As people age, health care expenses consume an increasing share of their budgets. Hospital, physician, and other acute care services tend to be high-cost and most elderly have had relatively recent personal medical experiences. Long-term-care costs have become a cause of widespread concern only in recent years.

Long-term care is most closely associated with nursing home care. Nursing homes are the dominant source of formally provided long-term care, comprising the second largest health care expenditure for the elderly, exceeded only by hospital expenditures. Long-term nursing home care is often needed when an individual can no longer return to his or her own home. The risk of needing such care, however, is very limited for most people.

Only when long-term care is more broadly defined do the links with housing become obvious. One definition of long-term care is help provided for people who have chronic conditions and need assistance for a long period in their regular daily activities such as getting dressed, going shopping, eating, or going to the bathroom. Although people get this help in a nursing home, they are at least as likely to get such help in their own home or in the home of a relative or friend. An often-quoted estimate is that about 80 percent of all long-term care is provided informally by family and friends. Estimates of the amount and cost of paid home and community care are more difficult to make because of the wide diversity of agencies and payers, but we do know that those expenditures are dwarfed by the amount spent on institutional care.[1] It is clear that housing is a critical ingredient in keeping the elderly in the community and out of institutions.

The housing component of long-term care, however, is primarily considered when rethinking long-term-care financing. The problem is at the heart of why long-term care is such a difficult public policy issue. People of any age may need long-term care because they are temporarily or permanently ill or disabled, but long-term care is needed mostly by the frail elderly. The needs of those aging in place are largely nonmedical and cover a broad range of health-related, social, and personal care needs. This means that virtually all aspects of a frail elderly person's daily living needs are potentially eligible for public assistance unless some limits are established.

This is a concern in the context of tight budgets, uneven personal resources among the elderly, and the need and desire for both personal preference and personal responsibility. Long-term-care financing programs, both public and private, have struggled to control expenditures. Typically the result has been to limit the definition of long-term care to health-related assistance, with heavy emphasis on the "medical model." Not only are housing considerations not included in such a definition, but home and community services are severely restricted.

There are signs of change, however. Home and community care benefits are in demand and some communities have developed both public and private programs to meet that demand. How to structure and finance these benefits has been a source of considerable debate. The various programs involved in financing long-term care are discussed below, to help in understanding the challenges and limitations involved in providing home- and community-based long-term care in residential environments. Also, some proposals are suggested for supporting housing that would tie that support to the funding of long-term-care insurance.

Current Public Financing Programs

Current public program support for long-term care in residential environments is clearly inadequate. Medicare support is limited to postacute skilled nursing and rehabilitation home health care received on an intermittent basis. Medicaid, the major public payer for long-term-care services, has an institutional bias and is limited to those who meet severe means tests. The remaining public support programs, such as those funded under the Title XX block grant program and the Older Americans Act, provide a variety of home and community benefits, but the programs are *ad hoc* in their focus and are limited in their scope and duration. Nevertheless, these programs represent an important part of what we know about financing long-term care in residential environments. They offer an opportunity to learn something from the real world, where lofty goals and limited resources collide.

MEDICARE

Medicare, the major source of health insurance for the elderly and disabled, primarily focuses on acute care. It pays for very little long-term care either in an institution or in the home. Home health care benefits are payable if a beneficiary needs part-time skilled nursing, physical therapy, or speech therapy. Personal care services provided by home health aides on a part-time or intermittent basis are covered if the patient is receiving one of the qualifying skilled services. Homemaker services can be provided only if they are incidental to personal care and do not substantially increase the time spent by the home health aide.

To qualify for these benefits the individual must be housebound and the needed services must be certified by a physician to be primarily skilled care. The services must be received from a home health agency approved by Medicare. In practice these restrictions result in only a limited amount of visits being covered. In 1984 persons receiving home health services under Medicare used an average of twenty-seven visits even though there were no statutory limits on the number of visits.[2]

The Omnibus Budget Reconciliation Act of 1980 lifted the one-hundred-visit cap under Medicare Parts A and B, the three-day prior hospital stay requirement, the deductible requirement for home health care, and the restrictions on proprietary home health agency participation.[3] Advocates of a broader role for Medicare in paying for long-term care argued that these changes were not enough. Other proposals for Medicare expansion currently being discussed are reviewed in the following paragraphs.

The only other assist to home care provided by Medicare is the coverage of durable medical equipment and hospice care. Medicare pays for up to 80 percent of the cost of medical equipment such as wheelchairs, dialysis machines, and oxygen pumps when the equipment is provided through an approved home health agency. Medicare also pays for hospice care benefits when the patient's life expectancy is expected to be six months or less. Under the new Medicare "catastrophic" insurance benefits, the 210-day limit on hospice benefits can be removed if the beneficiary's physician or hospice director recertify the patient as terminally ill.

The new Medicare Act also provides for a limited respite benefit and better transitional home health coverage. The latter benefit is in response to the effects of previous Medicare reform (the Prospective Payment System), which encouraged earlier hospital discharge. Discharging some patients after relatively short hospital stays created a greater need for transitional home health services. Since the home health care benefits were designed for those who could get by on intermittent care, it was possible for someone needing daily home care services after an early hospital discharge to go uncovered. A Medicare recipient is now able to receive up to thirty-eight consecutive days of home health assistance from a health aide or nurse in a given period, instead of the five days a week for up to two or three weeks that was previously allowed.

The respite benefit allows up to eighty hours a year from an outside aide for short spells to relieve family and friends. There is a substantial deductible. Eligibility requires the patient to have at least two dependencies in basic activities of daily living, and to have already met the Part B catastrophic limit of the deductible outpatient drug costs. Since both deductible amounts represent a significant out-of-pocket cost, the respite benefit is not likely to be widely used.

Medicare home care benefits clearly are most useful for transitional care. As such, they are the gateway benefits to other home and community service use once the patient's situation has stabilized. Unfortunately, they are not designed to assure that stabilization has occurred prior to the termination of benefits.

Several other provisions of the new Medicare Act are potentially important for future financing of long-term care in residential environments. The act calls for four demonstration projects to provide case management services to Medicare beneficiaries with high-cost illness and authorizes $5 million for each of the next five years for research on delivering and financing long-term-care services.

The provisions in the new Medicare Act most relevant to aging in place are several changes in Medicaid rules regarding the protection of income and assets of the spouses of institutionalized patients. Concerns about spousal impoverishment have become the topic of considerable discussion in the last several years.[4] The fear is that when one spouse is institutionalized, the couple's income and assets have to be depleted to poverty levels to enable the spouse in the nursing home to qualify for Medicaid. This simultaneously impoverishes the noninstitutionalized spouse. The state's welfare system, including Medicaid, then faces two problems rather than one, apart from the clearly inhumane effects of the law.

The new Medicare Act requires states to allow a Medicaid-eligible individual's spouse living in the community to receive sufficient income each month to allow his or her income to be at least 122 percent of the federal poverty level for a couple, effective September 30, 1989. The amount increases up to 150 percent by July 1, 1992, not to exceed $1500 per month unless a higher amount is determined necessary by fair hearing or court order. Also, states are required to divide all nonexempt resources equally in determining Medicaid eligibility for an institutionalized individual with a spouse who is living at home. The minimum amount protected is $12,000, with the option for states to go as high as $60,000 for the spouse's share. For those couples who kept their assets in joint accounts where each had complete access, this second provision may turn out to be more restrictive: It may preclude movement of resources into an account solely controlled by the spouse. The latter action has been a favorite recommendation of financial planners assisting couples faced with the previous impoverishment rules.

MEDICAID

The Medicaid program suffers from many of the same medical biases that exist in Medicare. Unlike Medicare, however, Medicaid is a means-tested program originally designed to pay the health
care bills of those who were poor or became poor because of large
medical bills. For the purpose of developing home and community
services, this is perhaps its major strength. Medicaid is a state-
administered program that requires selected services to be covered
by state payments matched by the federal government. States establish eligibility requirements, which vary widely. In addition to the
mandatory services, states can choose from a broader array of
optional services, again with significant federal funding (50 to 75
percent federal contribution depending on the per capita income of
the state). Because the program is responsible for all the health care
needs of those who are eligible under the Medicaid program, and
Medicare and private insurance cover little of the long-term-care bill,
the states have become the major public payers of nursing home
care. Medicaid is typically either the largest or the second largest
single item in state budgets (after education), and the fastest
growing item, which has prompted all states to try to contain its
rapid growth. This has stimulated many states, with the support of
the federal government, to experiment with alternatives to nursing
home care.

Two ways to offer home and community care benefits are
available to states under the Medicaid program. First, current statutory authority allows states to offer as optional benefits home
health services, personal care services, day care, private duty nursing, and case management. But if a state chooses to offer any of
these benefits, they must be provided to the entire categorically
eligible (aged, blind, and disabled) population on a statewide basis.
This requirement increases the cost and complexity of the program
too much for most states. Concerns cited in a recent review include:
insufficient infrastructure for such a broad effort; distinct differences
in need among Medicaid's varied long-term-care populations (for
example, developmentally disabled, chronically mentally ill, adult
disabled, and elderly); Medicaid eligibility rules that do not allow
limiting the availability of selected services to only a subset of the
elderly poverty population; and restrictions on the types of services
offered.[5]

The second option, the "2176 waiver" program, eliminates many of these concerns but has significant limitations of its own. The Omnibus Budget Reconciliation Act of 1981 included a Section 2176 that permitted states to apply for special Medicaid waivers that would allow them to pay for nonmedical services on a more selective basis—if the average cost to Medicaid was no greater than if the person had been placed in a nursing home. Services do not need to be provided on a statewide basis but can be targeted to selective groups of Medicaid recipients, and income eligibility levels can be the same as those used for determining eligibility of nursing home residents. Prior to this waiver authority, Medicaid payments for service to persons living in the community were generally restricted to being at least medical services. Under the 2176 waiver, services such as case management, respite care, personal care services, home modification, and transportation can be covered.

The implementation of this program by the Federal Health Care Financing Administration (HCFA) has been conservative. States have had to deal with a protracted approval process, strict limits on who will qualify, and close scrutiny of projected cost estimates. A criterion of budget neutrality, tied to an already restricted supply of nursing home beds, has served to keep participation limited. In 1987, thirty-seven states had operational 2176 waiver programs, but only about 59,000 elderly were being served.[6]

Section 4102 of the Omnibus Budget Reconciliation Act of 1987, a second, more recent waiver option, allows states to increase their long-term-care spending under Medicaid as long as the total (including that for nursing homes) does not exceed the base year amount by seven percent. After October 1, 1989, the growth rate will be the greater of two amounts: 7 percent, or a rate reflecting the growth in the state's population age seventy-five and older, the costs of providing long-term-care services, and a 2 percent "intensity factor."

For those states with an adequate base of Medicaid long-term-care services, this option may be helpful in meeting the needs of a growing elderly population while continuing to restrain the growth of institutional services.[7] The problem is that Medicaid benefits vary substantially among states; the poorest states generally have not expanded their base of services despite the higher federal match available to them.[8] However, Section 4102 does make it possible for states to move forward in innovative ways using the

Medicaid program to cover home and community care. It remains to be seen how HCFA will administer it. There is a long way to go before a significant amount of home and community benefits are financed by Medicaid.

OTHER GOVERNMENT PROGRAMS

At least eighty federal programs help persons with long-term-care problems, either directly or indirectly through cash assistance, in-kind transfers, or the provision of goods and services,[9] but most are very narrowly focused vis-à-vis eligible beneficiaries and benefits provided. Besides Medicaid, the federal programs most involved in financing home and community assistance for long-term-care needs are the Older Americans Act, the Social Services Block Grant (SSBG) Program, and the Supplemental Security Income (SSI) Program. These programs have different goals, legislative authorities, administrative structures, eligibility, and benefits. The states have been delegated much of the responsibility for administering these programs, and there is substantial flexibility in program design. This delegation of federal authority, along with the significant budgetary constraints of the programs, has prompted states to view these programs as limited opportunities to leverage their own revenues to meet the growing demand for long-term-care services.

Older Americans Act. The Older Americans Act has a broad mandate to improve the lives of the elderly, but its emphasis has been on supporting congregate and home-delivered meals programs. Title III of the act is the major vehicle for providing this support. Title III grants are made to state agencies on aging, which award contracts to local area agencies on aging to plan, coordinate, and advocate for services to meet the needs of the elderly. The amount a state receives is based on its share of the population sixty years and older as compared to all states. Services are provided to older persons without regard to income, but emphasis is on those with the greatest social and economic needs. However, since services are limited by the availability of funds, recipients who can afford to pay something are encouraged to do so. There is no automatic entitlement to program benefits.

The Older Americans Act has recently been extended, with Title III amended to include a separate authorization of funds for nonmedical in-home services for the frail elderly. Previously, there had been no separate authorization of funds for such assistance, and the limited funding had been used primarily for nutritional services. In fiscal year 1988, $834.4 million was authorized for Title III programs, with one-third specifically appropriated for the following social services: homemaker and home health aides; visiting and telephone reassurance; chore maintenance; in-home respite care and adult day care as respite for families; and minor home modifications not to exceed $150 per client.[10]

Social Services Block Grant Program. Title XX of the Social Security Act is a modest attempt to balance the medical orientation of Medicare and Medicaid with block grants to states for a wide spectrum of social services for the aged, the disabled, and children. The only requirements for the use of these funds are that they must be for social services, although medical care can be covered if it is "integral but subordinate" to the provision of social services. A state's share of the funds is based on its population, with the total amount available set by congressional authorization.

The program's funding is relatively small and has not kept up with inflation. For fiscal year 1988 Congress authorized $2.75 billion; for fiscal year 1985 through fiscal year 1988, the annual appropriation has been $2.7 billion.[11] Only a portion of the funds are used for the elderly. A recent survey of forty-four states found that this proportion ranged from 1 to 50 percent with the average amount being 18 percent.[12]

Supplemental Security Income Program. Title XVI of the Social Security Act authorizes the federally administered Supplemental Security Income (SSI) Program to provide minimum income levels for aged, blind, and disabled persons. In addition to providing low-income elderly with the basic federally allowed minimums of $354 per month for an individual and $532 for a couple, the program allows states to make supplementary payments. Most states have taken advantage of this authority because it allows them either to make payments to all SSI beneficiaries or to target them to selected SSI recipients.

Many states have used the SSI extra payment option to help keep low-income elderly from going into nursing homes by authorizing special supplements to those in residential care facilities (for example, adult foster care homes, board and care homes, and domiciliary care facilities).[13] A recent report by the Center for the Study of Social Policy found that forty-three states supported a diverse range of long-term-care services through their optional SSI programs.[14] However, the programs were small with a nationwide total of about 320,000 SSI recipients receiving assistance with long-term-care needs.

State programs. The use of state-only funds has recently been cited as one of the basic sources of financing for home and community long-term care by those states judged to be the most advanced in developing community care systems.[15] The significant role they have in each of the funding sources cited above (with the exception of Medicare) has encouraged states to experiment, taking advantage of program flexibility to accomplish long-term-care system reform. This experimentation has focused on expanded home and community care.

Home and community care is commonly preferred to institutional care. There is a strongly held belief that home and community services, once developed, can limit the rapid rise in nursing home costs without an equally large increase in alternative care costs. This belief, however, has been tested in numerous demonstrations and evaluations, and the results are not encouraging.[16] Home and community benefits tend to be an add-on cost to the system because they are difficult to target to those who will be able to use them effectively to delay or prevent the need for institutional care.

The preference for home and community care is nonetheless strong, and the use of state dollars for this purpose is becoming more common for three reasons:

- It allows for flexibility in program design without the need to meet federal Medicaid requirements.
- It allows for the use of existing programs and institutions that have grown up outside the Medicaid system with their own practical and political traditions.
- It is essential if the program of home and community-based services is to be available to the large group of elderly who are not Medicaid-eligible but who may need similar support.[17]

The importance of the last factor has prompted considerable discussion along two fronts: the need for some kind of universal long-term-care program, and the need to encourage more personal responsibility for financing through private sector initiatives.

Long-Term-Care System Reforms

For many, the long-term-care financing problem is best solved by expanding Medicare or by enacting a new national program that is federally financed and universal in coverage. Whether such a program is likely now or in the near future is uncertain.

Three bills introduced in Congress in 1987–88 illustrate this thinking. The Pepper/Roybal Long-Term Home Care bill (H.R. 3436) proposed a new home care entitlement under the Medicare program for chronically ill elderly, disabled persons, and children. Under this provision, a case management team would determine whether an individual was unable to perform two or more basic activities of daily living (bathing, dressing, eating, toileting, and transferring). Eligible persons would receive a care plan that provided nursing care; homemaker/home health aide services; medical social services; rehabilitation therapies; medical supplies; and patient and caregiver education, training, and counseling. Services would be provided by a Medicare-certified home health agency and would be reimbursable on a reasonable cost basis up to 62 percent of the average state Medicare rate for skilled nursing home services.

A system of consumer protection, provider training, and outcome-oriented provider inspection features was proposed to assure quality home care services. Financing for the program was to come from eliminating the cap on income exposed to the 1.45 percent Medicare payroll tax (which is $45,000) with the possibility of copayments if costs exceed revenues. The bill also would authorize demonstrations to test the expansion of the program to mentally ill and disabled persons otherwise not covered, the feasibility of including adult day care, and the use of alternative organizations and models for doing case management.

The bill introduced by Senator George Mitchell of Maine (S. 2305) also proposed to expand Medicare by adding long-term-care benefits. The proposal featured a home care benefit (including homemaker and chore-aide services), a respite benefit, and full protection for all nursing home stays that extended beyond two years. For the home care benefit there was a $500 annual deductible, a 20-percent copayment, and a cap on expenditures per day of 65 percent of the skilled nursing home charge. A 50-percent copayment on up to $2,000 of respite care was proposed. The nursing home benefit was to have a 30-percent copayment. The intent of the long deductible period on the nursing home benefit is to encourage private insurance; the Mitchell proposal, however, acknowledges the need by some for assistance with the deductible by suggesting protection against spousal impoverishment and Medicare buy-in of premiums for those at or below the poverty level. Like the Pepper/Roybal bill, financing would come primarily from raising the cap on the Medicare payroll tax. In addition, a $2 monthly premium would be assessed on everyone, plus an extra premium for those with higher incomes. Medicaid savings and a new 5-percent tax on gifts or inheritance above $200,000 would cover the rest of the estimated cost of about $18 billion per year at the outset. The Mitchell bill also incorporated some of the tax incentive ideas currently being proposed in a variety of other bills to encourage private insurance development. These include accumulating insurance reserves tax-free, deducting long-term-care expenses as medical expenses, and encouraging long-term-care options in employee benefit packages.

A bill proposed by Senator Edward Kennedy went even further. The proposed program would have two parts. Part A would cover the full cost of home care (including homemaker services, respite care, and adult day care) and the first six months of nursing home care. All individuals sixty-five and over would be covered and eligibility for services would be based on the need for assistance with one or more basic activities of daily living. It would be fully financed by federal funds. Part B would cover longer stays in nursing homes and be financed by a combination of public funds and private premiums. A copayment equal to 35 percent of the daily bill would be charged, with Medicaid as the gap filler for those with insufficient income. Enrollment could begin at age forty-five with premiums lower for those who begin before age sixty-five. The program would be financed by raising the Medicare payroll tax cap to $75,000 and increasing alcohol and cigarette taxes.

Each of these proposals is estimated to cost in the range of $16 to 20 billion a year at the start. This is an amount roughly equal to the federal deficit at the end of the Carter administration. Although the costs are formidable, particularly in light of the recently passed Medicare catastrophic act and the associated increase in premiums, there is a growing recognition of long-term care as an important political issue. It is also clear that home and community care benefits will be given serious attention in any contemplated reforms.

Federal, State, and Private Partnerships

Although a major new federal program to finance long-term care is a possibility, many states are studying financing alternatives on the assumption that a limited federal role in financing is likely to continue for some time. Alternatives to broad new entitlements may focus on improvements to Medicaid, such as more uniformity in eligibility standards, benefits, quality control systems, and reimbursements, with emphasis on expanding eligibility criteria for home and community benefits.[18]

Strategies to encourage the development and purchase of private long-term-care insurance by those who can afford it, subsidizing those who can only partially afford it, and assuring coordination with programs that are fully publicly funded also may relieve the burden on both consumers and government. Eight states (Connecticut, Massachusetts, Indiana, Wisconsin, New York, New Jersey, California, and Oregon) are currently participating in a new program supported by the Robert Wood Johnson Foundation to design and develop cooperative public-private long-term-care insurance partnerships.

In this program the states are considering numerous strategies to encourage the development of a private long-term-care insurance market.[19] Options that involve reorientation—rather than expansion—of current public responsibilities include: (1) educational campaigns to enhance public awareness; (2) regulatory review to encourage market flexibility while promoting consumer protection; (3) support for improved data development and sharing to minimize uncertainty; and (4) coordination of public cost and care management mechanisms (for example, preadmission screening, utilization review, case management, benefit coverage, and rate regulation) with those of the private market. More aggressive strategies involving direct market subsidies are also being discussed.

States are considering several different types of market subsidy. One approach offers a stop-loss guarantee by providing full protection from further asset spend-down for anyone paying through insurance for a set number of years. Another is some type of premium subsidy, including tax credits or deductions for a person who buys a specified level of insurance protection. Other proposals involve subsidizing the deductible period or copayment for those who must use the benefit. These types of subsidies are designed to increase the affordability of long-term-care insurance policies. Both asset waiver and premium subsidy strategies would target the consumer and vary on the basis of income.

Another example of a consumer-oriented subsidy strategy is to underwrite some portion of inflation in the cost of care that exceeds a "reasonable rate." Only a few insurers have attempted to address the problem of protecting benefits from inflation.

Subsidies to insurers could be in the form of premium tax breaks or public reinsurance programs to help insurers overcome their hesitancy to enter or expand the market. Assistance to market development might also be accomplished if the state paid the insurance premium for persons eligible for Medicaid or established special subsidized risk pools for those who would otherwise be uninsurable. This would serve to broaden the risk pool and spread administrative costs.

The small and underdeveloped nature of the current market has prompted the above proposals. Until there is more experience with insuring long-term care, progress will be slow and conservative. The limited market size and high premiums in turn tend to restrict the market to relatively high-income persons. By designing subsidies to encourage participation by persons otherwise unable to afford long-term-care insurance, the market size may be increased to include greater numbers of those most likely to spend down to Medicaid.

The Robert Wood Johnson Foundation Program to Promote Long-Term-Care Insurance for the Elderly has as a major emphasis the development of insurance mechanisms that cover home and community care. Successfully implementing any of the more aggressive support strategies is likely to require federal support in the form of waivers of current Medicaid requirements.

Current Private Financing Options

The past few years have seen a dramatic growth of interest in private sector financing initiatives for long-term care. At the heart of this interest is the idea that long-term care is an insurable risk. Although the major focus is on risk-pooling mechanisms, other ideas have been proposed, such as offering tax preferences for individual savings accounts dedicated to the purchase of long-term-care insurance, or linking the purchase of such insurance to home equity conversion options to take advantage of offsetting risks. Although an enhanced retirement resource base can certainly help pay for long-term care, cash accumulation and resource mobilization strategies can be more effective if linked to risk-pooling mechanisms.

PRIVATE LONG-TERM-CARE INSURANCE

Most current long-term-care insurance policies cover only the nursing home. The insurability of home and community benefits remains a major question for most insurers. Nonetheless, successful marketing of long-term-care insurance may well depend on progress being made in covering home and community care.

Much of the early development of long-term-care insurance focused on nursing home care, expanding the limited Medicare benefits to include multiyear coverage for intermediate and custodial care. For home health care, further liberalization of Medicare means removing the homebound requirement and increasing the coverage to include personal care and homemaker services without the strict ties to skilled care. Removing the homebound requirement involves covering community care benefits that are important services in the long-term-care continuum: day care, transportation, nutrition services, respite care, and chore services.

The problem insurers have with expanding the insurance package beyond Medicare's benefits is that long-term-care needs are complex and definitions are not uniform. Services tend to overlap in their purpose and there is little consensus about how such services should or could be packaged, staffed, and provided. In addition, the best approach to providing care often depends on the living circumstances of the individual, including the availability of family care and other informal support.

Many of these services are nonmedical and are required to assist with functional status deficits associated with the normal aging process. Insurers seriously question whether such services are insurable. They are concerned about being liable for the care of persons who no longer want to live independently. Insurers are inclined to rely on medical needs to define insurable events. The fear is that many people who would not seek institutional care would use home and community care benefits, leading to higher costs.

Traditionally, services are considered insurable if they cannot be paid for without significant financial difficulty, if the probability of needing them is low enough to allow the risk to be spread, and if the need is random enough that users cannot be identified in advance. Many long-term-care services do not satisfy these criteria without further clarification of how the risk will be managed, including the use of deductibles, copayments, payment caps, and case management. Most home and community services meet the above criteria only indirectly. They are considered insurable only because they are believed to be lower-cost substitutes for institutional services.

In spite of these difficulties, insurers recognize that consumers have a strong preference for home and community care. The response to date, however, has been cautious. The home care benefits are designed to be secondary to the nursing home benefit. Risk is controlled by limiting the amount paid per visit and the period of time the benefits are paid. Typically, both payment rate and time of coverage are half that provided for nursing home care, and risk is controlled by making the home care benefits available only after a paid nursing home stay. Because the nursing home benefits are usually payable only after a deductible period, this can be a major restriction. When time in the nursing home beyond the deductible period is required the benefits are not likely to be very useful. Few elderly people are discharged back home after an extended stay in a nursing home.

Taken together, these provisions are very restrictive. In most cases consumers should be cautious about choosing insurance if home and community benefits are the primary motivation for purchasing it. However, there is some justification for selected insurance features.

Limiting the amount payable per home visit to a percentage of the daily nursing home rate may reflect the fact that nursing home care has a room and board component that is not necessary when the patient is cared for at home. However, there are important economies of scale in providing care in a nursing home that are not possible with home care. Transportation costs for bringing caregivers to the home, for example, may offset some of the savings on room and board. Limiting the rate to the amount paid in the nursing home may be the most that could be hoped for at this time, although it might be in the insurer's interest to offer a richer home benefit in the early days following a nursing home discharge as a way to encourage such transitions.

To the extent that the amount payable per home care visit is less than what is required, the payment rate implicitly involves a copayment and/or continued involvement of family and other informal supports to make care at home possible. These factors are very important in controlling insurance-induced demand for home and community benefits, a major worry for insurers.

Limiting the number of visits may also be workable, if we assume that someone being cared for at home after a nursing home stay can get by with intermittent care, perhaps three or four visits per week. If the benefits are structured in a flexible way the beneficiary could vary the intensity of use to suit the need, perhaps using more in the early days after discharge and decreasing use as the situation stabilizes.

The real weakness in many of the current offerings is that home care is only covered if it follows a hospitalization of at least three days or a paid nursing home stay that has continued for an extended period. There are major problems with these requirements. The first one limits the benefit to those who can legitimize a hospital admission, which is a subset of those who need long-term care. Insurers are beginning to back away from this requirement.

With the nursing home stay requirement, the longer a person is institutionalized the less likely is his or her chance of successfully being discharged home, even when benefits are available. This approach assures that home care benefits are used as substitutes for nursing home care coverage but does so in a way that raises questions about the intended scope of the benefit.

One exception is the insurance policy that Prudential is developing for the American Association of Retired Persons. It offers the following features:

- Coverage includes nursing home, home health, and adult day care without prior institutionalization.
- Nursing home care is covered for 1,095 days (3 years) at $50 per day with a 90-day deductible.
- Home health and adult day care are covered for 730 visits at no more than 7 visits per week. Covered home care includes nurse and therapist services at $35 per visit, home health aide and homemaker services at $25 per visit, and adult day care at $30 per visit to an adult day care facility. A visit must be at least 3 hours. There is a 45-visit deductible for the home health and adult day care benefit.
- Benefit upgrades will be offered at least every four years to help protect against inflation.
- These services are covered only if nursing home confinement would otherwise be required and they must be recommended by a physician.

This later clause is the "but for" criterion and it is perhaps the critical consideration insurers have in offering home and community benefits. That is, they want to limit the use of home and community benefits to those persons who would be institutionalized but for the availability of these benefits. In the case of Prudential, insurers are willing to rely primarily on physician judgment rather than on a required nursing home stay.

Most insurers are not comfortable with relying on a physician's judgment as the primary basis for paying claims. In screening individuals, they would like systematic criteria that are administratively feasible, reliable enough to determine whether a person would otherwise need institutional care and sturdy enough to withstand a legal test. Insurers are increasingly looking toward the use of disability screening criteria based on limitations in basic activities of daily living such as bathing, dressing, getting to the toilet, and general mobility. They are also considering the use of case managers to help with assessment and care planning.

One of the more innovative designs has been developed by Blue Cross and Blue Shield of the Rochester, New York, area (Finger Lakes Long Term Care Insurance Company). This plan offers long-term home and community services as well as nursing home benefits at the custodial level of care. The policy includes nursing home benefits with options of three-, four-, or five-year coverage. Home and adult day health care visits of less than eight hours count only as half a service day, effectively allowing for the possibility of doubling coverage for those benefits. The nursing home benefit requires a 100-day deductible, but there is no deductible for the home and community benefit. No prior hospitalization is required for these benefits. The policy uses "preferred providers," paying 75 percent of the cost of nursing home and home health agencies that have contracted with Blue Cross. Selecting other providers drops the allowed reimbursement rate to 50 percent. The policy requires and pays for personalized care planning to determine the patient's needs, develop a service plan, approve services, assist in arranging services, and revise the plan as needed. Covered benefits include nursing supervision and services as well as aide service and routine medical supplies. Among the services specifically excluded are durable medical equipment, transportation, and services provided by immediate family or people who reside with the patient.

Another significant benefit in the Finger Lakes policy is the coverage of alternative level of care days in a hospital, charged at the rate of four service days per hospital day. This helps a patient who no longer needs hospital care but for whom appropriate alternative care is not immediately available. In areas where the supply of long-term-care services is limited, the need for such protection is important. The cost of a three-year policy purchased at age fifty-five is $59.43 per month and $86.52 if purchase is delayed until age sixty-five. The premiums and benefits are designed to be indexed for inflation.

There are many difficulties in offering home and community benefits, but insurers have begun to recognize that consumers have a strong preference for those services in lieu of institutional care. They appreciate that growth in the sale of long-term-care insurance probably depends on insurers making further efforts to cover such services. Some have begun to examine other arrangements such as social-HMOs and continuing care retirement communities, for both the lessons they teach about insuring home and community care and the market segment they represent in the personal preferences of some consumers.

MEDICARE HMOS

The emergence of Medicare HMOs may encourage long-term-care insurance development if certain barriers can be removed. As part of the Tax Equity and Fiscal Responsibility Act (TEFRA) of 1982, Medicare regulations were changed to allow HMOs to provide services to Medicare beneficiaries on a prospective, capitated, at-risk basis. The managed care environment, with the insurance risk integrated into the service delivery system, seems well-suited to the needs of older persons.

An initiative undertaken at Group Health in Puget Sound, Washington, one of the earliest participants in the Medicare HMO demonstration projects from which the TEFRA regulations were formulated, suggests the interest Medicare-HMOs may have in adding long-term-care benefits. Group Health entered into a joint venture with Metropolitan Life to offer long-term-care benefits as a separate product with its own underwriting criteria. Although disagreements about underwriting criteria have recently caused Group Health to seek a new partner, the latter is committed to offering their product.

By marketing it as a separate product, Group Health sidesteps a major barrier to the expansion of Medicare HMOs into long-term care. Medicare HMOs are not allowed to exclude any applicant on the basis of preexisting conditions.[20] This is a strong disincentive to directly integrate long-term-care benefits into the HMO benefit package if, as might be expected, they would attract the chronically impaired elderly. The current reimbursement formula does not reflect characteristics associated with patient needs. As such, it discourages Medicare HMOs from seeking to specialize in the provision of a comprehensive benefit package because of the fear of adverse selection. With open enrollment, healthy people might rationally stay in a lower-cost acute care plan until they become disabled.

To fulfill the potential of Medicare HMOs as long-term-care insurers, refinements to the reimbursement formula to reflect both acute and chronic illness needs should be considered. An alternative solution would be to permit HMOs to restrict coverage under a high option to those people willing to buy when they turn sixty-five years old.[21] People who chose the high-option plan could be allowed to move to a lower-coverage plan, but not the other way around. This would greatly reduce the risk of adverse selection.

Health status adjustments in the reimbursement formula might also reduce concerns about removing or liberalizing the limit of Medicare or Medicaid enrollees to 50 percent of the total. This would permit the development of HMOs that specialize as geriatric health care centers. Providing long-term care in a managed care environment is viewed by advocates as the most feasible way to insure home and community services.

SOCIAL HMOS

Under this model, a single provider organization assumes responsibility for a full range of ambulatory, acute inpatient, rehabilitative, nursing home, home health, and personal care services under a prospectively determined fixed budget.[22] Elderly persons who reside in the target marketing area are voluntarily enrolled through the marketing efforts of the social HMO. The social HMO consolidates the system at all levels: provider, population, finance, and risk. The model is currently being tested at the following four sites: Metropolitan Jewish Geriatric Center (MJGC), Brooklyn, New York (Elderplan); Kaiser Permanente Medical Care Program, Portland, Oregon (Medicare Plus II); Ebenezer Society, in Partnership with Group Health, Inc., Minneapolis, Minnesota (Seniors Plus); and Senior Care Action Network, Long Beach, California (SCAN Health Plan).

The social HMO model calls for a broad benefit package because one of its underlying assumptions is that substantial downward substitution of services is more likely when the financial incentives of prepaid capitation are combined with the opportunity to use a wide array of lower-cost alternatives. Each site provides all Medicare Part A and Part B services without the copayments and deductibles associated with these services. In addition, acute care benefits include dentures, prescription drugs, optometry, audiometry, eyeglasses, hearing aids, and preventive visits; some of these have copayments. All sites offer unlimited hospital days, and two sites have significantly extended "Medicare-type" skilled nursing facility (SNF) benefits.

The chronic care benefit package includes case management, home nursing and therapies, personal care and homemaker services, adult day care, medical transportation, hospice and respite care, and chronic care in an SNF or intermediate care facility. Sites also include or will arrange for home-delivered meals, electronic response systems, chore and escort services, and other necessary transportation.

The social HMO is financed by a pooling of public and private dollars. More specifically, for non-Medicaid eligibles, the social HMO receives a monthly capitation payment or premium from Medicare and a monthly premium from the enrollees themselves. In addition, there are various copayments that the enrollee is required to pay for long-term-care services. For Medicaid eligibles, the social HMO receives monthly capitation payments from both Medicare and the state Medicaid program. At one site, Seniors Plus, the county also provides financing for Title XX eligibles.

CONTINUING CARE RETIREMENT COMMUNITIES

The oldest long-term-care risk-pooling model in this country is the continuing care retirement community (CCRC), also known as a life care community. Relatively few CCRCs offer an unlimited chronic care guarantee.[23] For some this may simply reflect intended limits to the scope of the benefit package. For others, however, the limited guarantee is related to the difficulty of insuring the long-term-care risk, especially with the small risk pool that most communities represent.

Some CCRCs are actively exploring joint ventures designed to connect the long-term-care insurance component with an established insurance company, and a number of insurance companies are marketing products to meet this demand. This type of arrangement eliminates the need for the community to act as its own small insurance company. By reinsuring with a company that specializes in long-term-care insurance the opportunity exists for creating a larger risk pool. This reduces the reserves needed by the CCRC to guarantee long-term-care coverage for all of its residents. CCRCs also represent an opportunity to market long-term-care insurance protection on a group basis, where all parties can work together in a managed care environment to control the risk. This type of arrangement has the potential of increasing the number of retirement communities that are willing to offer some form of long-term-care protection.

Life Care at Home

Recognition of possible links among the concepts involved in free-standing LTC insurance, social HMOs, and CCRCs has stimulated another idea: continuing care at home. This is a program in which participants, living in their own homes, buy into a risk-pool arrangement that has a managed care component. Unlike traditional CCRCs, enrollees are not required to move to a "campus."

According to its proponents, this alternative accomplishes two purposes. By eliminating the housing costs of traditional CCRCs, similar retirement security can be achieved at a lower cost, thus making it affordable to more people. In addition, this alternative may appeal to persons who can afford a traditional CCRC, but who prefer to remain in their own homes.

The Health Policy Center at Brandeis University and the Friends for the Aging in Philadelphia have developed a life-care-at-home plan.[24] The prototype has received start-up funding from several foundations and is in the process of becoming operational. Three other sites are currently in the early stage of development under a Robert Wood Johnson Foundation demonstration grant.

Cash Accumulation

Cash accumulation vehicles dedicated to the payment of long-term-care expenses is another financing option that has been proposed. The idea is to allow individuals to make tax-deferred contributions to an account that can be used solely to pay long-term-care expenses.

To make this an effective public policy, it is important to target the account for the purchase of some form of LTC insurance rather than allow the account to be used for self-insurance. Self-insuring against the risk of catastrophic expenses is neither efficient nor realistic. It is also not good public policy because it requires much larger aggregate savings to provide reasonable protection — as compared with risk pooling — and consequently a much larger drain on tax revenues.

Another consideration is that IRAs already provide the option of tax-deferred saving for long-term care, and are more appealing because they are not limited to that purpose. They can be used for anything the owner chooses. If this type of account is to be optional, serious consideration must be given to incentives for participation. Tax deductions, the incentive in IRAs, will probably not be enough. Prior to the recent tax changes only about 17 percent of the people eligible to establish an IRA did so. People are likely to choose an IRA option first because it can be used to purchase LTC insurance as well as other things. Offering tax credits may be a better incentive than tax deductions because they are more valuable to people with low and middle incomes. Varying the amount of tax credit by income might be a way to encourage wider participation.

With any of the IRA-type strategies, public subsidies are involved and careful assessment of the costs and benefits are needed to evaluate their merits. Also, these approaches would be effective only in terms of the future; they do not address the current or near-term needs for long-term-care protection.

HOME EQUITY CONVERSION

Converting the equity in one's home to cash without having to move has received considerable attention as a potential source of funds for facilitating aging in place.[25] But activity in this area has been limited. Although housing is the major asset for most elderly persons, it remains a largely untapped source of funds because of market resistance on the part of both consumers and lenders. Recent developments, however, may stimulate more interest in this approach.

Congress recently approved a demonstration program that allows the Federal Housing Administration (FHA) to provide insurance backing to mortgage lenders who wish to offer equity conversion opportunities to consumers. The equity conversion arrangements covered by the program include reverse mortgages that pay a monthly amount for as long as the house is occupied as the principal residence (the "tenure model"), reverse mortgages that pay for a set number of years (the "term" model), and mortgages that allow for variable withdrawals (the "line of credit" model). The line of credit approach is new and thought to be a more appealing option for using home equity because it allows for withdrawals as needed. In terms of paying for long-term care, however, all these options have the drawback of being self-insurance with no risk pooling.

Direct integration of home equity conversion and long-term-care insurance might result in a more feasible and appealing option than can be expected when these are marketed separately. This integration could balance the risk that a person would remain in the home for an unexpectedly long period of time, thus incurring extra cost for the lender. That is, this risk would be offset by the risk that a person would leave home to enter a nursing home, thus incurring cost for the long-term-care insurer. There would be one profit margin and possibly a more efficient, less costly product for the consumer.

A key assumption behind home equity conversion arrangements is that people feel strongly about staying in their current home. If, on the other hand, this preference is not widespread and strongly held, then it may be economical and appealing for people to sell their current home and use some of the proceeds to buy or rent a less expensive residence, freeing the remainder for other uses.

Rethinking Housing and Long-Term Care

The link between housing and long-term care for the elderly is ripe for rethinking. Consider the following:

- Housing is by far the most significant asset of the elderly. An estimated 73 percent of the elderly own their own homes, and most of them have no mortgage debt.[26] In total the equity value has been estimated to be between

$548 billion and $700 billion. Without effective means of freeing this equity for their own use, many elderly are "house rich and cash poor," leaving their heirs as the major recipient of these resources.

- Under most circumstances the home is effectively exempt from any claim by Medicaid.[27] Therefore, the most significant asset of the elderly is not available to help pay the long-term-care bill, leaving Medicaid as the payer of last resort even when the elderly recipient may have had significant means to contribute.
- It is increasingly difficult for young persons to afford to enter the housing market. According to the National Association of Home Builders, the rate of home ownership has begun to decline with the most noteworthy decreases among those twenty-five to thirty-four years of age.[28] This has prompted numerous proposals to assist first-time home buyers, including allowing IRA funds to be used as a downpayment by first-time home buyers.[29]
- Homeownership tax deductions, valued at $38.8 billion in 1988, are increasingly mentioned as a potential source of tax revenues to help broaden the distribution of tax benefits to address the growing needs of the poor or at least to help reduce the federal deficit.[30]

This mix of factors may help establish linkages between housing and long-term-care public policies. For most people the best vehicle for saving is the purchase of a house. It is an appealing form of consumption and at the same time is an investment that can accumulate additional value. Linking housing investment to long-term-care needs may reinforce housing as an important part of long-term care, for both the services it provides and the asset accumulation it represents.

Public policies could be shaped to help bring about this linkage. Current or future tax benefits to facilitate saving for housing purchases could require that some of the equity value in the home be linked to purchase of long-term-care insurance. This would serve the multiple purposes of stimulating investment in housing, saving for long-term care, and reducing resistance to using home equity as a source of funds for the elderly in need of such care. Creative linkages can be imagined that would help to balance the concerns implicit in these arrangements.

LINK WITH CAPITAL GAINS

One change that could have an immediate impact would be to require that tax savings from the exclusion of up to $125,000 in capital gains on the sale of a home by persons age fifty-five and over be set aside for long-term-care needs. Under current tax law the maximum tax savings from this exclusion ranges from $18,750 to $35,000. Even half this amount (more in line with the median home value) could make a significant dent in long-term-care costs, especially if the tax savings are used to help purchase insurance. Targeting these savings to long-term-care needs represents no additional tax loss to the Treasury. And for consumers it is certainly more appealing than having this tax break eliminated. It simply reinforces the use of those funds for long-term-care needs, something that is otherwise easily overlooked.

LINK WITH DOWN PAYMENT

Another idea would be to allow first-time home buyers to use tax-free funds accumulated in an IRA for a down payment on a house, in exchange for a commitment to devote a proportion of the accumulated value to help pay for long-term care if needed. One of the challenges in developing a market for long-term-care insurance is motivating younger people to save for such expenses. And one of the concerns about allowing use of IRA funds for home purchase is that it involves trading housing for retirement income. This link might help on both issues.

LINK WITH PRINCIPAL PAYMENT

Another possibility would allow monthly principal payments on a home mortgage to be treated like IRA accumulations, in exchange for a commitment similar to that suggested above on long-term care from current homeowners. The deduction could be targeted to lower- and middle-income persons along the lines of the current IRA rules or broadened by allowing the deduction up to some limit, such as paying off the first $100,000 of a mortgage.

The incentive for saving in this form is more than just the tax deduction. On a $100,000, thirty-year, 10.25-percent mortgage, a payment of $25 extra per month can cut the life of the loan by four years and save nearly $39,000 in interest. Even before the recent change in the rules, participation in IRAs was low and skewed toward the higher-income brackets. The link to housing equity accumulation and earlier mortgage payoff may be a relatively appealing form of saving for low-income persons because the value of tax write-offs from interest payments is lower for them than for people in high-income brackets.

Also, for lower-income persons the savings are more likely to be new rather than just shifted from other sources. Encouraging an increase in savings may be especially important in garnering serious consideration for this proposal in the current fiscal environment. Any tax break to encourage savings in some form of long-term-care account represents a drain on the Treasury now in exchange for benefits in the future. This type of benefit-cost comparison will give discouraging results unless externalities (such as enhanced economic growth from increased savings and investment rates) can be introduced into the calculations.

Conclusion

Successful aging in place opportunities will require new thinking in this country. Federal assistance for housing through our current tax structure is a major benefit enjoyed by older Americans. Formalizing the links between our efforts to support housing as the major societal benefit and financing long-term care should be considered. This will require widespread availability and acceptance of home equity conversion mechanisms as a means of helping pay for long-term care in residential environments. Success in this area will allow better targeting of limited resources for those segments of the population unable to afford these benefits.

Notes

1. Lipson, D.J., and E. Donohoe. *State Financing of Long-Term-Care Services for the Elderly.* Volume I: Executive Report. Intergovernmental Health Policy Project. Washington, D.C.: George Washington University, 1988.

2. Kirby, W., V. Latta, and C. Helbing. "Medicare use and cost of home health services, 1983–84." *Health Care Financing Review,* 8, 1:93, 1986.

3. Pillemer, K.A., and A.S. Levine. "The Omnibus Reconciliation Act of 1980 and its effect on home health care." *Home Health Care Services Quarterly,* 14, 1982.

4. Tilly, J., and D. Brunner. *Medicaid Eligibility and Its Effect on the Elderly.* Public Policy Institute Report No. 8605. Washington, D.C.: American Association of Retired Persons, 1987.

5. Etheredge, L. "Financing and management of home and community-based services." In *State Long-Term Care Reform: Development of Community Care Systems in Six States.* Washington, D.C.: National Governors' Association, 1988, pp. 115–145.

6. Neuschler, E. *Medicaid Eligibility for the Elderly in Need of Long-Term Care.* Washington, D.C.: National Governors' Association, 1987.

7. Justice, D. (Ed.), *State Long-Term-Care Reform: Development of Community Care Systems in Six States.* Washington, D.C.: National Governors' Association, 1988.

8. Erdman, K., and S.M. Wolfe. *Poor Health Care for Poor Americans: A Ranking of State Medicaid Programs.* Washington, D.C.: Public Citizen Health Research Group, 1987.

9. O'Shaughnessy, C., and R. Price. "Financing and Delivery of Long-Term-Care Services for the Elderly." Congressional Research Service, Library of Congress, May 25, 1988.

10. Ibid.

11. Ibid.

12. Gaberlavage, G. *Social Services to Older Persons Under the Social Services Block Grant.* Public Policy Institute Report No. 8701. Washington, D.C.: American Association of Retired Persons, 1987.

13. See Chapter 4.

14. Center for the Study of Social Policy. *Completing the Long-Term-Care Continuum: An Income Supplement Strategy.* Washington, D.C.: Center for the Study of Social Policy, 1988.

15. Justice, *State Reform.*

16. Rivlin, A.M., and J.M. Wiener. *Caring for the Disabled Elderly.* Washington, D.C.: The Brookings Institution, 1988, pp. 190–99.

17. Etheredge, "Financing and management."

18. Erdman and Wolfe, *Poor Health Care.*

19. Meiners, M.R. "Enhancing the market for private long-term-care insurance." *Business and Health,* 5, 7:19–22, 1988.

20. Iverson, L.H., and C. Polich. *The Future of Medicare and HMOs.* Excelsior, Minn.: Interstudy, 1985.

21. Greenberg, J., W. Leutz, M. Greenlick, J. Malone, S. Ervin, and D. Kodner. "The Social HMO Demonstration: Initial operating experience." *Health Affairs,* Summer 1988.

22. Leutz, W., R. Abrahams, M. Greenlick, R. Kane, and J. Prottas. "Targeting expanded care to the aged: Early SHMO experience." *The Gerontologist,* 28, January 1988.

    Greenberg et al., "The social HMO."

23. Winklevoss, H.E., and A. Powell. *Continuing Care Retirement Communities: An Empirical, Financial, and Legal Analysis.* Homewood, Ill.: Richard D. Irwin, 1984.

24. Tell, E.J., A. Cohen, and S.S. Wallack, "Life care at home: A new long-term-care finance and delivery option." Health Policy Center, Brandeis University, unpublished manuscript, 1987.

    Moon, D.L. "The life care at home plan: Is it an affordable option in the future?" Unpublished paper presented at the Harvard University and Farnsworth Trust Symposium "Life Care: A Long-Term Solution," March 7, 1988.

25. Scholen, Ken. *The Role of Home Equity in Financing Long-Term Care: A Preliminary Explanation.* Report submitted to the Minnesota Housing Finance Agency. Madison, Wisconsin: National Center for Home Equity Conversion, February 28, 1986.

26. Jacobs, B. "The national potential of home equity conversion." *The Gerontologist,* 26:498, October 1986.

27. Office of the Inspector General, Office of Analysis and Inspections Department of Health and Human Services. *Medicaid Estate Recoveries: National Program Inspection.* Report Number OAI-09-86-00078. Washington, D.C.: Office of the Inspector General, 1988.

28. Apodaca, P. "Homeownership declines despite sales boom." *Investor's Daily,* 7, February 20, 1988.

29. Harney, K.R. "A bumper crop of (election year) bills." *Washington Post,* October 1, 1988, F28.

30. Mariano, A. "Affluent get thousands in subsidies." *Washington Post,* October 15, 1988, E1.

PART FOUR

Planning for the Future

CHAPTER NINE

Value and Ethical Issues in Residential Environments for the Elderly

BRIAN F. HOFLAND

The literatures of values and ethics, housing, and gerontology largely have ignored residential environments for the elderly. This chapter discusses many of the major value and ethical issues involved in developing and managing housing and services for the frail elderly.

Basic Value and Ethical Questions

A useful starting point is the identification of some of the major values and assumptions about aging and human life that guide the development of housing for older people.

ROLE OF ELDERLY IN SOCIETY

In an insightful article, philosopher and gerontologist Harry R. Moody presented four societal models of aging and examined their implications for education and curriculum development.[1] His analysis is relevant to housing and services for the elderly. The four models, forming a continuum from materialistic to holistic values, are (1) rejection; (2) social services; (3) participation; and (4) self-actualization.

241

Rejection. Model I, rejection, involves the avoidance, repression, and neglect of old people as a result of industrialization and its heavily materialistic emphasis. In an industrial society old age is devalued and old people are considered expendable. The thrust of the modern ethos is toward materialistic growth, change, and progress. The experience of old age includes the deterioration of the body and the acceptance of the ultimate limitations of material existence. Old people represent loss of productivity, unaccomplished goals and dreams, and the uncomfortable recognition of the boundaries of life. Old age conflicts with the prevailing values of modern life, resulting in an instinctive avoidance of old people and the death and consciousness of mortality that permeate their lives. Modern man shuns and fears old people because they symbolize his own fate. Implicit attitudes of repression, dread, and denial are reflected in the social institutions and mechanisms that modern life has developed to deal with the "problem" of aging.

Under the rejection model, older people are allowed to reside in the community as long as they can function independently or with the help of their families. But if they lose their capacity to function independently, they are moved to nursing homes. If housing is built especially for the elderly, it constitutes what Lawton and his colleagues have termed a "constant environment";[2] that is, it does not provide additional supportive services for residents who become more frail as they age. Only applicants who can live completely independently with the services provided are allowed to remain in such housing. As residents become functionally impaired, they are asked to leave and are moved to a nursing home. Old people are tolerated in the community only as long as they are like young people.

Given the negative perspective of this first model, there can be no rationale for supporting frail and dependent older people in the community. Human beings are primarily production units to be discarded when their usefulness is over.

Social services. Model II, social services, is an expression of political liberalism and the mechanisms of the welfare state. Government intervenes to meet the human needs of the casualties of industrialized society through transfer payments such as social security, food stamps, welfare, and through concrete service programs such as senior centers and expanded nursing home care. Old people require social services that are best provided by government bureaucracies and specialized professionals. The elderly become a constituency of sorts, with professionals and bureaucrats advocating ever more public funding to support a variety of expanded services and professional roles.

Although Model II redistributes resources to remove the worst excesses of Model I, it offers no basic challenge to the underlying attitudes and institutions. Old people still are not valued as integral members of society. Social services in this model are done *for* someone by a certified professional in a highly paternalistic way that often subtly leads the patient or client to become more passive and dependent, a phenomenon known as "learned helplessness." The social distance between professional and client tends to segregate old people and prevent them from sharing in many aspects of community life. Old people, perceived as something less than total human beings, are not seriously engaged in activities and projects that are respected and valued by the entire community. They contribute to the community's well-being as consumers rather than as producers, and through leisure rather than through work.

The housing of Model II is characterized by a goal of placing older people in the "least restrictive environment." If housing is specially built for the elderly, it constitutes what Lawton and his colleagues have termed an "accommodating environment,"[3] that is, one that is accorded additional supportive services as residents require them. However, because old people are perceived primarily in the roles of patient/client and consumer, services often are made available or even required whether residents need them or not. Thus services can have the effect of actually making residents more functionally dependent and lessening their sense of personal control.[4] In addition to a plethora of social services, housing management often provides an array of leisure-time activities either on-site or in conjunction with a nearby senior center. Activities can include square dancing, ceramics, crafts, bingo, card-playing, bus trips, and, in higher-priced housing, golf. These activities are often a source of pride to residents as indicators of their good life. However, these recreational activities appeal to these older people precisely because of their values and beliefs about the meaning of old age within human life as a whole.

Participation. Model III, participation, involves an expanded view of the dignity, self-determination, and societal integration that are possible for old people. Whereas Model II argues for a focus on the needs of old people in the name of social conscience, Model III rejects the "elderly mystique" of disability and passivity and proposes to enable older people, to the extent possible, to live their lives in the mainstream of society.[5] The "least restrictive environment" goal of avoiding nursing home placement is seen as a very limited one. Rather, the potential for growth, development, and continuing engagement are pursued through activities associated with a normal community life. Model III involves a recognition of sexuality, the right to work, and opportunities for making meaningful contributions to society. The changing demographics of an aging society have led to demands for rights for old people that previously had been denied to them, often through policies supposedly developed to protect them. Parallels with the civil rights, women's, mentally retarded, and independent living movements are strong. These political values are an implicit component of Model III.

The leisure pastimes and consumer role of Model II are seen as increasingly untenable and demeaning, particularly as the trend for very early retirement creates a segment of the population that will face a retirement period of up to thirty-five years. More than one retiree has concluded that "There are only so many golf games that you can play." The leisure-oriented senior centers with their crafts and games have been described scathingly by Maggie Kuhn, the founder of the Gray Panthers, as "giant geriatric playpens."

With Model III's emphasis on integration into the community, the passivity and segregation of Model II give way to societal involvement through second careers, volunteer activities, and other creative ways to participate in and contribute to society. Recently, for example, the New York State Catholic Conference's Commission on the Elderly thoughtfully outlined possible continuing roles for older persons within the parish.[6] There is a recognition that most older people are relatively unimpaired "well elderly" and that the older population is a heterogeneous group with diverse preferences on most issues. Personal autonomy of older people becomes a paramount concern.

Housing for old people in Model III involves an "accommodating environment" in the best and truest sense of the term. Person-environment congruence is achieved. Supportive services for old people are added to housing, but only as required and desired. The emphasis is not on the existence and expansion of these services but rather on *how* they are structured and delivered. Supportive services are implemented in partnership with old people.

Age-segregated congregate housing is not ruled out, for a segment of the older population prefers such housing due to increased safety, quiet, and opportunities for social interaction with peers,[7, 8] but neither is it particularly encouraged. When segregated housing exists, special efforts are made to foster the integration of the older residents into the surrounding community.

Most older people are homeowners and there is an emphasis on rehabilitating their houses or apartments so that these older people can age in place within their long-time community setting. The remodeling goes to where the older people are, rather than the people going to where the builders want them to go. Home health care and other supportive services are made available so that these individuals can remain in their own homes as long as desired, but the least restrictive environment objective is not an obsession. Older people are not kept in their own homes through strenuous efforts at the expense of their overall well-being. Alternative forms of supportive housing are available to older people who no longer can remain in their own homes but who do not require nursing home placement.

Under Model III, housing developers respond to the heterogeneity of the older population by building and marketing for multiple and distinct buyer profiles. Older people are involved in the design, decoration, and operation of housing.

Self-actualization. Model III underlies current efforts at social reform. It involves a more holistic perspective of old age than the earlier two models but stops short of challenging modern society's basic values. Its major goal is normalizing the life of old people in terms of housing, work, politics, and social life. The standard for fulfillment and self-esteem emulates those for earlier life stages. This insistence on continuity still denies the aging process.

Model IV, self-actualization, challenges the fundamental values of modern life by suggesting that old age brings special possibilities. Model IV is characterized by emphasis on spiritual values. It establishes goals of spiritual growth not yet on the agenda of social policy or debate. It is difficult even to describe these goals, because old age in modern thought has few positive attributes.

However, in Vedic civilization in ancient India, the human life span was seen as a series of stages, each with its own demands, role, and potential for growth. The first stage was that of child and student, followed by the role of householder. Householders maintained a home, raised children, and practiced a trade or profession. Once children were grown, the householder had the option of renouncing work and family responsibilities to pursue a spiritual life. Through meditation and other spiritual practices under the guidance of a guru or master, the elder experienced transcendence and spiritual growth in pursuit of the ultimate goal of enlightenment. Each stage of life had its own distinct meaning, with old age personifying the supreme meaning of self-realization. The oldest generation commanded considerable respect because of its embodiment of wisdom and the flow of generations.

In contrast, modern Western societies have a strictly materialistic vision of life and death, with old age symbolizing decay rather than the cyclical nature of life. Modern culture lacks a holistic vision of life and this spiritual desiccation underlies the despair of old age. Indeed, in perhaps the closest approximation of Model IV that can be found in Western culture, Erikson presents a schema for psychological development across the life span in which the last stage of life involves a resolution of a crisis between the conflicting dimensions of ego integrity and despair.[9] The key psychological issue in old age, then, is whether the old person can look back on his or her life in its totality with a sense of completeness, acceptance, and serenity.

The implications of Model IV for housing for older people are unclear because the model is not yet visible in current society. But it is possible to conjecture that the baby-boom cohort, with its interest in self-improvement and development, will move toward the self-actualization model. Housing might be developed under the concept of a spiritual community, designed to incorporate the collective practice of meditation and other spiritual practices in an effort to develop individual and group consciousness. From the marketing perspective and terminology of Wolfe, "being experiences" involving self-development would be cultivated.[10] In addition, supportive services provided would include diet, exercise, and health promotion and disease prevention activities under a holistic medicine model.[11] The word "spiritual" as it is used here is not to be equated with "religious," but instead with "holistic." The same spiritual technique could be practiced by individuals of many different religious faiths. At the same time, religion would be an important aspect of this holistic view of life and housing for the elderly under Model IV, which could be centered on religious themes as well.[12] Perhaps by the year 2020 an exemplar of housing under Model IV will exist.

THE RESPONSIBILITY OF SOCIETY TO THE ELDERLY

Ethics is the study of morality. Morality comprises rules of conduct about what we ought and ought not do. It also encompasses expectations of character, that is, what sorts of persons we should strive to be. From an ethical perspective, then, public policy has to ask not only what the rules of conduct should be—how society should act, through its governmental agencies—but also what implications public policy has for our character as a people.

A basic question is: What are our responsibilities as a society to the elderly? For example, to what extent should the younger generation be expected to transfer resources to the elderly population? What sort of people should we want to be? Are current public policies consistent with these aspirations?

In responding to these questions, McCullough applied the important ethical principle of justice to the public policy context.[13] The formal definition of justice states that each person should receive what is owed to that person. There are competing theories of how to decide what is owed to someone. A model of merit maintains that people should earn what is owed to them. A model of need states that people who are vulnerable and needy not by choice but by accident of circumstance should, in fairness, have that state of need redressed. A model of choice postulates that a just solution is to let individuals make free marketplace choices and to accept the consequences of those choices. Finally, a model of promoting the general good avers that outcomes should be examined to see how they benefit those who are affected by them. Rawls took the position that any attempt to produce general social benefit should improve the condition of the least well-off first.[14] The impaired and poor elderly are a relevant example.

Most current public policy is made under economic models of choice wherein people are allowed to make their own choices and the marketplace works things out. The belief is that if individuals demonstrate enough initiative, they will not be in need. Because they have a materialistic, quantified character that can be expressed in the dollars-and-cents language of cost-benefit or cost-effectiveness comparisons, economic values tend to dominate public policy debate, including that regarding the elderly. They tend to ignore all perspectives of justice except that of the marketplace.

This situation is inappropriate for several reasons.[15] First, some of the obligations of the younger generation to the elderly generation are based on entitlements. For example, the elderly have contributed to the Social Security program from which they are entitled to receive certain returns. Second, filial responsibility or the obligation of children to care for and meet the needs of their elderly parents is a reasonable societal expectation. All adults have bene-fitted as children from society's structure and programs and they have an obligation to repay this debt to their elders through the transfer of resources to the elderly population. Repayment is not a matter of choice, because one is a child not by choice. The obligation is one of justice. Third, many older persons are vulnerable for reasons not of their choice, but through widowhood, poor health, or inade-quate income. By imposing only a choice theory of justice, one could miss an important reality. Finally, there is a responsibility to remedy a history of injustice. Black and female elderly Americans have a higher rate of impoverishment than white and male elderly Amer-icans, respectively, partially because of historic circumstances that did not allow these groups the same opportunity to save for their old age.

If these additional factors are placed in policy formulation, then economic values cannot be justified as the fundamental ethical consideration and are only one set of values against which other competing values, for example, entitlement and filial responsibility, must be balanced in a complex process. For example, a substantial number of elderly individuals live alone in deteriorating dwellings and are at high risk for physical and functional decline. These individuals more easily could remain in their own homes through the rehabilitation of existing housing stock and through the devel-opment and financing of an array of community-based and in-home care services. These actions clearly would meet the needs of this group and would prevent relocation and institutionalization. We can and should properly value the equal opportunity of elderly individ-uals to live independently in the general community. Moreover, we should not exploit their vulnerability, which stems from circum-stances that are not the result of their own choices. One does not choose the death of a spouse as a means to live alone or choose health problems and frailty. It may well turn out, however, that a combination of home modification/repair and supportive home-delivered services will add to the cost of providing housing and services to the elderly and will not result in a net savings. If one simply held to a fiscal cost-benefit analysis and an economic theory of justice, then one would conclude that there is no obligation to provide such housing assistance and services to the elderly. Alternatively, if one took a far broader view of social justice, it might be obligatory to enact and carry out such public policies.

Issues of intergenerational justice and interdependence also must be considered. The interdependence of the generations means that the broad obligations of the younger to the older generation are not incompatible with economic models of justice, provided that one takes a sufficiently comprehensive and long-term perspective.[16] In this vein, Struyk urged policymakers and housing professionals to see "the big housing picture."[17] For example, the elderly are over-represented in the major cities and within cities are disproportionately concentrated in physically declining neighborhoods. Thus the elderly, with their relatively low rates of home maintenance and repair, are concentrated in neighborhoods with high rates of deterioration and abandonment. It could be argued that housing rehabilitation assistance to elderly homeowners in such neighborhoods represents a poor public investment. However, the low rate at which the elderly change residences often makes them a neighborhood's bulwark against further decline. Public programs to improve the housing of these elderly would not only upgrade their immediate environment and living conditions but also improve the area's housing stock and encourage others in the neighborhood to invest in their own homes. From this longer-term perspective, rehabilitation assistance to these elderly homeowners represents a good public investment.

Chapter 7 of this book underscored the distressingly fragmented, shortsighted, and static nature of most public policy for older adult housing. Public policy has largely ignored the dynamic nature of the older person's fit with the environment and has either lacked a firm value base or has resulted from the unsatisfactory and incomplete resolution of competing value claims. What have been missing are an ethical framework to guide public policy formulation and a sense of the civic virtues and duties of citizens that incorporates the principle of justice.

THE RESPONSIBILITY OF THE FOR-PROFIT SECTOR

If society has obligations in justice to the housing of the elderly that must be incorporated into public policy, what then is the responsibility of the for-profit sector? Traditionally the business of business has been making money without an explicit focus on the public interest. More recently, however, a new sense of corporate responsibility for the public good has developed.[18-21] The corporate culture provides the framework of shared beliefs and values that identifies a group of individuals as a corporation. It is the collective purpose that channels the actions of those individuals, giving the corporate collective a kind of moral agency.[22] Thus, corporations are seen as members of the moral community with responsibilities to all of society and with a broader constituency than stockholders alone.

Bowie outlined three arguments in support of this broad view of corporate responsibility.[23] First, the right to make a profit is not absolute. Business and profit-seeking are already controlled and limited by laws and regulations. However, the law is a minimum standard of what *must* be done. Ethical standards are higher and prescribe what *ought* to be done. For example, a building could be constructed to meet the letter of the law regarding building codes, yet violate the spirit of the law and represent shoddy workmanship. Second, the rights of stockholders are not absolute. The fact that stockholders are the legal owners of a firm does not give them unlimited rights to do what they want with the firm. Just as a landowner cannot denude, strip mine, and pollute a piece of his or her land, neither can stockholders of a firm do anything with their property without regard to the consequences for the public good. In fact, stockholders represent but one player in a corporation. Other stakeholders are the employees, managers, customers, suppliers, and the community in which a company or company facility is located. These other players often have as great a stake in the firm as the stockholders, and the corporate manager has a moral responsibility to them also. Third, businesses, like all citizens, have duties of citizenship to society. Corporations benefit from a host of societal programs and institutions, including family and educational training of workers and the infrastructure of utilities, transportation, and communications. The obligations of justice that apply to individual citizens apply also to corporations.

What must a corporation do to be morally excellent and exhibit an appropriate level of responsibility to the community? First, it must develop a clear set of corporate values and foster an ethical point of view. The corporation must recognize responsibilities to clients, employees, and the community as well as to stockholders. Consultation with the corporation's legal department would be only the first step in determining what is morally right; officers also must develop the capacity to be on the alert for ethical issues and formulate clear strategies and structures within the corporation to make appropriate moral choices.[24] Next, the corporation must enhance and encourage the moral autonomy and excellence of each individual within the corporate culture so that sufficient opportunity is given to personalize the corporate moral objectives within specific areas of responsibility. Finally, the morally excellent corporation must shift the primary motivation for its conduct from a profit to a service orientation.[25] Management should emphasize the production and marketing of quality goods and services that customers truly need, foster a positive working environment for employees, and treat suppliers and contractors fairly and honestly. In doing so, the company will make a profit.

For-profit corporations that provide housing to the elderly need to implement these principles to develop corporate moral excellence. What are some of the implications of moral excellence for these corporations? First, these companies have a responsibility to provide housing that is high-quality in terms of physical structure and workmanship. Second, these companies need to take a longer-term perspective on the impact that the housing will have on the lives of the older residents. Aging in place has serious repercussions for elderly residents as they become older, frailer, and functionally more dependent. Companies have a moral responsibility to think through these issues so that they do not market housing to older adults that is highly inappropriate from a ten- to twenty-year perspective; for example, two-story housing with stairs that cannot be used safely by a mobility-impaired elder. The housing should be designed so that it is an accommodating environment with the potential for supportive services to be added as required and desired. Otherwise, developers may be fulfilling their minimal legal responsibilities of what must be done, but not their ethical responsibilities of what ought to be done. Third, the moral autonomy and excellence of all employees, including on-site managers, should be encouraged within the parameters of the corporate culture.

THE RESPONSIBILITY OF THE NONPROFIT SECTOR

The discussion about the ethical responsibilities of the for-profit sector can be generalized to the nonprofit sector. However, the nonprofit sector ultimately must be held even more accountable for its obligations in justice to further the public good. By accepting an exemption from taxes, each nonprofit organization essentially has entered into a contract with society in which it has agreed to maintain a longer-term perspective and actively work to improve the public good.

Ethical responsibilities of for-profits often are expressed in the negative. Corporations should not pollute the environment or otherwise actively harm society. In contrast, the nonprofit sector is held to a higher standard: Its moral responsibility is to work actively to promote the social good by striving to foster social justice. From a more exacting, Rawlsian definition of justice, it should attempt first to benefit those who are least well off.[26]

Therefore, nonprofit providers of housing to the elderly have all of the responsibilities of the for-profit sector with the additional obligation to more actively work to improve society through housing and housing services and to focus on those elderly individuals who are poor and frail. In a disturbing trend today, some nonprofits, including those in housing, are beginning to act very much like for-profit entities, focusing on market share and upscale clients. From an ethical perspective this is irresponsible and a violation of a nonprofit organization's moral obligation to society.

Management Issues

Each of the four models of aging outlined earlier in this chapter — rejection, social services, participation, and self-actualization — has implications regarding the existence and nature of housing initiatives for the elderly. In addition, the principle of justice calls for administrators to develop systems that enhance the lives of older residents.

Model III, participation, currently is at the forefront of social reform for older adults, with its emphasis on integration of residents into the larger community, societal involvement through meaningful roles, and honoring individual preferences and personal autonomy. This model raises numerous policy issues with ethical dimensions for managers of senior housing. It applies to board and care facilities, congregate housing facilities, CCRCs, and apartment complexes and other naturally occurring retirement communities with a high percentage of older residents.

PROPERTY MANAGER VERSUS CASE MANAGER

Property managers for senior housing deal with day-to-day operations. Responsibilities include renting up vacant units, maintaining waiting lists, overseeing lease or contractual compliance, supervising maintenance and administrative personnel, doing governmental regulatory paperwork, preparing operating budgets, resolving tenant issues, and keeping the owner/sponsor informed of the building's status and needs.[27] In congregate housing and CCRCs, property managers deal with residents, but often not explicitly for supportive services. Larger facilities often have an on-site service coordinator to address service or case management dimensions. Core case management activities include: working with the housing owner/sponsor and property manager to ensure that the facility's physical aspects reflect the residents' needs; outreach efforts to identify potential residents; screening of tenant applications to assure eligibility and need for the housing; interviewing and intake/selection of applicants; assessing individual resident service needs; developing and implementing a supportive service plan for each resident; coordinating and monitoring the delivery of these supportive services; periodically reassessing residents' service needs; developing and executing appropriate termination procedures; and integrating the facility into the local community.[28] The full-time or part-time service coordinator also handles information and referral and counseling.

Many apartment houses and public housing facilities, however, have one on-site manager, a property manager. As residents age in place, the changing profile of the resident population and the presence or absence of needed services have direct implications for these managers, most of whom are not trained to address the social and health needs of older people.[29] These professionals have no formal responsibility for case management, but they select and terminate residents. Moreover, tenants may seek out the manager as an information and referral source for supportive services or for counseling on personal matters. In addition, if elderly tenants need support services and are not getting them, a crisis situation may occur that the manager must resolve. For example, residents may lie undiscovered in their apartments after falling ill. An isolated and depressed tenant may develop disruptive alcohol or drug abuse problems. The question is not whether managers should take on a case management role, but how they can improve their performance in that role or delegate aspects of it to other appropriately trained professionals.

A recent survey of 278 Wisconsin housing managers for older people indicated that many managers experience anxiety about the case management dimensions of their jobs, including concerns about the residents' health, ability to care for themselves, social isolation, falls and safety, and confusion.[30] Another study reported that housing administrators consistently judged fewer tenants as needing services than did the tenants themselves or social service professionals.[31] Managers need training in the human service aspects of their jobs so that they are able to recognize tenant needs more readily. It is not necessary for each housing manager to become a skilled case manager, but at the very least he or she should be aware of available community resources and develop mechanisms to link residents with those resources as needed.

FORMAL CONTRACTS

Contracts with residents are a major management issue. Although few formal analyses of housing contracts exist, two types of housing have been examined: continuing care retirement communities (CCRCs) and nursing homes.

CCRC contracts are ethically complex because they involve large sums of money, a variety of services, and an explicit focus on long-term accommodating environments. Guidelines for the regulation of CCRCs developed by the American Association of Homes for the Aging focus largely on legal and ethical concerns regarding the refund and fiduciary management of entry fees.[32] The CCRC contract should specify clearly all financial arrangements, including conditions for entry fee refund and for contract cancellation, all services provided to the resident without additional charge, and services available at additional cost. The basis and procedure for changes in the fee structure should also be specified, including the consequences of a resident's marrying or permanently moving to a personal care unit or nursing home bed while at the facility.

CCRC contracts also should clearly specify the responsibility of the CCRC to resume services following care in another facility, conditions under which a resident may be dismissed or discharged, and the conditions under which a resident may be transferred to another living unit or level of care. The CCRC's annual statement should disclose significant information including ownership and control, conflict of interest, relationships with other organizations, and finances. Also, CCRC advertising should not misrepresent the relationship that the community has to a respected community organization such as a church or imply another organization's financial responsibility toward the CCRC that does not actually exist. Conversely, organizational ties that do exist should be explicitly acknowledged.

A legal and ethical analysis by Ambrogi of a stratified random sample of California nursing home admission agreements offers some findings and recommendations that are generalizable to other housing agreements.[33] A primary consideration in any consumer contract is its readability and comprehension by the consumer. A basic principle of contract law is that a contract should be knowingly and voluntarily entered into. Most of the agreements in the Ambrogi sample had features that obscured the meaning of the contract, including language incomprehensible to nonattorneys, small print size, colored paper, noncontrasting ink, and provisions written on both sides of thin paper. It was recommended that agreements should be printed in black type of not less than twelve-point size on one side of plain white paper of not less than twenty-pound bond. The contract should be written in clear, coherent, and unambiguous everyday language.

Nearly all of the agreements in the Ambrogi sample also contained misleading, illegal, or unenforceable clauses, of which the facility was or should have been aware. For example, about 25 percent of the agreements in the contained clauses seeking to immunize the facility from liability for "acts or omissions" that by law were the facility's responsibility. Although such clauses are unenforceable, they can misinform or intimidate residents and discourage them from pursuing a valid claim against the facility. Other personal rights often violated in the examined agreements included confidentiality of—and residents' access to—records, the right to receive visitors of all ages at reasonable times, privacy with respect to photographs taken by the facility for publicity purposes, the use of appliances and personal furnishings, and the establishment of grievance and appeal procedures for violations of facility rules.

INFORMAL CONTRACTS

Upon admission to a housing facility, the older resident enters into an informal as well as a formal contract with the management regarding rules and regulations and the delegation of decisions to management. The informal contract often plays a larger role in the day-to-day life of the resident. Problems may arise because the "clauses" of the informal contract have not been mutually agreed upon and made explicit. Collopy made a useful and relevant distinction between direct and delegated autonomy in the lives of older adults.[34] Direct autonomy is a matter of deciding or acting on one's own as a self-sufficient agent. In delegated autonomy, by contrast, the individual gives authority to others to decide and act for him and freely accepts these decisions and activities of others. As a practical matter, all of us delegate large sections of authority over our lives to others as part of living within the larger society and to save time. For example, most individuals freely give to others the responsibility for calculating and deducting payroll taxes, accept decisions about which side of the road to drive on, and authorize others to make decisions for them concerning the investment and management of stock portfolios.

The transference of decision-making authority to others has considerable potential for misunderstanding. In senior housing, residents and management may not perceive direct and delegated autonomy in the same way. For example, sexual liaisons between older unmarried residents in board and care facilities sometimes are actively discouraged or forbidden by the manager, to the anger and dismay of the residents involved: Who put the manager in charge of the residents' sex lives? Less dramatically, a congregate housing facility may have requirements about the daily number of congregate meals that must be attended by residents and the seating of residents at those meals. If these expectations were not communicated explicitly as part of the admission process, or if decisions were reached unilaterally without resident involvement, then the meal requirements may be the object of much dissatisfaction and resistance. Conversely, residents of a congregate housing facility may have strong expectations about a high level of personal involvement and decision-making by on-site management staff in their personal lives and problems, expectations that may not be shared by staff members. Again, an explicit mapping of direct and delegated autonomy may prevent this type of misunderstanding.

A number of key questions highlight the conflicts of direct and delegated autonomy.[35] Do elderly residents and managers share common expectations about what decisions and activities will remain under the direct autonomy of the residents? Do the older residents know and accept the conditions and times when others will decide or act for them? Do managers have the same understanding? Is the potential for conflict in these areas openly admitted and examined? Is the delegation of authority tacit or is it negotiated mutually by residents and management? Even if all these questions are dealt with in an ethically satisfactory manner, the issue of informal contracts for housing for the elderly is not resolved entirely. As residents age in place and become increasingly frail and dependent, and their capacity for direct autonomy declines, these delineations of direct and delegated autonomy will have to be periodically renegotiated and redrawn. This requires periodic functional and needs assessments of residents and the development of a system for renegotiating the informal contracts.

ADMISSION DECISIONS

Admission decisions are a major management concern in housing that involves shared space and activities. Important features in the successful selection of residents include a clear definition of the population to be served, the use of referrals from appropriate sources, and careful screening of prospective residents to assess their service needs.[36] A multidisciplinary assessment team that meets regularly can be used to assist on-site managers in the assessment and selection process. Community social service agencies should be represented on this assessment team as well as mental health and home health care providers and other local agencies that offer services needed by residents. Residents also should be represented. The service coordinator, if there is one, or the housing manager should lead the assessment team. The use of such a team assures a diversity of perspectives in admission decisions, increases the probability that appropriate decisions will be made, avoids the situation of tough decisions being solely the responsibility of the manager, and involves current residents in important decisions affecting their community.

Criteria must be developed for determining an applicant's suitability for a facility based on functional capacity, social need, relevant asset and income limits, and age. These criteria should be clearly stated in any promotional materials for the facility and communicated to referral sources.

In congregate settings, selection should be based on these criteria and the likelihood that the resident will remain in the facility for a reasonable period of time barring unexpected acute illness. Congregate residents generally must be capable of independent living, but may require one or more supportive services to maintain high-quality living conditions. Applicants who require maximum assistance with activities of daily living or who require constant supervision are not appropriate.[37] The dilemma for the congregate housing manager and assessment team is to balance the needs of the marginally independent individual applicant against the needs of the overall resident community. Both the assessment team and the applicant need to face some difficult questions and respond honestly.

Board and care facilities offer more services and serve a frailer resident population than congregate facilities. Therefore, the use of a professional assessment team and the matching of the applicant's needs with the available service package is even more critical.

The admission process for all facilities should include a time when the resident and manager sit down and read the housing contract, discuss it, answer questions, and sign it. For some residents the time of admission is fraught with the confusion and stress of relocation and loss of home; it is important that documents not be signed without the full informed consent of the resident.[38] There also should be an open discussion of relevant informal contracts regarding everyday life at the facility. In addition, a tour of the facility or a weekend trial visit for prospective residents would be helpful. These actions uphold the autonomy of the resident, lessen resident ambiguity and anxiety about the clauses and rules of formal and informal contracts, and avoid misunderstandings that result in later problems.

TERMINATION DECISIONS

Termination decisions regarding residents can be particularly important and difficult from an ethical perspective. Can the facility continue to support the needs of an individual resident without ignoring or harming the quality of life of other residents? How is management's responsibility to the individual resident balanced against its responsibility to the entire community of residents? Can management accept the moral responsibility for prolonging the stay of a resident who is at the margins of support of the facility's service package, thus risking harmful consequences for that resident?

The assessment team used for resident selection also should be used for termination so that decisions are arrived at from multiple professional and resident perspectives. The involvement of secretaries and maintenance personnel also might be encouraged. These staff members are in daily contact with residents and may be able to contribute important information and insights. In addition, other professionals might be consulted as needed, including private physicians, psychiatric social workers, and county conservators. In all cases, the confidentiality of the residents under consideration must be maintained.

In a board and care facility termination issues are difficult because they often occur as the result of acute illness or extreme fragility, when the resident is particularly vulnerable. Because such a facility is intended to be an alternative to nursing home placement, it is important that the manager make every effort to continue to support the resident. These facilities, however, do not have the intensive service capabilities of nursing homes and hospitals, and the manager has a moral responsibility to match the seriously ill or frail resident with one of these more appropriate settings. Moreover, the shared environment of board and cares can mean that serious health or behavior problems of a resident can disrupt or even endanger other residents.[39] In these instances the manager has to consider the legal and ethical obligations to the resident community.

In congregate housing facilities, termination issues usually center on behavioral and health problems and the definition of "independent living." Reasons for termination most frequently given by surveyed on-site and management staff included: persistent resident drinking or other substance abuse problems and an unwillingness to seek or accept treatment; accident problems with safety considerations for the tenant and other residents; major physical health problems requiring professional care and daily supervision not available at the facility; refusal to accept supportive services when clearly needed; substantial inability to live cooperatively and in common with other residents; serious psychological problems; serious confusion; senility; incontinence; and wheelchair confinement.[40] Some of these reasons involve safety and situations that cannot be resolved through traditional community services. Other problems such as incontinence or wheelchair use may be unacceptable to management because they present an unwanted frail image. The value structure underlying termination decisions, however, should not be formed from a rejection model of aging.

In all facilities, counseling, discussion, and negotiation with the resident under consideration for termination are extremely important. To the extent possible, the resident should be involved in the decision; termination should not result from a manager's unilateral directive. Residency termination policies should be provided in the formal contracts or leases so that the informed consent of residents is upheld and both residents and their families know what to expect. The conditions for termination should be stated as clearly as possible, but with enough flexibility built in so that situations still can be dealt with on a case-by-case basis. Residents and their families need specificity and clarity sufficient to plan ahead for the possibility of a future move.[41, 42]

The periodic assessment of a resident's functional level, medical history, and receipt of formal services could help to identify person-environment mismatches, provide residents with the services needed, and avoid termination decisions made in a crisis environment. A factor that clearly can complicate the termination process for congregate housing managers, however, is the frequent lack of alternative housing options other than inappropriate nursing home placement.

Sheehan and Wisensale found that the family role in providing assistance to public housing residents was an extremely important factor in influencing management decisions about tenants' continued residence.[43] Frail tenants with supportive services provided by families and community agencies frequently were allowed to remain in apartment units, but frail tenants without such support were required to move out. Without specific provisions to assure support services in senior housing, residents without families or financial means will be particularly vulnerable to termination. This situation violates the ethical obligations of housing managers/ sponsors and society to these vulnerable elderly.

THE MANAGER AS ADVOCATE

The housing manager's underlying conception of resident autonomy within a participation model of aging shapes definition of professional roles and the manner in which admission and termination procedures are developed and implemented. Collopy's distinction between negative and positive autonomy is illuminating here.[44] The manager who holds a notion of negative autonomy refuses to interfere in a resident's self-determination. The manager essentially says, "I respect the autonomy of this resident so much that I will leave her alone so that she is free to make any decision that she chooses as long as she doesn't violate her housing contract. She is an adult and doesn't need any meddling from me in any way." This manager primarily is a property manager. On the other hand, the manager who holds a positive notion of autonomy steps forward and provides resources for the enhancement of resident autonomy. This manager says, "I respect the autonomy of this resident so much that I will do everything within my ability to empower and support her in fulfilling her potential within this setting so that she can be as autonomous as possible." This manager assumes case management responsibilities and is an advocate for the resident.

The danger of a negative sense of autonomy within the senior housing setting is that it quickly reverts to the characteristics of either a rejection or a social services model of aging as the resident ages in place. In the former case the resident is treated as an autonomous consumer who freely chooses a particular housing setting. As the resident ages and becomes frailer, she is left alone with no supportive services and effectively is abandoned so that she must move from the facility. In the latter instance services are provided, but in a custodial way that leads to learned helplessness. There is no sense of obligation to empower the resident to become a participating member of the community in a meaningful way.[45]

The housing manager who is an advocate for residents also faces ethical issues. Given limited resources and time, housing managers cannot be responsible for open-ended obligations to residents. Recognition of autonomy may present ever-expanding opportunities in the life of the resident, but it should not exact limitless obligations on others. Also, managers must be careful not to interfere with the choice and behavior of residents in the name of "enhancing" their autonomy and "empowering" them. This heavy-handed approach to positive autonomy would smack of the paternalism of a social services model of aging.

ETHICAL PROBLEMS INVOLVING THE FAMILY

Senior housing residents have been found to maintain intense relationships with their children.[46] The family often provides a powerful support network. Planners of housing services should consider developing social services geared to relatives of residents that maintain and strengthen stable family relations and support networks for functionally impaired residents.

Efforts to use the family support network, however, beg a larger ethical question facing the housing manager.[47] Who is the client—the resident or the family? The principle of respect for autonomy emphasizes the obligation to consider the resident as the client. The family should be involved as much as possible in all aspects of housing services for the older resident, but only with the consent of the resident. The preferences of the resident must be upheld regarding the degree of decision-making authority delegated to the family. The issue can become more difficult for the manager when the family is paying part or all of the bill or as the resident becomes increasingly impaired.

It seems right that the problems of residents should fall first to family members, not housing managers. The family members have benefited from the care and support of the older person in the past, and they have a moral obligation to provide some care in return. However, if the family in effect abandons the older relative or if there is no family, the manager has a moral obligation to do all that needs to be done in resolving any problems and participating in decision-making about the resident's status. In a sense, the manager becomes a surrogate family member.

RESIDENT COMPETENCY ISSUES

A very complicated and troubling issue for on-site managers is declining or fluctuating competency of residents. When does the resident begin to pose a threat to her own safety and to others through actions that are the result of declining competency? What should the manager do in response to this situation? How does the manager balance the desire to do good for the resident against obligations to respect the resident's autonomy, and obligations to other residents?

Competency is a legal term implying formal determination of individual competency or incompetency by a court. A variety of standards have been proposed for the determination of competency with no clear consensus emerging as to the best one.[48] In most states, the term "competency" implies an either-or situation in which an individual is either competent or incompetent. A more appropriate term may be "decisional capacity," which implies a continuum of abilities.

For some older people capacity fluctuates according to the time of day, setting, mood, physiological health, reaction to pre-scribed and nonprescribed drugs (including drug interactions), and clinical depression.[49] Relocation to new housing or the loss of a loved one also can have an adverse impact on capacity. What appears to be irreversible declining capacity may in fact be the result of a highly reversible condition. Therefore, before a resident is labeled and treated as incapacitated, it is important that she receive a thorough physical and psychological assessment.

When a resident declines in capacity, it is important for the manager to understand that incapacity on one dimension does not imply incapacity on all dimensions. For example, a resident may not have the capacity to drive a car or balance a checkbook but nevertheless function well on all other aspects of residential living. It is critical for the manager to be aware of supportive community services, including protective services, available to residents, and to assist residents to obtain these services. For example, a resident with no family who has great difficulty managing her financial affairs could benefit from the services of a representative payee who is delegated the authority to handle the resident's financial affairs. This would allow the resident to remain in the residential setting. Guardianship should be the intervention of last resort in any situation involving resident capacity, because court determination of incompetency and the appointment of a legal guardian result in the ultimate loss of autonomy, with the resident regressing to the legal status of a five-year-old.[50]

When serious illness strikes, the older person may be unable to make decisions, but the values and preferences built up over a lifetime might indicate the resident's preferences in treatment decisions. Efforts are needed to identify the preferences of residents regarding a variety of issues, so that their autonomy can still be upheld when impairment to decisional capacity arises.[51] Whenever possible and with the consent of the resident, family members should be encouraged to take an active role in helping residents to articulate values and discuss treatment and care preferences. The establishment of a value history and the formulation of advanced directives such as living wills and durable powers of attorney for health care should be part of standard admission and orientation procedures for all residential facilities for older adults.

RESPONSIBILITIES OF RESIDENTS

What are the responsibilities of residents, both to management and to other residents? Jameton argues that responsibility is part of autonomy and a limiting feature to it.[52] All people have obligations as an expression of human dignity and membership in the community. The commitment of individuals to their obligations is a central feature of their individual values and autonomy. From the perspective of a participation model of aging, it is important that residents of senior housing clarify their responsibilities in cooperation with managers and other residents and receive assistance in meeting the responsibilities that they assume.

The responsibilities of residents to managers include upholding the terms of formal leases or contracts such as timely payment of rents or fees. Although a manager has a responsibility to make as explicit as possible the informal contracts associated with the facility at the time of the resident's admission, the resident has a responsibility to learn the rules and culture of the facility. Residents and managers should treat each other with respect and courtesy. Where the design and operation of a facility is based on a participation model of aging, residents have a responsibility to involve themselves in the governance and operation of a facility through appropriate participatory mechanisms.

Residents may assume a number of responsibilities to other residents, including assisting with access to care, giving advice, helping with activities of daily living, and serving on residents' councils. In fact, one of the presumed benefits of senior housing is that it provides increased opportunities for social interaction and mutual support among residents. Several studies, however, failed to document high levels of such interaction and support, particularly among more impaired residents.[53-55] Informal support among residents becomes critical as residents age in place, because such help may mean the difference between residency continuation or termination for a seriously impaired individual. Attempts to enhance such informal supports must consider the perspective of both the impaired and the healthier, more independent older resident.[56] Frail residents may choose to withdraw from social relationships and informal supports because they wish to avoid being labeled as "poor dears" with subsequent loss of integrity and autonomy. Healthy and independent residents may try to limit their involvement with frailer residents because they wish to conserve physical strength and engage in only truly reciprocal relationships. Managers should not assume that the mere existence of senior housing will guarantee helping relationships among neighbors. But it is important for managers to support and enhance such relationships.

Because responsibility expresses the bonds of human relationships, it is essentially a communitarian notion. Responsibility is an extremely important concept in residential environments within a participation model of aging. Together with the concept of autonomy, it forms the basis for morally principled community.[57]

A Research and Training Agenda

Research that is useful to the formulation, consideration, and resolution of value and ethical considerations is at a rudimentary stage. Research is needed on the preferences of older adults regarding the design, operation, and management of housing. The work of Moos and his colleagues provides a laudatory example.[58, 59] Knowledge of preferences could be used by developers, planners, and managers to shape multiple and distinct buyer/renter profiles and to develop housing and systems that truly meet the desires and needs of older residents.

Also helpful would be research paralleling Ambrogi's analysis of nursing home admission agreements, which critically examined the legal and ethical dimensions of leases and formal contracts from various forms of senior housing.[60] Are the legal rights and autonomy of older residents abridged and compromised in these contracts? Older adults entering board and care facilities are particularly vulnerable in the admission process because they generally are frail and functionally dependent.

A variety of needs for ethical training and guidelines exist. Education on ethical issues would enable housing policymakers to better fulfill society's obligations to social justice. Similarly, trustees and officers of for-profit and nonprofit providers of senior housing could benefit from ethical guidelines and training. Housing managers badly need good training programs and materials that provide information on the aging process, specific service needs of older adults, and existing community resources to call on for help in meeting residents' supportive service needs. Useful existing materials include a series of primers for senior housing managers recently developed by the Center for Health Services at the University of Wisconsin–Madison that examines a variety of resident health issues,[61] and a series of booklets on elderly housing published by the Council of State Housing Agencies and the National Association of State Units on Aging.[62] On-site managers also require guidelines and training for each of the microlevel on-site management issues discussed in this chapter: formal and informal contracts; case management and advocate roles and conflicts; admission and termination decisions; capacity issues; and enhancement of residents' abilities to assume responsibilities and create a strong sense of community.

Residents and their families also could benefit from information on the aging process and services available. Seltzer and her colleagues, for example, developed and tested a case management training program for family members of older adults. This program involved the collaboration of family and social worker on the development of a case management service plan for the older person, information on community resources and entitlements, and regular personal or telephone contact between the social worker and the family member.[63] Family members were not asked to deliver additional services but rather to increase their involvement in service coordination. Training resulted in those family members performing a significantly greater number of case management tasks for older relatives than family members in a control group. The investigators concluded that the training program should also be offered to the older adults themselves so that they can become case management partners.

All guidelines developed should be evaluated carefully as to their relevance and effectiveness. Given the complexity of ethical issues in residential environments for the elderly, guidelines and training materials should use descriptive and case study, rather than "cookbook" approaches. Rather than offer highly specific prescriptive answers, such materials should outline a process that can be adapted to a variety of individual cases and help professionals to ask the right questions.

Conclusion

At first blush, it may seem paralyzing to consider each of the value and ethical issues that arise in housing policy for the elderly. However, awareness and discussion of these issues often will enhance the satisfaction of both professionals and residents by clarifying issues and identifying options. There are many difficult obligations to fulfill and decisions to make in developing and managing senior housing as well as in living in these environments. Making the implicit ethical issues and underlying values explicit will improve the quality of decisions and services and illuminate a clearer picture of the higher goals that are possible for policymakers, developers, professionals, and residents.

Notes

1. Moody, H.R. "Philosophical presuppositions of education for old age." *Educational Gerontology,* 1:1–16, 1976.

2. Lawton, M.P., M. Greenbaum, and B. Liebowitz. "The lifespan of housing environments for the aging. *The Gerontologist,* 20:56–64, 1980.

3. Lawton, et al. "Lifespan."

4. Krause, N. "Understanding the stress process: Linking social support with locus of control beliefs." *Journal of Gerontology,* 42, 589–93, 1987.

5. Cohen, E.S. "The elderly mystique: Constraints on the autonomy of the elderly with disabilities." *The Gerontologist,* 28, Supp.:24–31, 1988.

6. Commission on the Elderly. *The Older Person and the Parish.* Albany, N.Y.: New York State Catholic Conference, 1984.

7. Cranz, G. "Evaluating the physical environment: Conclusions from eight housing projects." In V. Regnier and J. Pynoos (Eds.), *Housing the Aged.* New York: Elsevier, 1987, pp. 81–104.

8. Regnier, V., and L.E. Gelwicks. "Preferred supportive services for middle to higher income retirement housing." *The Gerontologist,* 21:54–58, 1981.

9. Erikson, E. "Eight ages of man." In E. Erikson (Ed.), *Childhood and Society.* New York: Norton, 1963.

10. Wolfe, D.B. "A new model for marketing health care and senior housing services." *Journal of Health Care Marketing,* 8:2–4, 1988.

11. Chopra, D. *Creating Health.* Boston: Houghton Mifflin, 1987.
    Chopra, D. *Return of the Rishi.* Boston: Houghton Mifflin, 1988.

12. Bishops of the State of New York. *A Treasure to the Church.* Albany, N.Y.: New York State Catholic Conference, 1987.

13. McCullough, L. "Ethics and aging: Public policy dilemmas." Paper presented at the 36th Annual Conference of the Council on Foundations, Washington, D.C., April 1985.

14. Rawls, J. *A Theory of Justice.* Cambridge: Harvard University Press, 1971.

15. McCullough, "Ethics and aging."

16. Kingson, E.R., B.A. Hirshorn, and J.M. Cornman. *The Ties That Bind.* Washington, D.C.: Seven Locks Press, 1986.

17. Struyk, R.J. "The big housing picture." *Generations,* IX:18–20, 1985.

18. Bowie, N. "Corporate management: Doing good and doing well." *Hastings Center Report,* Supp. 17:17–18, 1987.

19. Newton, L.H. "The internal morality of the corporation." *Journal of Business Ethics,* 5:248–58, 1986.

20. Hoffman, W.M. "What is necessary for corporate moral excellence?" *Journal of Business Ethics,* 5:233–42, 1986.

21. Fahey, C. "Corporate ethical decision making in health care institutions." *Hospital Administration Currents,* 31:19–26, 1987.

22. Hoffman, "Corporate moral excellence."

23. Bowie, "Corporate management."

24. Hoffman, "Corporate moral excellence."

25. Bowie, "Corporate management."

26. *Justice.*

27. Mollica, R., and B. Ryther. *Congregate Housing.* Washington, D.C.: Council of State Housing Agencies and the National Association of State Units on Aging, 1987.

28. Ibid.

29. Ryther, B. *Aging in Place . . . Training for Managers.* Washington, D.C.: Council of State Housing Agencies and the National Association of State Units on Aging, 1987.

30. Bowers, B. "A profile of Wisconsin housing managers and their perceived needs." Paper presented at the 40th Annual Scientific Meeting of the Gerontological Society of America, Washington, D.C., November 1987.

31. Lawton, M.P., M. Moss, and M. Grimes. "The changing service needs of older tenants in planned housing." *The Gerontologist,* 25:258–64, 1985.

32. American Association of Homes for the Aging. *Guidelines for Regulation of Continuing Care Retirement Communities.* Washington, D.C.: American Association of Homes for the Aging, 1987.

33. Ambrogi, D.M., and F. Leonard. "The impact of nursing home admission agreements on resident autonomy." *The Gerontologist,* 28, Supp.:82–89, 1988.

34. Collopy, B.J. "Autonomy in long-term care: Some crucial distinctions." *The Gerontologist,* 28, Supp.:10–17, 1988.

35. Collopy, B.J. "The conceptually problematic status of autonomy." Unpublished monograph, 1986.

36. Ryther, B. *Board and Care Homes.* Washington, D.C.: Council of State Housing Agencies and the National Association of State Units on Aging, 1987.

37. Mollica and Ryther, *Congregate Housing.*

38. Ambrogi and Leonard, "Admission agreements."

39. Ryther, *Training for Managers.*

40. Bernstein, J. "Who leaves—who stays: Residency policy in housing for the elderly." *The Gerontologist,* 22:305–13, 1982.

41. Ibid.

42. Sheehan, N.W. "Aging of tenants: Termination policy in public sector housing." *The Gerontologist,* 26:505–9, 1986.

43. Sheehan, N.W., and S. Wisensale. "Discharge policies in senior housing." Paper presented at the 40th Annual Scientific Meeting of the Gerontological Society of America, Washington, D.C., 1987.

44. Collopy, "Status of autonomy."

45. Cohen, "Elderly mystique."

46. Kaye, L.W., and A. Monk. "Patterns of social network reciprocity in elder congregate housing. Paper presented at the 40th Annual Scientific Meeting of the Gerontological Society of America, Washington, D.C., 1987.

47. Seltzer, M.M., J. Ivry, and L.C. Litchfield. "Family members as case managers: Partnership between the formal and informal support networks." *The Gerontologist,* 27:722–28, 1987.

48. Stanley, B., M. Stanley, J. Guido, and L. Garvin. "The functional competency of elderly at risk." *The Gerontologist,* 28, Supp.:53–58, 1988.

49. Caplan, A.L. "Let wisdom find a way." *Generations,* X:10–14, 1985.

50. Iris, M.A. "Guardianship and the elderly: A multiperspective view of the decisionmaking process." *The Gerontologist,* 28, Supp.:39–45, 1988.

51. Caplan, "Wisdom."

52. Jameton, A. "In the borderlands of autonomy: Responsibility in long-term-care facilities." *The Gerontologist,* 28, Supp.:18–23, 1988.

53. Ehrlich, P., I. Ehrlich, and P. Woehlke. "Congregate housing for the elderly: Thirteen years later." *The Gerontologist,* 22:399–403, 1982.

54. Stephens, M.A.P., and M.D. Bernstein. "Social support and well-being among residents of planned housing." *The Gerontologist,* 24:144–48, 1984.

55. Sheehan, N.W. "Informal support among the elderly in public senior housing." *The Gerontologist,* 26:171–75, 1986.

56. Ibid.

57. Jameton, "Borderlands of autonomy."

58. Brennan, P.L., R.H. Moos, and S. Lemke. "Preferences of older adults and experts for physical and architectural features of group living facilities." *The Gerontologist,* 28:84–90, 1988.

59. Moos, R.H., S. Lemke, and T.G. David. "Priorities for design and management in residential settings for the elderly." In V. Regnier and J. Pynoos (Eds.), *Housing the Aged.* New York: Elsevier, 1987, pp. 179–205.

60. Ambrogi and Leonard, "Admission agreements."

61. Center for Health Services. *Health Issues for Housing Managers.* Madison, Wis.: Center for Health Sciences, University of Wisconsin, 1987.

62. Council of State Housing Agencies and the National Association of State Units on Aging. *State Initiatives in Elderly Housing: A Series of Models.* Washington, D.C.: CSHA and NASUA, 1987.

63. Seltzer, et al., "Family members."

CHAPTER TEN

Designing a Humane Environment for the Frail Elderly

LEON A. PASTALAN

N*ot too long ago,* four federal agencies—the Department of Health and Human Services, the Administration on Aging, the Department of Housing and Urban Development, and the Department of Agriculture—entered into an unusual agreement for the' purpose of improving the design of facilities for the elderly so that older people may live with dignity in environments that take their needs into consideration.[1] Although this initiative may not itself produce any major innovations, particularly since no funds were allocated for such improvements, it does evidence increasing public recognition of the special needs of elderly persons in the design of their environment.

No matter where an elderly person lives, be it at home, in an extended-care facility, or temporarily in an acute-care hospital, the physical environment should maximize the person's independence, choices, opportunities for social interaction, privacy, safety, and security.[2] We must be sensitive to the interplay of a whole array of factors in the person-environment interaction, such as: (1) reduced physical activity and autonomic nervous system dysfunction and ambient temperature (sedentary elderly people generally require a higher ambient temperature to avoid hypothermia); (2) the "senile gait" and other mobility problems and barriers to accessibility to

273

buildings and to destinations within buildings (walls, stairs, elevators, curbs, uneven sidewalks, and so on); (3) visual impairment and legibility factors within buildings (room numbers, signs, arrows, lighting, colors, and textures); (4) cognitive disorders and orientation to spaces regarding their order and predictability (that is, ease of finding desired destinations); and (5) increased physical vulnerability and the need for a building secure enough to keep out intruders or uninvited visitors.[3]

Design goes beyond the mere physical dimensions of an appropriately configured and appointed space. It has also much to do with those more elusive qualities of autonomy, privacy, environmental mastery, and sense of place. These qualities do not flow automatically from well-designed spaces, but depend greatly on administration and staff. The attitude of staff and how it manages the delicate balance between residents' needs and the delivery of services can to a great extent determine the quality of life of those residents.

This chapter examines some important aspects of environmental design and related management and quality of life issues as they pertain to the housing environment.

Design Issues

The first design issue concerns the quality of the physical elements of the environment, such as temperature-humidity levels, lighting, and acoustics. It has been demonstrated, for example, that certain temperature-humidity levels have a health impact. When humidity levels are below 30 percent, as frequently happens in the winter when buildings are heated, there is a marked increase in the incidence of upper respiratory illnesses. This is a good example of how good design and management sensitivity can mean better health for the residents. By closely monitoring humidity levels management can make adjustments as called for in an accommodating environment.

Adequate lighting levels for activities of daily living must be part of the overall design for a building. It is known, for instance, that a lighting level necessary to perform a given task doubles approximately every thirteen years after the age of twenty-five.

Designers must be aware of the latest research on lighting arrangements and standards for older persons, and a knowledgeable staff must see to it that appropriate levels are actually used by replacing burned-out lightbulbs, replacing fixtures with those having the same capacity, and matching activities and appropriate lighting levels.

Acoustics is another area that requires informed design decisions. Background noise from air conditioners, appliances, television, and so on interferes with conversations and other forms of social interaction. Since presbycusis (loss of hearing of high-frequency sounds and decibel loss) is a common age-specific hearing change attending the elderly, it is important to specify the correct materials and surface treatments to better support activities of daily living. The primary design concept here is to eliminate noise and accentuate meaningful sounds.

Accessibility to buildings and locations within buildings must be assured for optimum use of buildings and participation in programs and activities. Parking areas and drop-off points should be barrier-free and as close by as possible. Connections between buildings should be covered and wheelchair-accessible to facilitate visits with neighbors and participation in activities located beyond immediate living areas. And accessibility within a building to all the important activity areas such as dining, therapy, and multiple-use spaces should be incorporated in the design.

With increasing problems of agility and balance, easy access between different areas in the living unit becomes more important for older persons. Areas difficult to reach not only create inconvenience but also endanger residents' safety and well-being. However, easy physical access must not be achieved at the expense of visual privacy in areas such as bedrooms and bathrooms. To maintain their dignity with visitors, residents need to control visual access to areas where the more private activities such as personal hygiene and sleeping take place. As a result, careful consideration must be given to minimizing physical distance and barriers between public and private areas in the unit while maximizing visual privacy.

Visual impairments among the elderly are common, and among the frail elderly, even more common. Frequent difficulties encountered are glare from uncontrolled natural light and unbalanced artificial light sources; lack of contrast between figure and ground; color changes; and limited depth perception. Design solutions must include control of glare yet provide sufficient light. They must provide strong contrast between lettering and background—preferably highly reflective lettering on a darker, more absorptive background; avoid blue and green colors in public areas as well as combinations of greens and blues on adjoining surfaces such as walls and floors; cue stairs and other changes in walking surfaces to help overcome problems of depth perception.

Order and predictability of residential spaces to make it easier to find desired destinations is important for frail elderly persons, particularly in larger, more complex living arrangements. In design terms, the goal is to organize spaces for their predictive value. The idea is that, in general, a space should have a single and unambiguous use. The various spaces should be cued with landmarks that act as focal points for functionally different areas. For example, surfaces can be color-coded to visually signal functionally different spaces and, similarly, they can be textured for the tactile sense. The aim is to load the spaces with sensory cues so that they more effectively serve as points of reference and avoid ambiguous messages.

Safety and security always have high priority in living arrangements for the elderly. A few of the many safety elements needed in the residential environment are appliances that can be operated easily and safely; stairways that are adequately lighted and have secure handrails; stairs that are appropriately cued; and safe and convenient bathing equipment and nonskid floor surfaces in the bathroom. The building must have reliable locks and bolts, and whenever possible twenty-four-hour-a-day security personnel should be available along with an emergency system for each unit so that assistance can be summoned when needed.

Storage and display space also are important design considerations. Older persons over their lifetime typically have accumulated many objects that reflect personal tastes and life-styles. Some objects are still used, if only occasionally, and some are associated with past events, persons, or periods in a long life. As older persons increasingly tend to reminisce, they place great value on these belongings and do not want to part with them. As a result, they need areas in the living unit to display as well as store their possessions. These items range from plants and photographs to suitcases and spare chairs and require a wide variety of display and storage areas. Problems of mobility and agility suggest that stored items be easily accessible and located closest to the area of their use.

Outdoor extensions of the living unit are a very positive feature and should be part of the overall design. Many older persons, either by choice or physical limitation, spend most of their time in their living units. With such a restricted home range, outdoor extensions of the private unit take on added importance. They provide a change of environment close at hand, an area to grow flowers and personalize, and they can perceptually increase the size of a living space. Outdoor extensions provide secure and protected environments for casual socializing with others. As a result of all these factors, outdoor extensions such as patios and balconies are highly desirable. When provided they must meet residents' needs for privacy, yet not compromise residents' views of pathways and opportunities to socialize.

There is also a need to design larger social spaces where residents with limited energies and capacities can still meet and make new friends. Older residents often have no job or immediate family to draw them into active community participation. As these former group ties weaken, older persons become increasingly dependent on people in their residential environment for social support and friendship. Older residents also often find it difficult to go out of their way to make friends. For these reasons older residents would benefit from situations that provide opportunities to meet their neighbors and other residents. Walking to and taking part in recreation and community activities provide many opportunities for daily social interaction. To achieve this the activities center must be located to maximize opportunities for meeting. This is especially true for housing settings where there is no off-site recreation and commercial center within walking distance.

In addition to programmed spaces for socializing and gardening, older persons have a need for more quiet and secluded outdoor areas. They occasionally retreat to these areas when they are in a contemplative mood, want to take a walk without meeting others, or need a change of scenery from their small unit. An important aspect of retreats is that they offer additional choices to older residents. Although the goal of a retreat is to provide a nice quiet place, the process of getting there may be just as important to older residents as the destination itself.

Although older residents often differ from each other in background, life-style, and attitude, older persons as a whole, as indicated above, have special environmental needs that differ from those of other age groups.

Some environmental needs can be met by more responsive housing design. Some design elements that must be better planned are small details such as height and location of steps, type of doorknob, and location of electrical outlets and light switches. Although it is true that architects address such small-scale elements in the final stages of a design, it is also true that if larger-scale design issues fundamental to the whole conceptual design approach have not been responsive to older person's needs, the small elements will do little to make residents' lives more comfortable.[4]

Some of the more elusive environmental qualities of autonomy, environmental mastery, privacy, and sense of place were mentioned earlier. These qualities do not flow automatically from design but depend greatly on the human or staff side of the environmental equation.

Spatial Experiences

Two years ago I completed a study with Dr. Valerie Polakow entitled "Life Space over the Life Span."[5] In this study we explored the spatial experiences of older people in a life review process, in terms of how these memories and reminiscences shape the environmental perceptions of elderly residents living in perhaps their last home, a retirement center. We discovered that when elderly residents traced their environmental biographies over a lifetime, the process yielded many insights into fundamental life themes of autonomy, privacy, solitude, environmental mastery, and sense of place. When these themes are violated, as frequently occurs in living arrangements for the elderly, it is vital that we pay special attention to the changing relationship between the older person and his or her environmental context. This changing relationship is steeped in a life history of emotional attachment to place and a rich reminiscence of past possibilities of action. How does the legacy of eighty or ninety years of living affect one's current environmental perceptions and sense of well-being?

These are some of the questions we raised in exploring the environmental autobiographies of our informants. In listening to the stories ot their everyday lives, the dramas, and the metaphors that have fashioned their spatial meanings, we realized that it is their voices that should strongly be influencing design. Of course, the attitudes and behavior of social and health personnel responsible for the humane management of people and space and the provision of care in planned residential settings also are important.

Autonomy and Dependence

Living in an institutional setting promotes dependence on organizational rituals, restricts spatial and temporal autonomy, and limits personal choices. Residents must eat prepared meals at specified times or forgo lunch or dinner. They are given no voice in the design of their rooms, or in the design of appliances (refrigerators can be too low, and central speakers too loud), or in the location of the bathroom, which may be too far to go to at night. Yet once these types of external institutional accommodations are made, residents report a feeling of increased autonomy because barriers to mobility or fears of safety are lessened.

Mr. Jones describes how he used to want a larger room, but now, as a stroke victim confined to a walker, he appreciates the confining dimensions of his room. "Now I don't mind – I can go anywhere in the room with a cane – if the room was two feet bigger I couldn't make it without a walker."

For Mr. Jones the experience of living in a ready-made community far outweighs the necessary accommodations and surrender of personal control over his temporal and spatial landscape. For him, the environment is action – people-centered – and, as he remarks, "Being busy keeps me alive." Mr. Jones functions as an invaluable helper-of-others in this center and he, too, realizes the acute dilemma of many of the residents like himself.

"You get people who've been in houses with furnishings and you put them in a room smaller than this (he gestures at the size of his tiny room) and they've lived in a big house for thirty years. They've lost a husband or wife. They get pretty homesick – I try and help them. Sometimes they lose their way – you can tell if they're lost by looking in their eyes. Then I say come on, I'll take you *home.*"

It is clear that Mr. Jones recognizes the center as home – for himself and many others. He is actively engaged in the world of the center, having disengaged from life on the outside. As he wisely points out, "I know it's not going to get better—but there's a lot I *can* do—here you've got people and you're not alone."

There were others living at the center who did not feel their autonomy was affected at all. For instance, Mrs. McGregor told us: "I treat my room as an apartment. I come and go as I please, I invite visitors or not, and I participate in those activities that interest me. Of course, one has to be firm sometimes about one's choices. The closeness of so many people can be a problem sometimes."

Being with others and engaging in the social world of the center, which stands outside the larger social world, appears to foster opportunities for autonomy within a structure of dependence. At this point, the capacity to act on and transform one's given landscape becomes critical.

There is a need for fostering active participation by residents in transforming the spatial landscape they have accepted as their last *home* into something of their own. How to increase the sense of participation and personal autonomy is a challenge for designers and managers of space.

Privacy and Private Spaces

Privacy and private space as perceived by our study participants over their lifetime was most interesting.

Privacy was discussed in relationship to private space.[6] Solitude was the primary focus.[7] Most of the participants indicated that as children they did not have their own private room or space; bedrooms typically were shared by siblings. Mr. Smith said, "As long as I lived at home I never had my own room and always shared it with my brothers." Mrs. Smith made the observation that their younger children had such spaces after the older children in the family left home. It seems that the number of the children in the family and the birth order were very important when it came to having or not having a room of one's own—one's own private space. Mrs. McGregor reported that her bedroom remained her private space throughout her entire adult life until coming to the Retirement Center. She reports, "Even here my room is a bedroom so it seems natural to be sewing and writing in it. It serves as a place of refuge just as my bedroom has all my adult life."

Most of the participants as adults really did not have spaces that were exclusively theirs. Frequently, to attain a state of solitude, many participants would go outdoors for long walks or to a nearby park. As children, most had to find private spaces out of doors in order to play or be alone. Mr. Smith remembered that his childhood home consisted of one all-purpose room, a kitchen, and bedrooms. You went outdoors if you wanted to play or be alone.

Privacy and Autonomy

Autonomy is closely related to the issue of privacy.[6] Our society professes a fundamental belief in the uniqueness of the individual, in the basic dignity and worth of each human being. Social scientists have linked the development and maintenance of this sense of individuality to the need for autonomy—the ability to make one's own choices and decisions. Autonomy is protected by privacy and is threatened by those who are not, for one reason or another, discretionary in their intrusion and usurpation of privacy and individual choice. People who are dependent on others for their welfare are particularly vulnerable to losing their autonomy. Unfortunately, there seems to be a general feeling among those who provide supportive services that the assistance being rendered compensates for the intrusion on or loss of autonomy.

Living arrangements at the center we studied range from independent cottages complete with kitchens, garages, and yards to individual rooms that serve as both sleeping and living areas. Some of these units have toilets; others do not. This physical context has a very important effect on the sense of autonomy at the center.

Some informants in our study had very perceptive views on the subject of autonomy. Those who lived in the detached cottages indicated that they "like it there rather than in the center because we can pick and choose when to have company or see someone or not. We don't feel pressured to engage in programmed activities." "We feel the administration and staff should have more understanding of people's choices regarding participation in activities with strangers." "At the center, there is only a thin wall separating one life from another; here in this cottage we have several hundred yards. This distance has made it possible to have more choice."

Participants were very perceptive in understanding the role that the physical environment plays in maintaining autonomy. There is also the observation of Mrs. Smith that as her health changes for the worse, "I may have to move to the center and then I will have less to say about what I do, where I go, and who I see."

Place Bonding and Displacement

As a person develops a sense of place over time, he or she attaches special meanings to certain activities and events that in turn are strongly identified with particular spaces. This process is known as place bonding. For example, a house in which a child grows up has many connotations of identity, and if that person involuntarily leaves or if the house is destroyed, a profound sense of loss—the experience of displacement—occurs.

This theme was articulated by some of the participants. For example, Mrs. McGregor observed: "We lost the farm during the Depression and along with it my walks along the river, the serenity of the trees and quiet places. I always enjoyed the out of doors." Mrs. Black also experienced a sense of loss: "My father developed a serious illness and as a result could not keep up with the demands of his position and was transferred to a less demanding situation and as a result lost the lovely house we lived in." Mrs. McGregor commented that "It was a lot easier for me to decide to come to the Retirement Center than some others because I didn't own my own house. I rented for a long time and so I didn't feel as attached as perhaps those might who owned their houses for a long time." Mr. Smith commented wistfully, "To be in the Upper Peninsula (Michigan), to enjoy the woods and the water, there's no place like it. That's my home, that's where I feel best, the big timber, the big country."

A sense of displacement seemed to be common among our participants. Perhaps the most difficult displacement occurs when one enters a more sheltered situation. For most people moving to such a place means giving up their home of long duration and accommodating to a quite different life-style. More than giving up one's home, this change frequently means giving up significant personal possessions. For example, Mrs. Black said, "I accumulated during the course of my adult life a number of possessions that had special meaning to me. For instance, I had a platform rocker that had been in my family for four generations. I played on it a great deal and I also sat in it and read in it as a child growing up. I also had a coin and stamp collection and a very unique collection of vases. When I came here I gave most of these and other things away because there really wasn't enough room here and I was afraid I'd lose them."

At the same time, possessions that are brought along to the Retirement Center are frequent reminders of other times, events, and places. They seem to provide tangible evidence of a meaningful past. As a person continues to age and the gap between the demands of the environment and the individual's competence widens, he or she begins to experience a loss of autonomy or mastery over necessary environmental elements. As this gap increases, a resident's sphere of life-sustaining and life-enriching stimuli diminishes. And as more and more energy is expended in satisfying even the minimum of life-sustaining needs, a person forgoes life-enhancing activities. It is vital that those who serve the frail elderly address the issue of how the physical environment can enrich personal growth.

Personal Growth

Personal growth is also related to the issue of adjustment in relocating from private housing to planned housing. People coming from private homes typically live in a single detached dwelling unit located on a lot that provides a spatial buffer in terms of proximity to others. Moving into planned housing presents a radical change since proximity is reduced, density is increased, and the spatial buffer may be no more than a thin wall. Although there are a number of potentially positive elements in such a situation—an increased friendship pool, greater proximity, and easier access to planned activities—not everyone can make the adjustment without help. We need to know more about the factors that are involved in the adjustment process and how housing counselors and managers may apply them to assist in the successful adjustment of all residents to planned retirement housing.

Institutional Time

It is difficult to separate design of physical space from management of physical space in planned housing. This is particularly true as it relates to the institutional time frame, that is, the scheduling of institutional rituals and program demands. These should be reexamined and made more flexible and individualized to better accommodate the diverse needs of residents in these special and planned environments.

Conclusion

Listening to the voices of older persons has taught us the importance of environmental biography. It is within these symbolic meaning structures that current satisfaction/dissatisfaction needs can be located. Those who are concerned about the well-being of older persons can derive important metaphors from this approach that yield significant insights about elderly people and their environments.

Notes

1. Christie, K. "Four federal agencies sign agreement to promote better design for older Americans." News release, National Endowment for the Arts, February 14, 1985.

2. Lawton, M.P. "An ecological theory of aging applied to elderly housing." *Journal of Architectural Education*, 31:8–10, September 1977.

3. Pastalan, L.A., and L.G. Paulson. "Importance of the physical environment for older people." *Journal of the American Geriatrics Society*, 33, 7:874, 1986.

4. Pastalan, L.A. "The physical environment and the emerging nature of the extended care model." In E.L. Schneider, et al. (Ed.), *The Teaching Nursing Home*. New York: Raven Press, 1985; pp. 19–55.

   Pastalan, L.A. "Designing housing environments for the elderly." *Journal of Architectural Education*, 31:11–13, September 1977.

   Pastalan, L.A. "Environmental design and adaptation to the visual environment of the elderly." In R. Sekuler, D. Kline, and K. Dismukes (Eds.), *Aging and Human Visual Foundation*. New York: Alan R. Less, 1982.

   Pastalan and Paulsen, "Physical environment."

5. Pastalan, L.A., and V. Polakow. "Life space over the life span." *Journal of Housing for the Elderly*, 4, 1:73–85, 1986.

   Suransky, V.P. *The Erosion of Childhood*. Chicago: University of Chicago Press, 1982.

6. Pastalan, L.A. "Privacy as an expression of human territoriality." In L.A. Pastalan and D.H. Carson (Eds.), *Spatial Behavior of Older People*. Ann Arbor: University of Michigan, 1970.

7. Solitude is considered here as a state of privacy in which an individual is separated from the group and freed from the observation of others.

8. Tuan, Y. *Space and Place: The Perspective of Experience*. Minneapolis: University of Minnesota Press, 1977.

CHAPTER ELEVEN

Knowledge Resources and Gaps in Housing for the Aged

M. POWELL LAWTON

Aging in place remains a relatively unexamined area, considering its major and growing significance for the country. The state of the art in the scientific study of the housing of older people—and of long-term care in residential environments—has not progressed in the past decade at the rate one might have expected given the spurt of knowledge in this field between 1965 and 1975. There are at least three main reasons for this lull. First, in the past eight years federal housing initiatives have virtually been eliminated. Without the continued production of assisted housing for the elderly, one major motivation for (and federal funding to support) formulating and testing service-relevant hypotheses is lost. Moreover, there are no longer rewards for producing higher-quality housing: When saving money is the overarching value, no room is left for experimentation, yet experimentation with new models is needed to stimulate research that fosters more innovation.

Second, although the drought in federal housing initiatives has not affected the activity of private developers, the latter by and large have not supported very much research other than relatively short-term and narrowly focused market research. The substantial investment in research and development that is normal in some other industries certainly does not occur among private developers of housing for the elderly. Increased research, accompanied by willingness to share information obtained by privately funded research, will be necessary to bring knowledge relevant to higher-income consumers up to the level of that obtained from government-funded research on lower-income people.

A third reason for the paucity of research may be attributable to the research community itself. We seem to have run out of variations on our old themes of the 1970s and are marking time while we await new methodologies and ideas. The one growth area in research has been studies in the economics of housing. It is possible that research in this area has grown recently because it is relatively new: It started about a dozen years ago. Although there are good examples of humanistically oriented economic research,[1-3] most of it has focused on reducing the cost of housing.

This chapter discusses three aspects of research on aging in place: (1) currently available data sets, many of them inadequately analyzed; (2) some important gaps in information, most of which should be addressed by government statistical agencies; and (3) research methodology.

The Meaning of Aging in Place

Aging in place represents a transaction between an aging individual and his or her residential environment that is characterized by changes in both person and environment over time, with the physical location of the person being the only constant.

There are several important aspects of this definition. First is the transactional aspect, which implies a system that is indivisible into separate entities of person and environment. Both person and environment are fluid, one changing as the other changes, with cause and effect being difficult to separate. Even the location where aging in place occurs is dynamic, in the sense that it is maintained through a continuing process of active decisionmaking. That is, the decision to remain in place is one made frequently or one continuously reaffirmed, not a static one-time decision. The need is to search for topics and research methods that recognize the constantly changing nature of aging in place.

It is not only a person's physical condition that changes over time through the process of biological aging: Three other types of change also occur. First is a psychological change in the person: self-directed change. The ecological model of Lawton and Nahemow[4] and its elaborations[5,6] note the elevation in competence that comes as the result of successful problem solving. Second, all residential environments are constantly changing as a result of physical wear, the actions of the natural environment, and the behaviors of other people. Finally, there are the alterations to the environment made by the older inhabitant, who may make it more stimulating, more supportive, more challenging, more private, and more secure according to his need.

Aging in place is thus an extremely complex phenomenon, rather than the static one conveyed by the image of a passive person experiencing biological aging in an unchanging physical setting. As a framework for discussing the knowledge base, it is necessary to know about multiple competences and other characteristics of the person, and the attributes of environment including microenvironment, dwelling, neighborhood, and community. Further, our knowledge must enable us to track both person and environmental context over time. Finally, the transactional aspects may be the most difficult of all to measure. These aspects include the ways in which—and the extent to which—the environment affects intrapersonal processes such as cognition; affect; motivation; behavior in relation to the external environment; impacts of this behavior on the environment; and feedback of the changed environment to another cycle of person-environment (P-E) transactions.

Sources of Data

The review of data sources in this section is guided by the transactional principle. Data are not considered relevant to research on aging in place unless the set meets two minimum requirements: It contains information on (1) older people, and (2) on some characteristics of the environments they inhabit. It should be evident that many important data sets do not meet these criteria. For example, most of the Health Interview Surveys (HIS) and the National Health and Nutrition Examination Surveys (NHANES) of the National Center on Health Statistics (NCHS) contain virtually no environmental information other than region of the country and household structure.[7, 8] Similarly lacking in environmental data are other surveys such as the National Council on the Aging's Myth and Reality of Aging[9] and Aging in the Eighties,[10] Shanas's National Surveys of the Aged,[11] and the Longitudinal Retirement History Survey of the Social Security Administration.[12] Morgan's Panel Study of Income Dynamics[13] contains only basic housing type, cost, and living arrangement items, although one wave (1975) had a special housing and neighborhood supplement.

The following section will first discuss existing data and then data needs and gaps.

DATA SETS CONTAINING BOTH OLDER PERSON AND ENVIRONMENTAL DATA

Unplanned housing. The richest data on a nationally representative sample is more than twenty years old, but its potential for exploring person-environment transactions has still not been adequately realized. The 1968 National Senior Citizens Survey contains interview records of almost 4,000 people age sixty-five and over.[14] The content includes data on social relationships, work and retirement, activities, health, self-perception, and psychological well-being. Almost half of the data is devoted to the physical, locational, and resource characteristics of the housing unit and neighborhood. Three years later, samples of 300 people who had changed residences and 200 who stayed in place were reinterviewed. The data are in the Inter-University Consortium for Political and Social Research (ICPSR) archives, and its component unit, the National Archive of Computerized Data on Aging (NACDA).

How relevant are twenty-year-old data? Advances in our ability to address contemporary social problems usually come from contemporary data, particularly those that provide a longitudinal or historical picture of current trends. But it is also true that important basic knowledge is not bound to contemporary events.

The major source of housing data is the Annual Housing Survey (the Biennial American Housing Survey since 1981) of the U.S. Department of Housing and Urban Development (HUD) and the Bureau of the Census.[15] The AHS began in 1973 and from 1974 through 1983 the same basic format and core sample were used.

Dwellings were the sampling unit, with each unit being resurveyed at each wave and the sample being adjusted for lost and new units to maintain the national representativeness of each separate survey. The national samples consist of about 60,000 units, including 12,000 or more with a householder sixty-five or over. In addition, there were originally sixty samples from Standard Metropolitan Statistical Areas (SMSA) (now reduced to forty) that are repeated in cycles of three or four years. The sample sizes for SMSAs vary from 4,000 to 13,000 and the survey content was revised in 1985. The AHS core provides the most extensive data in existence on the physical and financial characteristics of dwellings, including about thirty physical features that are clear indicators of housing quality and information on the householder's previous dwelling unit for those who had recently moved. An overall rating of housing quality and a series of ratings on neighborhood quality and services are the only subjective variables included. Household structure and demographic characteristics are the major person variables. There are no indicators of health or psychological well-being. However, one-time or occasional supplements have been used in some years to augment the core questions. The most notable supplement relevant to the aged appeared in the 1978 AHS, when a group of questions on functional health and housing modifications to enhance access and safety were included. The 1985 AHS began a new dwelling-unit sample constructed from the 1980 Census of Population and Housing. Although the 1974–83 AHS surveys are longitudinal with respect to dwelling units, combining these samples in this way makes the data difficult to analyze. ABT Associates in Cambridge, Massachusetts, has constructed and made available for purchase a merged longitudinal data file for both the national and SMSA samples.

Almost no use of the merged longitudinal AHS data file has been made with respect to the elderly. The aging in place phenomenon could be addressed in depth with such an approach. However, since the sampling unit is the dwelling rather than the person or household, one may study (1) older households who have remained in place; (2) older households whose unit has been removed from the sample (although the data do not follow them to their new dwelling); (3) older households occupying a dwelling unit added to the sample in a given year, usually a newly constructed unit (plus a small set of data on the householders' previous dwellings); and (4) older households occupying an old unit for the first time. If the householder changes, only that fact is ascertainable, and the amount of information on nonhouseholder occupants is very small. There are thus limitations on the types of longitudinal studies that can be done.

The decennial census itself has a few housing items in the basic schedule and seventeen additional ones in the sample (one in six) interview. In 1980 the complete-count items included number of dwelling units, access to unit, plumbing, number of rooms, tenure, condominium, acreage, value, rent, persons in unit, and persons per room. The retention of housing items in the 1990 census was opposed by the Reagan administration, but most appear to have survived.

Aging in place along with changes in location are among the phenomena included in a broader category called "housing adjustments." Struyk and Newman designed what was to be the pilot for a multiple-site longitudinal study of housing adjustments. The first site study was completed in 1979 on a sample of 1,070 older residents of Houston, Texas. Newman merged these data with the 1979 Houston SMSA Annual Housing Survey data. Although still short on subjective assessments of either environment or psychological state, this data set is the largest one to contain information on adjustments such as home alterations, changed room uses, and community service use, in addition to many other residential variables. (The data tape is not available from HUD, but has been cleaned and is available at cost with codebook from the Institute for Policy Studies at Johns Hopkins University, attention Dr. Sandra Newman.) Struyk and Katsura also assembled a smaller seven-city sample from the larger Community Development Block Grant evaluation that they were able to follow over five years.[16] The data tape has been archived by the National Institute on Aging.

The Experimental Housing Allowance Program (EHAP) was one of the largest social experiments undertaken by the federal government. Face-to-face interviews with housing consumers were done in three different substudies. The Demand Experiment included 3,600 people from the Pittsburgh and Phoenix areas who were offered subsidies. The Supply Experiment made subsidies available to income- and housing-eligible applicants in two small cities on their initiative. These data sets are among the most complete in housing and economic data. They also contain a few subjective data items. A few publications have appeared on the elderly subsamples,[17] but for the most part the data lie unused and cannot be found in

HUD archives. (The data from the Supply Experiment, gathered from 1973 to 1978, are well documented and are available from RAND Corporation, with codebook and software, at cost — RAND Corporation files #250-257.)

Other HUD-contracted data sets were gathered from 1,350 older homeowners in a pilot home-repair program demonstration reported by Rabushka and Jacobs,[18] and further analyzed by Struyk and Devine.[19] Subjects were surveyed regarding their housing and their perception of housing; independent quality evaluations were made by professional housing experts. The data, unfortunately, do not seem to be available at present. A later demonstration program was begun in Baltimore in 1981, with a sample of 1,024 older people;[20] that data set also is available from Sandra Newman at Johns Hopkins. The full demonstration program in nine additional cities was evaluated by Urban Systems of Cambridge, Massachusetts, but the data were not saved either by the contractor or by HUD.

The Survey of Low-Income and Disabled (SLIAD) was a longitudinal evaluation of the Supplementary Security Income (SSI) Program, done on a sample of 5,940 low-income elderly and disabled people in 1973 and 1974. Although somewhat short on housing data, the evaluation is rich in health, income, and social data and allows those who moved to be compared with those who did not. Some analyses may be found in Struyk and Soldo.[21] The data are available from the Social Security Administration and the Inter-University Consortium for Political and Social Research.

The National Long-Term-Care Survey (NLTCS) began in 1982 (see Chapter 1). The 5,580 nationally representative subjects were sampled from a universe of Medicare beneficiaries meeting a disability criterion. The data set contains some basic neighborhood, housing, and household information as well as items on housing modifications for livability and safety. The NLTCS was repeated in 1984 and 1989. The latter survey contained partial longitudinal samples plus new age cohorts, which will afford a look at housing adjustments over time.

The Health Interview Surveys (HIS) performed biennially for the National Center for Health Statistics by the Bureau of the Census included an aging supplement in 1984 that added some housing content; one of the questions asked whether the residence was in a "retirement community."[22] This supplement, in turn, was repeated under National Institute of Aging support as the National Longitudinal

Study on Aging in 1988 and may continue. Both the NLTCS and the HIS supplements are available from the NCHS and the ICPSR.

The American Association of Retired Persons (AARP) performed a nationally representative telephone survey of 1,500 older people specifically directed to their housing needs.[23] It has extensive data on housing characteristics, preferences, and attitudes and some data on health. This data set is available on request for uses approved by AARP.

DATA SETS FROM SPECIFIC PLANNED HOUSING TYPES

None of the data files from large multiple-site surveys of planned housing are available from the ICPSR or easily obtainable from their sources. All have been done either on contracts or grants from the government or generated privately. Lack of demand for their use by investigators other than the original ones is certainly part of the reason why they have not been offered for more general use.

Congregate housing. HUD contracted with Urban Systems of Cambridge, Massachusetts, in 1975 to do an evaluation study of a stratified national sample of twenty-seven HUD-subsidized congregate housing sites.[24] The study was completed in 1976 and a descriptive monograph was published. However, the original data are not available either through HUD or Urban Systems. In addition, an evaluation of the first year of operation of the Congregate Housing Service Program (CHSP) was done by Sherwood et al.[25] This program included fifty-five sites (both public housing and Section 202 facilities) where supportive services were targeted to older tenants at risk of institutionalization. The data set is rich in both environmental-level and personal-level variables, and the longitudinal design is ideal for the examination of aging in one specific type of residence.

Public housing. Public housing has been studied by several investigators. Two such studies focused on management and were performed under contract to HUD by the Urban Institute. Neither focused on the elderly alone, and the amount of information on elderly-designated projects is not known.[26] Neither HUD nor the Urban Institute have been able to locate the original data.

Another such study included a great deal of data on management and physical facilities, and subjective perceptions of management, social environment, and physical environment in thirty-seven public housing sites.[27] Individual interviewing was done on 1,907 tenants, including a large subset of old people. Although the data have not been prepared for public use, an inquiry to Dr. James Anderson at the Housing Research and Development Program, University of Illinois, would yield information on their availability.

My colleagues and I studied a nationally representative sample of one hundred public housing and fifty Section 202 housing sites in 1970.[28] We gathered extensive data on the physical, social, and management characteristics of the site, plus a very brief interview with 3,000 tenants and a more extended interview with 900 of them. Three-year follow-up interviews were done on about 1,000 of the public housing tenants. We are preparing this data set for deposit in the ICPSR archive.

Continuing care retirement communities (CCRCs). CCRCs, or life care communities as they formerly were called, are one variety of privately sponsored planned housing for the elderly that provide housing and services for residents ranging from housekeeping, laundry, and meals to nursing home care. Chapter 6 contains an extensive discussion of CCRCs. Since there is no central registry of any privately sponsored housing, it is virtually impossible to draw a representative sample of such environments. The first systematic look at life care came from the study of nonprofit CCRCs by Winklevoss and Powell,[29] a study that focused primarily on the actuarial aspects of life care and CCRC financial stability. Subsequently, the American Association of Homes for the Aging (AAHA), in cooperation with Ernst and Whinney, undertook a survey of CCRCs.[30] Eleven hundred facilities were identified, 683 were considered to meet AAHA criteria as CCRCs, and 400 responded to the first survey questionnaire. Future plans involve collecting data regarding tenants and opening the data base for use by researchers, as well as annually updating the survey.

In addition, AAHA, in collaboration with the American Association of Retired Persons (AARP), produced a *National Continuing Care Directory.*[31] Because many CCRCs do not fall under any licensing jurisdiction and there is no central registry, construction of such a list requires combing publications and local media for announcements about such environments. A new edition of the *National Continuing Care Directory* was published in 1988.

The accounting firm of Laventhol and Horwath gathers extensive operational data on a sample of for-profit and nonprofit CCRCs and publishes annual reports of summary data. The 1987 survey showed extensive organizational and financial data on 173 facilities.[32] These data exist in a computer file with code book, and Laventhol and Horwath has indicated its willingness to consider requests from outside users for access to the data. Such data are clearly not representative of any known universe of housing environments and for that reason must be used with caution.

An unusual data file has been created by the Foundation for Aging Research in Clearwater, Florida. A continuing series of studies of both community-resident aged and members of retirement communities (including a subset of about 1,000 in longitudinal assessment) begin in 1980 and is now producing interesting trend data.[33] The data are gathered for prospective sponsors of housing, and of course the respondents represent constituencies of particular interest to a series of clients rather than any representative or easily characterized group. The data have been merged and weighted in such a way as to give a broad, though not nationally representative, picture of older people still living in the community. These data are unique in focusing on topics of relevance to aging in place, such as wishes for services and amenities, preferences for design alternatives, and evaluations of different means for taking care of one's combined health and housing needs. This data set is not available for general use, but the periodic reports show a good model for useful data that many organizations might consider collecting.

INFORMATION GAPS

Federal housing programs. HUD has always been remarkably short of information on its own programs. HUD formerly published directories of public housing, which listed every project within every housing authority, together with a small amount of information about each project. Although occupancy reports are still filed, directories are no longer published. The Section 202 program also no longer publishes directories of its own sites. As the only federal program still producing new units, the 202 program would seem to have particular reason to provide such updated listings. However, the 202 central office can produce on request an updated computer printout of 202 projects in operation, under construction, and under contract.

HUD program monitoring dropped off precipitously during the years of the Reagan administration. A task force is currently in operation at HUD, however, to develop an occupancy reporting system for public housing. Although it is likely to contain only the most basic information, anything is an improvement over zero level.

It should be easy and it is certainly important for HUD to begin again to publish reports containing annual basic data on the units in its various programs — Sections 202, 221(d)(3) and (d)(4), 232, and 236 — designated for older people. Even programs no longer developing new units, for example, Section 236 and public housing, are experiencing changes, such as the abandonment of some units and switches from family- to elderly-designated housing, which should be reported. Outside support for the effort to reinstitute a reporting system in public housing would seem to have a good chance of success, and such an effort is already beginning. It would be desirable to make the reporting mandatory and to specify some additional information to be included or collected that would be useful for planning public policies to deal with aging in place. It would not be a large burden on the management of elderly housing facilities to supply information annually on such tenant character-istics as age, sex, minority status, household or marital status, length of tenure, and turnover by reason. Although some index of health would obviously be desirable, this information is much more difficult to produce; age and reason for separation (or separation destination such as nursing home, hospital, and so on) are partly acceptable proxies.

With such a system for public housing, and the alertness of 202 management to the aging in place phenomenon, it would seem feasible to press for a similar system for the latter program. The programs that are less likely to have service-oriented management (some Section 8, 221, Farmers Home Administration, and others) may be more difficult to persuade. The appeal to them could be that data on their own housing will be useful to them in their own planning. It would also give them an opportunity to compare their own data with those of comparable facilities in their region and elsewhere in the country. The examples reviewed above of the private sector's recognition of the necessity for planning data might be persuasive in arguing for such an expenditure of energy.

Data deficiencies mirror the governmental fragmentation of responsibility among departments of housing, health, mental health, social services, welfare, and taxes. For that reason, relatively few data collection efforts exist that effectively cross bureaucratic boundaries to provide clear insights into the aging in place phenomena. The absence of housing data from the health surveys, of health data from the housing surveys, of psychological data from others, has already been noted. The past decade has demonstrated, however, that groups of experts working together on these issues can have a positive effect. The Council of Professional Associations on Federal Statistics, for example, has had considerable input into the decennial census, as has the Gerontological Society of America. The National Center for Health Statistics convened a multidisciplinary group in 1975 to study and recommend what was called a "minimum data set for long-term care." A series of meetings with recommendations has followed. This effort has neither produced the perfect and final compilation of data needs nor has it been startlingly successful in establishing the standard for all federal efforts. But it has clarified information measurement and data requirements in important ways.[34] People within and outside the government have continued to press for adoption of this recommended data set. Another outcome was the formation within the federal government of an Interagency Statistical Committee on Long-Term Care for the Elderly, chaired by Joan Van Nostrand of the National Center for Health Statistics, which issued a very useful compendium of federal data sources.[35] In 1984 the Gerontological Society of America established a Task Force on Data on Aging, also chaired by Joan Van Nostrand. This group of concerned scientists has been able to influence both the decision to carry out some surveys and their content. Their first analysis of needs and the survey of such federal statistics on the aging[36] was updated in 1986. This should be repeated every year.

There also is a federal Interagency Forum on Aging-Related Statistics. A representative of HUD—Duane McGough, the director of the American Housing Survey—is on this committee. One reason for the decision to begin producing AHS tables for the aging was the request for them that came to this group from the National Institute on Aging and the Administration on Aging. It thus would seem to be a good time for a more concerted effort by nongovernmental people in pressing for the inclusion of environmental content in nonhousing surveys. The National Research Council has just completed a study of all federal statistics with recommendations to increase financial support for such data. Because this effort could be useful far beyond the governmental sector, gathering potential information from nongovernmental sources will be discussed before any concerted action is taken.

Moves toward filling knowledge gaps. The compilation of this list of data sets and organizations thought to have a stake in further data development may help to sensitize both organizations and individual experts to the need for better data and access to it. Much of the information reviewed above is in less than perfect form. A prospective user may have to work hard to determine the exact location of the data set, get permission to access the data, and figure out the intricacies of coding and programming. Such problems, however, are unlikely in the ICPSR archive data. Data sets established as public-use tapes by the government also are usually reasonably clean and useable. One-time surveys, on the other hand, have often been set aside without being documented for subsequent use by other researchers. Data bases created for in-house use by sponsoring organizations may be the most difficult to access. In some cases a request for an external use of the data may be the stimulus for a major improvement in the sponsor's ability to use its own data base.

HUD is the obvious location for a housing data archive. At one time it did begin such an archive, but only after the loss of many of the early data files. Continuity and commitment were never sufficient to establish an ongoing structural archive. It seems incredible, in fact, that few of the HUD-initiated data are now available from HUD. Outside pressure from both nonprofit and proprietary groups as well as developers might be successful in motivating HUD to reassume this initiative.

The time may be right for a scientist-contractor to perform the second step—procuring some of the more obscure data sets and cleaning and cataloguing them in codebook form. Such operations are routinely performed by the ICPSR. The assembly of this archive might be a possible project for its related unit, the National Archive of Data on the Aging. A special funding effort would be required for such a focus on the housing issue.

Another phase would convene the professional organizations (including those named on the preceding pages) with an interest in housing and management data for a discussion of joint needs and an exploration of resources, with the goal of formalizing and linking some of their activities. One of the best-developed of the current systems, AAHA's CCRC data base, quickly became a very expensive enterprise for AAHA alone and now requires outside funding to continue. There will be a limited supply of such outside funding for individual organizational activity, however. It thus seems essential for the long term that collaborative activity and sharing of the product occur. Thus an early multiorganizational meeting of professional organizations with government and social science participation would seem very useful.

Planning should also begin for the evolution of a *recommended housing data set*. Such a set should be conceived in hierarchical fashion. That is, the task should be to produce a complete and exhaustive set of categories of content that reflects the current state of the art in attainable data. Regular revisions would be required to reflect changes in the kinds of information seen as desirable. However, this complete category system should be organized so that the categories themselves are designated in priority order, and within each category, the most important features designated. The important subproduct of this effort would be the *minimum housing data set*. This would be a very short list of categories together with suggested operationalized measures, which could be incorporated into a non-housing survey for the purpose of linking housing and the focus of the survey, be it health, long-term care, income maintenance, or other issues.

The evolution of such a minimum housing data set would require a substantial effort from a multidisciplinary group, including extended staff work in assembling background material from the existing environmental measurement literature. Thus, there is no basis at present for making even a preliminary recommendation. Nonetheless, it may be worthwhile to illustrate in the table following how such an effort might proceed. The table names only a few examples, not necessarily in order of importance, of entries that might appear in a recommended data set. Entry candidates for a minimum data set, that is, those of highest priority, might include the following:

Category	Data item
Focus of data set	
Individual dwelling unit	Housing type (detached, row)
Apartment building	Number of units
Perspective	
Objective physical description	Housing deficit, as in AHS
Subjective evaluation	Housing satisfaction, as in AHS
Type of information	
Physical material	Masonry
Physical configuration	Three-story stairway structure
Organizational sponsorship	Nonprofit religious sponsor
Social/medical service type	Congregate housing
Financial data	Annual rent
Subjective rating	Preferences for Services
Managerial	Manager's housing training

1. Dwelling unit: number of rooms, number of floors, number of units in structure, number of people in household
2. Community: population, section of country
3. Subjective environment: four-point rating scales of housing satisfaction and neighborhood satisfaction as used in AHS
4. Organizational environment: subsidized versus market rate, nonprofit versus for-profit, congregate versus non-congregate.
5. Financial data: estimated value of outstanding mortgage (owners), monthly rent (renters)

Methodological Needs

The previous section assumes that descriptive information is intrinsically useful for planning and research. The need for such data is clear and the methods for gathering it are straightforward. However, social-scientific research on person-environment relations must go beyond pure description. The subdiscipline of person-environment relations was created by people who put traditional social-scientific research methods and concepts together with architectural and other design methods and concepts to specify the principles behind such relations and ultimately to produce better environmental design.

It is not the purpose of this chapter to review such methodologies. A comprehensive treatment of person-environment (P-E) research methods has been published recently,[37] including a chapter devoted to such methods in gerontological P-E research.[38] Rather than repeat such a review, this short section will express a strong sense of dissatisfaction with today's state of development of such methods and speculate about how the quality of research might proceed again from its present plateau.

P-E RESEARCH

Two major strategies characterized most of the P-E research performed during its first two decades of flourishing activity: the search for environmental features associated with positive psychological outcomes, and the approach characterized as "asking the consumer."

The most influential research findings were those that showed how such features as new planned housing,[39] larger-sized kitchens,[40] generalized housing quality,[41] neighborhood amenities,[42] and service-rich housing[43] could be differentially related to increased life satisfaction or housing satisfaction. Somewhat less frequent, but still notable, were attempts to relate desirable behavioral outcomes to such environmental features.

In retrospect, these approaches clearly represent stimulus-response (S-R) conceptions of the person-environment transaction, that is, unidirectional causal effects of an environmental feature on some behavioral or psychological outcome. There has always been a strong cognitive stream in P-E research, but more so in general P-E research than in gerontological applications. The S-R conception does not take adequate account of the many factors that may moderate the environment-person causal effect, that is, the cognitive and affective responses by which the "objective" environment is made meaningful to the person. We have ample evidence of how a person's interpretation of an external environmental attribute may be the overwhelming determinant of the person's response.

What S-R research may show us are a few very strong effects, where the strength of the environmental effect is great enough to show through despite the variation that may be introduced by individual and other factors. I have argued in favor of not neglecting the direct effects of the external environment.[44] It seems at this point, however, that the number of effects with such strength are limited and that we are running out of influences of this type that are productive to put to empirical test.

The consumer preference stream of research[45] was a welcome addition to gerontological research because of the recognized need to moderate high-handed judgments of "experts" regarding what is good for a particular consumer group. Of course, consumer-preferential research had been used in applied social science for many decades before environmental researchers in gerontology picked it up; the advantages and disadvantages of this type of research are well known.[46] We certainly have not exhausted the usefulness of this type of research. For example, two very disturbing reports have recently appeared showing radical disagreements among experts in applied P-E activity about the preferences of older consumers.[47]

However, the payoff in terms of incremental increase in general P-E knowledge is diminishing as we unsuccessfully struggle with the old issues of how to ask a preference question meaningfully, how a nonuser can construe accurately the object being judged, how to interpret the effects of response sets, and so on.

Thus, the two stocks in trade of the P-E researcher with a social-scientific orientation seem not to offer much potential for significant new information. Even within the P-E research network, an original split remains, and is perhaps even more evident now than before, between the design-oriented and the social-science-oriented researchers. Despite the many productive research efforts that have bridged the disciplinary gap, there seems to be a persistent tendency for quantitative research to grow more esoteric in its reliance on discipline-specific research methods, and for qualitative research to grow in a multitude of poorly articulated ways.

Most of the interesting ideas about behavioral design have come from the qualitative components of research studies. Classic examples are Cooper's study of the Easter Hill public housing,[48] Howell's articulation of "previewing space" and other transactional design elements,[49] Newman's basic work on defensible space,[50] and Osmond's conceptions of sociopetal and sociofugal space in mental hospitals.[51] It is probably not coincidental that these examples all have involved collaboration between design professionals and scientists. Unfortunately, there have been very few such research efforts in gerontological research.[52] It is possible that a deliberate attempt to fortify the multidisciplinary character of future research teams will provide the empirical researcher with a better supply of creative and design-relevant ideas.

Greater utilization of the anthropological perspective in such multidisciplinary research should be encouraged. The search for meaning in people's relationships to their environment is a goal in itself for the anthropologist,[53] but the analysis of personal themes as observed in qualitative gerontology[54] may also lead to an evaluative perspective that will produce better environments.

ARE NEW METHODS AVAILABLE?

I do not believe we are in a position to scrap S-R methods, consumer preferential surveys, behavior mapping, time budgets, or any other of our traditional armamentaria. Although the frustration over repetition and diminishing returns is real, I have no truly new approach to suggest. What follows are suggestions for appropriate foci of new research, not new and better methods.

The previous mention of the design orientation, qualitative methods, and anthropology as desirable research team components fits into the need to treat P-E transactions with the complexity intrinsic to the topic. The black box between stimulus and response is easier to see into with the use of methodologies that are attuned to identify the striking instance, the exception to the rule, the latent meaning, the undercurrent usually obscured by a social veneer, and the leveling of individuals that is inherent in social-scientific quantitative methods. Some of the underlying complexity may be better understood if observers are attuned to these kinds of data. For example, qualitative observation of ongoing behavior in a specific physical space by an architect, a service professional, and a behavioral scientist working together may capture the richness of behavior but also allow appropriate controls on idiosyncratic or biased interpretation of what is taking place.

In sum, research on environment and aging has experienced a lull in productivity and creativity. We need new conceptualizations and a renewed emphasis on individual differences in need and on multidisciplinary design research.

We have failed to retain much valuable data collected in past studies. We must recoup and preserve what we can.

We must determine proactively the direction of future knowledge integration and archiving.

Finally, the federal government *must* make a major effort to improve its data gathering and reporting on the phenomena of aging in place.

Notes

1. Newman, S., and R.J. Struyk. *Housing and Supportive Services: Federal Policy for the Frail Elderly and Chronically Mentally Ill.* Washington, D.C.: Urban Institute, 1988.

2. Newman, S.J., J. Zais, and R.J. Struyk. "Housing Older America." In I. Altman, M.P. Lawton, and J. Wohlwill (Eds.), *Human Behavior and the Environment: The Elderly and the Physical Environment.* New York: Plenum, 1983, pp. 17–56.

3. Struyk, R.J., and B.J. Soldo. *Improving the Elderly's Housing.* Cambridge, Mass.: Ballinger, 1980.

4. Lawton, M.P., and L. Nahemow. "Ecology and the aging process." In C. Eisdorfer and M.P. Lawton (Eds.), *Psychology of Adult Development and Aging.* Washington: American Psychological Association, 1973, pp. 619–74.

   Lawton, M.P., and L. Nahemow. "Social science methods for evaluating the quality of housing for the elderly." *Journal of Architectural Research,* 7:5–11, 1979a.

5. Lawton, M.P. "Behavior-related ecological factors." In K. W. Schaie and C. Schooler (Eds.), *Social Structure and the Psychological Aging Processes.* Hillside, N.J.: Lawrence Erlbaum, 1989, pp. 57–78.

6. Lawton, M.P. "Environmental change: The older person as initiator and responder." In N. Datan and N. Lohmann (Eds.), *Transitions of Aging.* New York: Academic Press, 1980, pp. 171–93.

7. National Center for Health Statistics. *Plan and Operation of the Health and Nutrition Examination Survey, 1971–1973.* Washington, D.C.: Department of Health, Education, and Welfare, 1973.

8. National Center for Health Statistics. "The National Health Interview Survey design, 1973–84, and procedures, 1975–1983." In *Vital and Health Statistics,* Series 10, No. 18 (PHS), 85-1320. Rockville, Md.: U.S. Public Health Service, 1985.

9. National Council on the Aging. *The Myth and Reality of Aging in America.* Washington, D.C.: National Council on the Aging, 1975.

10. National Council on the Aging. *Aging in the Eighties: America in Transition.* Washington, D.C.: National Council on the Aging, 1981.

11. Shanas, E. *The Health of Older People.* Cambridge, Mass.: Harvard University Press, 1962.

Shanas, E. *National Survey of the Aged.* Final report to the Administration on Aging. Washington, D.C.: U.S. Department of Health, Education and Welfare, 1978.

Shanas, E., P. Townsend, D. Wedderburn, H. Friis, P. Milhoj, and J. Stehouwer. *Old People in Three Industrial Societies.* New York: Atherton, 1968.

12. Irelan, L.M., and K. Schwab. "The Social Security Administration's Retirement History Study." *Research on Aging,* 3:381–86, 1981.

13. Morgan, J.N., and associates. *Five Thousand American Families — Patterns of Economic Progress.* Vols. 1–9. Ann Arbor, Mich.: Institute for Social Research, 1968–83.

14. Schooler, K.K. *Residential Physical Environment and Health of the Aged.* Final report. USPHS Grant EC 00191. Waltham, Mass.: Brandeis University, Florence Heller School for Advanced Studies in Social Welfare, 1970.

15. Office of Policy Development and Research. *Annual Housing Survey, 1981.* Washington, D.C.: U.S. Department of Housing and Urban Development, 1983.

16. Struyk, R.J., and H.M. Katsura. *Aging at Home: How the Elderly Adjust Their Housing without Moving.* Washington, D.C.: The Urban Institute, 1985.

17. Connell, T.L. "An overview of the elderly experience in the experimental housing allowance program." In M. P. Lawton and S. L. Hoover (Eds.), *Community Housing Choices for Older Americans.* New York: Springer Publishing Co., 1981, pp. 299–313.

18. Rabushka, A., and B. Jacobs. *Old Folks at Home.* New York: Free Press, 1980.

19. Struyk, R.J., and D. Devine. "Determinants of dwelling maintenance activity of elderly households." In M.P. Lawton and S.L. Hoover (Eds.), *Community Housing Choices for Older Americans.* New York: Springer Publishing Co., 1981, pp. 221–44.

20. Chen, A., and S. Newman. "Validity of older homeowners' housing evaluations." *The Gerontologist,* 27:309–13, 1987.

21. Struyk and Soldo, *Improving the Elderly's Housing.*

22. National Center for Health Statistics, "The National Health Interview."

23. American Association of Retired Persons. *Understanding Senior Housing.* Washington, D.C.: AARP, 1987.

24. Urban Systems Research and Engineering Inc. *Evaluation of the Effectiveness of Congregate Housing for the Elderly.* Final report. Contract No. 2255R. Washington, D.C.: Department of Housing and Urban Development, 1976.

25. Sherwood, S., J.N. Morris, C.C. Sherwood, S. Morris, E. Bernstein, and E.J. Gornstein. *Evaluation of Congregate Housing.* Final report. HUD Contract #HC-5373. Boston: Hebrew Rehabilitation Center for the Aged, 1985.

26. Sadacca, R., S.B. Loux, M.L. Isler, and M.J. Drury. *Management Performance in Public Housing*. Washington, D.C.: The Urban Institute, 1974.

27. Francescato, G., S. Weideman, J. Anderson, and R. Chenowith. *Design and Management Factors in HUD-Assisted Housing*. Washington, D.C.: U.S. Department of Housing and Urban Development, 1979.

28. Lawton and Nahemow, "Social Science Methods."

    Lawton, M.P., L. Nahemow, and J. Teaff. "Housing characteristics and the well-being of elderly tenants in federal-assisted housing." *Journal of Gerontology*, 30:601–607, 1975.

29. Winkelvoss, H.E., and A.V. Powell. *Continuing Care Retirement Communities*. Homewood, Ill.: Richard Irwin, 1984.

30. American Association of Homes for the Aging. *Continuing Care Retirement Communities*. Washington, D.C.: AAHA, 1987.

31. American Association of Homes for the Aging. *National Continuing Care Directory*. Washington, D.C.: AARP Books, 1986.

32. Laventhol and Horwath. *Retirement Housing Industry 1987*. Philadelphia: Laventhol and Horwath, 1988.

33. Parr, J., and S. Green. "Consumer factors in facility programming." Paper presented at the Conference on Design and Development of Retirement Living Environments," Orlando, Florida, September 1987. Clearwater, Fl.: Foundation for Aging Research.

34. U. S. National Committee on Vital and Health Statistics. *Report to the Secretary on a Minimum Long-Term-Care Data Set*. Washington, D.C.: U.S. Department of Health and Human Services, 1980.

35. National Center for Health Statistics. *Inventory of Data Sources on the Functionally Limited Elderly*. Rockville, Md.: NCHS, 1980.

36. Storey, J. *Availability of Federal Data on the Aged*. Washington, D.C.: Gerontological Society of America, 1985.

37. Bechtel, R.B., R.W. Marans, and W. Michelson. *Methods in Environmental and Behavioral Research*. New York: Van Nostrand Reinhold, 1987.

38. Lawton, M.P. "Methods in environmental research with older people." In R. Bechtel, R. Marans, and W. Michelson (Eds.), *Methods in Environmental and Behavioral Research*. New York: Van Nostrand Reinhold, 1987, pp. 337–60.

39. Carp, F.M. *A Future for the Aged*. Austin: University of Texas Press, 1966.

40. Lawton and Nahemow, "Social science methods."

41. Schooler, K.K. "The relationship between social interaction and morale of the

elderly as a function of environmental characteristics." *The Gerontologist,* 9:25–29, 1969.

42. Carp, F., and A. Carp. "Perceived environmental quality of neighborhoods." *Journal of Environmental Psychology,* 2:4–22, 1982.

43. Lawton, M.P. "The relative impact of congregate and traditional housing on elderly tenants." *The Gerontologist,* 16:237–42, 1976.

44. Lawton, M.P. "Competence, environmental press and the adaptation of older people." In M.P. Lawton, P.G. Windley, and T.O. Byerts (Eds.), *Aging and the Environment: Theoretical Approaches.* New York: Springer, 1982, pp. 33–59.

45. For example, Regnier, V.A. "Programming congregate housing." In V.A. Regnier and J. Pynoos (Eds.), *Housing the Aging.* New York: Elsevier, 1987, pp. 207–26.

    Sherman, S.R. "Satisfaction with retirement housing: Attitudes, recommendations, and moves." *Aging and Human Development,* 3, 339–66, 1972.

    Sherman, S.R. "Provision of on-site services in retirement housing." *International Journal of Aging and Human Development,* 6:229–47, 1975.

    Turner, L.F., and E. Mangum. *The Housing Choices of Older Americans.* Washington, D.C.: National Council on the Aging, 1982.

46. Lawton, "Methods in environmental research."

    Marans, R. "Survey research." In Bechtel, Marans, and Michelson (Eds.). *Methods in Environmental and Behavioral Research,* pp. 41–81.

47. Brennan, P.L., R.H. Moos, and S. Lemke. "Preferences of older adults and experts for physical and architectural features of group living facilities." *The Gerontologist,* 28:84–90, 1988.

    Duffy, M., S. Bailey, B. Beck, and D.G. Barker. "Preferences in nursing home design." *Environment and Behavior,* 18:246–57, 1986.

48. Cooper, C. *Easter Hill Village.* New York: Free Press, 1975.

49. Howell, S.C. *Designing for Aging: Patterns of Use.* Cambridge, Mass.: MIT Press, 1980.

50. Newman, O. *Defensible Space.* New York: Macmillan, 1972.

51. Osmond, H. "Function as the Basis of Psychiatric Ward Design." *Mental Hospitals,* 8:23–30, 1957.

52. For one such collaboration, see Walsh, D.A., I.K. Krauss, and V.A. Regnier. "Spatial ability, environmental knowledge, and environmental use: The elderly." In L.S. Liben, A.H. Patterson, and N. Newcombe (Eds.), *Spatial Representation and Behavior Across the Life Span.* New York: Academic Press, 1981, pp. 321–57.

53. Rubinstein, R.L. "The home environments of older people: Psychosocial processes relating person to place." *Journal of Gerontology,* in press.

54. Rowles, G.D. *Prisoners of Space?* Boulder, Colo.: Westview Press, 1978.

Schulamit, R., and G.D. Rowles. *Qualitative Gerontology.* New York: Springer-Verlag, 1987.

Index